METHODS IN MOLECULAR BIOLOGY™

Series Editor
**John M. Walker
School of Life Sciences
University of Hertfordshire
Hatfield, Hertfordshire, AL10 9AB, UK**

For other titles published in this series, go to
www.springer.com/series/7651

Cancer Susceptibility

Methods and Protocols

Edited by

Michelle Webb

*Faculty of Medical and Human Sciences, School of Clinical Laboratory Sciences,
University of Manchester, Manchester, UK*

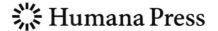

Editor
Michelle Webb, Ph.D.
Faculty of Medical and Human Sciences
School of Clinical Laboratory Sciences
University of Manchester,
Manchester, UK
Michelle.Webb@manchester.ac.uk

ISSN 1064-3745			e-ISSN 1940-6029
ISBN 978-1-60761-758-7		e-ISBN 978-1-60761-759-4
DOI 10.1007/978-1-60761-759-4
Springer New York Dordrecht Heidelberg London

Library of Congress Control Number: 2010930786

© Springer Science+Business Media, LLC 2010
All rights reserved. This work may not be translated or copied in whole or in part without the written permission of the publisher (Humana Press, c/o Springer Science+Business Media, LLC, 233 Spring Street, New York, NY 10013, USA), except for brief excerpts in connection with reviews or scholarly analysis. Use in connection with any form of information storage and retrieval, electronic adaptation, computer software, or by similar or dissimilar methodology now known or hereafter developed is forbidden.
The use in this publication of trade names, trademarks, service marks, and similar terms, even if they are not identified as such, is not to be taken as an expression of opinion as to whether or not they are subject to proprietary rights.
While the advice and information in this book are believed to be true and accurate at the date of going to press, neither the authors nor the editors nor the publisher can accept any legal responsibility for any errors or omissions that may be made. The publisher makes no warranty, express or implied, with respect to the material contained herein.

Cover Illustration Caption: Figure 1 from Chapter 3.

Printed on acid-free paper

Humana Press is a part of Springer Science+Business Media (www.springer.com)

Preface

Over the past 2 decades, spectacular advances have been made in understanding the molecular genetics of cancer. One of the major objectives of modern day cancer research is to identify genes that when mutated result in an increased susceptibility to the disease. This knowledge can be translated into clinical practice where screening for a predisposition becomes part of an at-risk patient's surveillance and management strategy. An example where this has been successful is in the management of hereditary breast cancer. Following the identification of the breast cancer susceptibility genes, *BRCA1* and *BRCA2*, in the early 1990s, genetic screens that estimate a patient's risk have now become available. While this success is now being extended to other cancer disorders, more genes need to be identified, characterized, and screens need to be developed. A book that brings together the most recent technological developments for identifying and screening cancer susceptibility genes is therefore very timely. The book is separated broadly into two parts. The first part, gene identification, informs scientists working at identifying novel cancer susceptibility genes, while the second part deals with mutation screening technologies that aid scientists and clinicians working to translate this knowledge into the clinic.

Manchester, UK *Michelle Webb*

Contents

Preface v
Contributors ix

PART I IDENTIFYING CANCER SUSCEPTIBILITY GENES

1 The Identification of Colon Cancer Susceptibility
   Genes by Using Genome-Wide Scans 3
   Denise Daley

2 Prioritizing Candidate Genetic Modifiers of *BRCA1* and *BRCA2*
   Using a Combinatorial Analysis of Global Expression and
   Polymorphism Association Studies of Breast Cancer 23
   Logan C. Walker and Amanda B. Spurdle

3 Microarray-Based Comparative Genomic Hybridization
   (Array-CGH) as a Useful Tool for Identifying Genes Involved
   in Glioblastoma (GB) 35
   *Yolanda Ruano, Manuela Mollejo, Angel Rodríguez de Lope,
   José Luis Hernández-Moneo, Pedro Martínez, and Bárbara Meléndez*

4 Multiplex Amplifiable Probe Hybridization (MAPH) Methodology
   as an Alternative to Comparative Genomic Hybridization (CGH) 47
   Ludmila Kousoulidou, Carolina Sismani, and Philippos C. Patsalis

5 Utilizing *Saccharomyces Cerevisiae* to Identify
   Aneuploidy and Cancer Susceptibility Genes 73
   Erin D. Strome and Sharon E. Plon

6 Computational Identification of Cancer Susceptibility Loci 87
   *Marko Laakso, Sirkku Karinen, Rainer Lehtonen,
   and Sampsa Hautaniemi*

7 Digital Candidate Gene Approach (DigiCGA) for
   Identification of Cancer Genes 105
   Meng-Jin Zhu, Xiang Li, and Shu-Hong Zhao

PART II SCREENING CANCER SUSCEPTIBILITY GENES

8 The Use of Denaturing High Performance Liquid Chromatography
   (DHPLC) for Mutation Scanning of Hereditary Cancer Genes 133
   Deborah J. Marsh and Viive M. Howell

9 Enhanced Mismatch Mutation Analysis: Simultaneous Detection of
   Point Mutations and Large Scale Rearrangements by Capillary
   Electrophoresis, Application to *BRCA1* and *BRCA2* 147
   *Claude Houdayer, Virginie Moncoutier, Jérôme Champ, Jérémie Weber,
   Jean-Louis Viovy, and Dominique Stoppa-Lyonnet*

Contents

10 Economical Protocol for Combined Single-Strand Conformation
    Polymorphism and Heteroduplex Analysis on a Standard Capillary
    Electrophoresis Apparatus.. 181
    Piotr Kozlowski and Wlodzimierz J. Krzyzosiak

11 Mutational Screening of *hMLH1* and *hMSH2* that Confer Inherited
    Colorectal Cancer Susceptibility Using Denature Gradient Gel
    Electrophoresis (DGGE) 193
    Tao Liu

12 s-RT-MELT: A Novel Technology for Mutation Screening.............. 207
    Jin Li and G. Mike Makrigiorgos

13 Zoom-In Array Comparative Genomic Hybridization (aCGH)
    to Detect Germline Rearrangements in Cancer Susceptibility Genes 221
    Johan Staaf and Åke Borg

14 Development of a Scoring System to Screen for BRCA1/2 Mutations......... 237
    Gareth R. Evans and Fiona Lalloo

15 Use of Splicing Reporter Minigene Assay to Evaluate
    the Effect on Splicing of Unclassified Genetic Variants 249
    *Pascaline Gaildrat, Audrey Killian, Alexandra Martins,
    Isabelle Tournier, Thierry Frébourg, and Mario Tosi*

16 Functional Analysis of Human BRCA2 Variants Using
    a Mouse Embryonic Stem Cell-Based Assay 259
    Sergey G. Kuznetsov, Suhwan Chang, and Shyam K. Sharan

17 Developing Functional Assays for BRCA1 Unclassified Variants 281
    Michelle Webb

Index.. 293

Contributors

ÅKE BORG • *Department of Oncology, Clinical Sciences, CREATE Health Strategic Centre For Translational Cancer Research, Lund University, Lund, Sweden*

JÉRÔME CHAMP • *Service de Génétique Oncologique, Institut Curie Hôpital, Paris, France*

SUHWAN CHANG • *Center for Cancer Research, Mouse Cancer Genetics Program, National Cancer Institute at Frederick, Frederick, MD, USA*

DENISE DALEY • *Department of Medicine, St. Paul's Hospital, University of British Columbia, Vancouver, BC, Canada*

GARETH R. EVANS • *Medical Genetics Research Group and Regional Genetics Service, St Mary's Hospital, University of Manchester and Central Manchester and Manchester Children's University Hospitals NHS Trust, Manchester, UK*

THIERRY FRÉBOURG • *Faculty of Medicine Department of Genetics and Institute for Biomedical Research, Rouen University Hospital, Inserm U614, IFRMP, University of Rouen, Northwest Canceropole, Rouen, France*

PASCALINE GAILDRAT • *Faculty of Medicine Department of Genetics and Institute for Biomedical Research, Rouen University Hospital, Inserm U614, IFRMP, University of Rouen, Northwest Canceropole, Rouen, France*

SAMPSA HAUTANIEMI • *Computational Systems Biology Laboratory, Institute of Biomedicine and Genome-Scale Biology Research Program, University of Helsinki, Helsinki, Finland*

JOSÉ LUIS HERNÁNDEZ-MONEO • *Department of Neurosurgery, Virgen de la Salud Hospital, Toledo, Spain*

CLAUDE HOUDAYER • *Service de Génétique Oncologique, Institut Curie Hôpital, Paris, France; Faculté de Sciences Pharmaceutiques et Biologiques, Université Paris Descartes, Paris, France*

VIIVE M. HOWELL • *Royal North Shore Hospital, Kolling Institute of Medical Research, University of Sydney, Sydney, NSW, Australia*

SIRKKU KARINEN • *Computational Systems Biology Laboratory, Institute of Biomedicine and Genome-Scale Biology Research Program, University of Helsinki, Helsinki, Finland*

AUDREY KILLIAN • *Faculty of Medicine Department of Genetics and Institute for Biomedical Research, Rouen University Hospital, Inserm U614, IFRMP, University of Rouen, Northwest Canceropole, Rouen, France*

LUDMILA KOUSOULIDOU • *Department of Cytogenetics and Genomics, The Cyprus Institute of Neurology and Genetics, Nicosia, Cyprus*

PIOTR KOZLOWSKI • *Laboratory of Cancer Genetics, Institute of Bioorganic Chemistry, Polish Academy of Sciences, Poznań, Poland*

WLODZIMIERZ J. KRZYZOSIAK • *Laboratory of Cancer Genetics, Institute of Bioorganic Chemistry, Polish Academy of Sciences, Poznań, Poland*

SERGEY G. KUZNETSOV • *Center for Cancer Research, Mouse Cancer Genetics Program, National Cancer Institute at Frederick, Frederick, MD, USA; Institute for Molecular Medicine Finland, University of Helsinki, Helsinki, Finland*

MARKO LAAKSO • *Computational Systems Biology Laboratory, Institute of Biomedicine and Genome-Scale Biology Research Program, University of Helsinki, Helsinki, Finland*

FIONA LALLOO • *Medical Genetics Research Group and Regional Genetics Service, St Mary's Hospital, University of Manchester and Central Manchester and Manchester Children's University Hospitals NHS Trust, Manchester, UK*

RAINER LEHTONEN • *Department of Biological and Environmental Sciences, Metapopulation Research Group, University of Helsinki, Helsinki, Finland*

JIN LI • *Division of Genomic Stability and Division of DNA Repair and Medical Physics and Biophysics, Department of Radiation Oncology, Harvard Medical School, Dana Farber Cancer Institute and Brigham and Women's Hospital, Boston, MA, USA*

XIANG LI • *Key Laboratory of Agricultural Animal Genetics, Breeding and Reproduction of Ministry of Education, Huazhong Agricultural University, Wuhan, China*

TAO LIU • *Cancer Centre Karolinska, Karolinska Institute, Stockholm, Sweden*

G. MIKE MAKRIGIORGOS • *Division of Genomic Stability and Division of DNA Repair and Medical Physics and Biophysics, Department of Radiation Oncology, Harvard Medical School, Dana Farber Cancer Institute and Brigham and Women's Hospital, BostonMA, USA*

DEBORAH J. MARSH • *Royal North Shore Hospital, Kolling Institute of Medical Research, University of Sydney, Sydney, NSW, Australia*

PEDRO MARTÍNEZ • *Department of Genetics, Virgen de la Salud Hospital, Toledo, Spain*

ALEXANDRA MARTINS • *Faculty of MedicineDepartment of Genetics and Institute for Biomedical Research, Rouen University Hospital, Inserm U614, IFRMP, University of Rouen, Northwest Canceropole, Rouen, France*

BÁRBARA MELÉNDEZ • *Molecular Pathology Research Unit, Virgen de la Salud Hospital, Toledo, Spain*

MANUELA MOLLEJO • *Department of Pathology and Molecular Pathology Research Unit, Virgen de la Salud Hospital, Toledo, Spain*

VIRGINIE MONCOUTIER • *Service de Génétique Oncologique, Institut Curie Hôpital, Paris, France*

PHILIPPOS C. PATSALIS • *Department of Cytogenetics and Genomics, The Cyprus Institute of Neurology and Genetics, Nicosia, Cyprus*

SHARON E. PLON • *Department of Molecular and Human Genetics, Baylor College of Medicine, Houston, TX, USA*

ANGEL RODRÍGUEZ DE LOPE • *Department of Neurosurgery, Virgen de la Salud Hospital, Toledo, Spain*

YOLANDA RUANO • *Molecular Pathology Research Unit, Virgen de la Salud Hospital, Toledo, Spain*

SHYAM K. SHARAN • *Center for Cancer Research, Mouse Cancer Genetics Program, National Cancer Institute at Frederick, Frederick, MD, USA*
CAROLINA SISMANI • *Department of Cytogenetics and Genomics, The Cyprus Institute of Neurology and Genetics, Nicosia, Cyprus*
AMANDA B. SPURDLE • *PO Royal Brisbane Hospital, Queensland Institute of Medical Research, QLD, Australia*
JOHAN STAAF • *Department of Oncology, Clinical Sciences, CREATE Health Strategic Centre For Translational Cancer Research, Lund University, Lund, Sweden*
DOMINIQUE STOPPA-LYONNET • *Service de Génétique Oncologique, Institut Curie Hôpital, Paris, France; INSERM U830 Institut Curie Centre de Recherche, Paris, France*
ERIN D. STROME • *Department of Molecular and Human Genetics, Baylor College of Medicine, Houston, TX, USA*
MARIO TOSI • *Faculty of Medicine, Department of Genetics and Institute for Biomedical Research, Rouen University Hospital, Inserm U614, IFRMP, University of Rouen, Northwest Canceropole, Rouen, France*
ISABELLE TOURNIER • *Faculty of Medicine, Department of Genetics and Institute for Biomedical Research, Rouen University Hospital, Inserm U614, IFRMP, University of Rouen, Northwest Canceropole, Rouen, France*
JEAN-LOUIS VIOVY • *Laboratoire Physicochimie-Curie, UMR/CNRS, Institut Curie Centre de Recherche, Paris, France*
LOGAN C. WALKER • *PO Royal Brisbane Hospital, Queensland Institute of Medical Research, QLD, Australia*
MICHELLE WEBB • *Faculty of Medical and Human Sciences; Medical Genetics Research Group, The University of Manchester, Manchester, UK*
JÉRÉMIE WEBER • *Service de Génétique Oncologique, Institut Curie Hôpital, Paris, France*
SHU-HONG ZHAO • *Key Laboratory of Agricultural Animal Genetics, Breeding and Reproduction of Ministry of Education, Huazhong Agricultural University, Wuhan, China*
MENG-JIN ZHU • *Key Laboratory of Agricultural Animal Genetics, Breeding and Reproduction of Ministry of Education, Huazhong Agricultural University, Wuhan, China*

Part I

Identifying Cancer Susceptibility Genes

Chapter 1

The Identification of Colon Cancer Susceptibility Genes by Using Genome-Wide Scans

Denise Daley

Abstract

Recent studies have indicated that in ~35% of all colorectal cancer (CRC) cases, the CRC was inherited. Although a number of high-risk familial variants have been identified, these mutations explain <6% of CRC cases; therefore, further genome-wide scans will need to be conducted in the future. There are two popular approaches to genome-wide scans, namely linkage and association. The linkage approach utilizes several hundred markers (typically between 300 and 500 markers) throughout the genome and identifies candidate regions shared among affected family members. Candidate regions are then scrutinized for the presence of susceptibility loci. Linkage studies require no prior information and can provide new avenues for future research, but the regions identified are often large and include many candidate genes. The second and more recent approach is the genome-wide association study (GWAS) in which hundreds of thousands of markers called single nucleotide polymorphisms (SNPs) are used to identify the SNPs associated with traits of interest by employing family-based or case-control association methods. GWAS studies require no prior information and, because they use hundreds of thousands of SNPs, they can target specific candidate genes and/or narrow regions for investigation. Study design considerations, methodology, and the execution of linkage and genome-wide association studies that use both family and case-control designs are covered in this chapter.

Key words: Colorectal cancer, Genome-wide association, Linkage, Single nucleotide polymorphism, Study design, Case-control, Family-based study designs

1. Introduction

In the numerous colorectal cancer (CRC) linkage and genome-wide association studies performed (1–12) in recent years, several regions of the genome have been identified as harboring CRC susceptibility genes, but there is considerable variability in the regions identified from study to study. It has been estimated that, for CRC, the common variants identified to date account for <1% of the familial risk and that known variants account for <10% of the heritability (8). CRC is a heterogeneous disease both in its genetic (allelic and locus) origins and in its phenotypic presentation; this heterogeneity presents significant challenges to the design and analysis of genome-wide scans. The purpose of this chapter is to identify the different study designs that may be used in genome-wide scans and to outline the steps in the analysis, from power calculations to the selection of markers for follow-up studies, while indicating key references (13–15), programs, and texts for the reader.

2. Study Designs

For any genome-wide scan, the key material is the study population on whom the scan is to be conducted. There are two broad categories of study designs: family-based and case-control. This section will outline not only the strengths and weakness of each of the designs, but also highlight the design considerations that influence the selection of the methods, such as the type of genome-wide scan (linkage or association), the analytical approach, and the quality control (QC) measures.

2.1. Family-Based Study Designs

Family-based study designs have several key advantages including the ability to perform segregation analyses to determine if a trait has a genetic component, to determine the mode of inheritance (16), and to protect against population stratification. Additional advantages that are often overlooked include the ability to study maternal exposures, maternal–fetal genotype interactions and imprinting effects (the phenomenon whereby the effect of a particular allele on disease risk varies according to the parental source of the allele), these effects are of particular interest to geneticists studying cancers with childhood onset. There are several types of family designs (multigenerational, founder populations, affected sib-pairs, discordant sib pairs, and trio designs), most of which are quite versatile, supporting both linkage and association designs. The aspects and attributes of each of the family-based designs are outlined below:

1. *Multigenerational family pedigrees* are identified in a variety of ways by using predetermined criteria known as ascertainment criteria. The ascertainment criteria may consist of a single affected individual (proband), multiple affected individuals, affected individuals in two or more generations, or established criteria such as the Amsterdam or Bethesda criteria (17). The purpose of the ascertainment criteria is to increase the power of the study by enriching the sample for familial cases with shared genetic susceptibility. Although multigenerational family studies

are well suited for use in studying diseases with a young age at onset, their use can be quite challenging for cancer researchers due to the later age at onset. Additionally, there are higher recruitment and phenotyping costs associated with family-based designs when compared to case-control designs. However, once ascertained and with appropriate correction for the ascertainment schema, this design is very powerful and facilitates the use of other nested designs, such as trios, affected sib-pairs, discordant sib-pairs, and other affected relative pairs (18).

2. *Founder populations* are subpopulations, started with a limited number of individuals (founders), who have lived in geographical or cultural isolation for many generations, with either limited or no migration into the group. Founder-population studies of common diseases are widely used in genetic-mapping studies; the design strengths include genealogies that link together many generations and a reduction in genetic, allelic, and environmental diversity (19–21). Well-known examples of founder populations include French Canadian, Finnish, Old Order Amish, Hutterite, and Ashkenazi/ethnically Jewish populations. Ashkenazi and ethnically Jewish populations are arguably among the more important of founder populations for cancer geneticists, as there are Ashkenazi-specific variants for two known breast-cancer genes (*BRCA1* [OMIM 113705] and *BRCA2* [OMIM 600185] (22), for the genes that predispose to colorectal cancer, including *FAP* (23) and for the mismatch repair genes (24–26). There are variants that had been first identified in, and thought to be specific to, Ashkenazi populations, but which were later identified as general CRC susceptibility variants (3, 27–29).

3. *Affected sib-pairs* are widely used in the study of genetic traits. The basic premise of the design is that, if siblings share a common disease phenotype, they do so because of shared genetic susceptibility. Genetic markers that are physically linked together on a chromosome tend to be inherited together (30). The degree to which siblings share markers (allele sharing) can be compared to that expected by chance (on average, siblings will share 50% of markers); alternatively, when the sample includes both concordant (whether affected or unaffected) and discordant (one affected; one unaffected) sib-pairs, the estimates of allele sharing can be used in the Haseman–Elston regression equation (31). Regions with increased allele sharing can then be prioritized for follow-up studies based on the degree of excess allele sharing and subsequently scrutinized for disease loci. The choice of the ascertainment scheme for affected sib-pair designs requires consideration, as the recruitment of parents and unaffected siblings increases the analytical power but also increase costs (32, 33). A limitation of the

affected sib-pair design is the lack of a control group; this may result in incorrect inferences about the linkage between a marker and a disease trait (34). Because regions of the genome may demonstrate excess allele sharing among all types of sibling pairs, such observations may be better explained by transmission distortion and relative fitness (34–36). Matched-sibling controls provide protection against these problems, making the test statistics more robust to Type I error (34). It has been suggested that studies should include discordant or concordantly unaffected sib-pairs to confirm linkage or association when using this design (36).

4. *Discordant sib pairs* are widely used in the study of both binary (dichotomous outcomes such as affected or unaffected) and quantitative traits (examples include height, weight, tumor markers). For binary traits, discordant sib-pairs consist of one affected and one unaffected sibling. For quantitative traits, the extreme discordant sib-pair design is favored, as it is the most powerful of the sib-pair designs (33, 37) in detecting genetic variants for quantitative traits. The increase in power is obtained by selecting the extreme discordant sib-pairs from the distribution; for example, one sib is in the top tenth percentile of the distribution and the other sib is in the bottom tenth percentile.

5. *Trios*, comprising parents and an affected child, are well suited for studies of diseases with a young age at onset. The study design allows for the use of a specialized, family-based method of association, the Transmission Disequilibrium Test (TDT) (38). The TDT uses parents who are heterozygous for the candidate allele and evaluates the frequency with which the candidate alleles are transmitted to affected offspring. If an allele is associated with the trait of interest, it will be transmitted more frequently than would be expected under the null hypothesis (i.e., alleles are transmitted equally). The family-based tests of association, as implemented in the FBAT package of programs (39–48), builds upon the original TDT (38), permitting the analysis of haplotypes, binary and quantitative traits, as well as covariates and gene–environment interactions (39, 48, 49).

2.2. Case-Control Designs

This design, based upon association, is the study design most frequently used today, having been reinvigorated by Risch and Merikangas (50). The advantages of the design include lower recruitment needs and reduced costs for phenotyping and genotyping; in addition, for genes with modest effect, the case-control association design is more powerful than linkage. One may ask about cohort designs; given the costs of genotyping for genome-wide scans, many researchers are using a nested case-control design for their genome-wide scans: one such example is the 1958 British Birth Cohort that is included in the Wellcome Trust Case Control Consortium (51). Although case-control designs are subject to population stratification, there are easily implemented methods to account for stratification (52) (see Subheading 3.6).

3. Methods

The first step in the design and analysis of any genome-wide scan is the development of a detailed timeline and plan of analysis. The initial analysis plan should be developed at the time the genome-wide scan is being considered, as the analysis plan is dynamic and may change over time; although steps may need to be repeated, it is important that there be a plan in place. The analysis plan should outline each of the steps to be performed and should include a decision tree that specifies the next steps, based upon the outcome of the previous step. Each analysis plan will be slightly different, depending upon the study design, the hypothesis to be tested, and the resources available, but the common steps are described in the following section.

3.1. Power Calculations

Accurate estimates of sample sizes are essential to the planning, postassessment, and follow-up stages of a genome-wide scan.

1. There are several readily available programs that allow users to easily estimate the power of an association study (case-control design) (53, 54).
2. Power calculators for linkage studies include SIMLINK (55, 56), SLINK which is part of the LINKAGE package (57), and DESPAIR (58) which is mainly used for sib-pair studies.
3. There are numerous power calculators for the TDT designs (59–61).

3.2. Parameters for Power Calculations

Determining the sample size required for a successful genome-wide study (linkage or association) requires the specification of several parameters. The exact parameters will vary depending upon the study design (family-based or case-control) and type of genome-wide study. The reader is encouraged to evaluate many different models and parameter settings in order to have a realistic perspective of the true power of the study. Some of the parameters that may be required include the following:

1. Sample size (number of cases/controls, or number and type of families, sib-pairs, etc.).
2. Genetic model (see Subheading 3.3 for further details).

3. Minor allele frequency (MAF) of the disease allele.
4. Penetrance is the probability of getting the disease, conditional on genotype. This can be either estimated from the data (family studies only) or specified by the user.
5. Prevalence of the disease in the population.
6. The effect size can be estimated as an Odds Ratio (OR), as an attributable risk fraction, or as a sibling reoccurrence risk (λ_s), depending upon the study design.
7. The number of markers to be tested.
8. Linkage disequilibrium (LD) between marker and disease allele (see Note 1).
9. Allele frequency difference between marker and disease allele (see Note 1).

If the sample size or the number of markers to be tested is fixed, then the user can input these parameters and determine the power of the study relevant to the other parameters.

3.3. Genetic Model

There are two general genetic models, namely Mendelian and complex, which can be used to describe and model the genetic contribution for the trait of interest.

1. Mendelian traits result from a mutation in a single gene, which is both necessary and sufficient to produce the disease phenotype. A subset of Mendelian traits will also have effect modifiers. Effect modification occurs when the main genetic liability is conferred by a single gene, but differences in phenotype, penetrance, or age at onset are explained by the effects of additional loci. Linkage studies are well suited to the identification of Mendelian traits.
2. Common complex traits are generally thought to be the result of complex inheritance patterns, involving both genetic and environmental risk factors. The underlying genetic susceptibility of complex traits can be further subdivided into two broad categories:
   (a) Oligogenic is the term used to describe diseases and traits that result from mutations in a relatively small of number of genes, each of which has its own mode of inheritance (i.e., additive, dominant, or recessive). Hirschsprung disease (HSCR) [OMIM 142623] is an example of an oligogenetic disease: it is caused by mutations in eight different genes (62) and there is interaction (epistasis) between loci (62). Association studies are well suited to identify susceptibility alleles for oligogenic traits, provided the risk alleles are relatively common and have modest effect sizes.
   (b) *Polygenic* is the term used to describe diseases and traits that result from mutations in a relatively large number of

genes, each having a very small contribution to the overall risk. As each of the genes involved contributes relatively little to the overall genetic liability of the disease, these traits are not well suited to either linkage or association studies.

3.4. Mode of Inheritance

The genetic model and mode of inheritance can either be estimated from family data by using segregation analysis or be specified by the user. Several categories that describe autosomal and X-linked modes of inheritance (see Note 2) are discussed below:

1. *Additive*: Each risk allele contributes to the disease risk in an additive/linear fashion, with the heterozygote risk being intermediate to risk of the two homozygotes.
2. *Dominant*: One copy of the risk allele is sufficient for the occurrence of the disease, with the heterozygote and homozygote (risk allele) genotypes having the same risk or OR.
3. *Recessive*: Two copies of the risk allele are necessary for the occurrence of the disease, and only the homozygote (risk allele) genotype has increased risk.
4. *Multiplicative*: Each risk allele contributes to the disease risk in a multiplicative fashion. For example, if the OR = 3 for the heterozygote genotype, then the OR = 9 for the homozygote genotype.
5. *X-linked*: Traits that are located on the X chromosome demonstrate unique inheritance patterns. X-linked traits can be inherited in a recessive or dominant pattern; however, because males have only one X chromosome, they are more likely to be affected if the mode of inheritance is recessive, as they only need to inherit a single affected chromosome from their mother. Females, however, need to inherit an affected chromosome from both mother and father. If the father has an X-linked trait, then he passes this trait to all of his daughters but not to any of his sons, as he donates a Y chromosome to each of the sons. Hemophilia (OMIM 306700) and color-blindness (OMIM 303900 and 303800) are examples of X-linked recessive traits, and Fragile X (OMIM 300624) a form of mental retardation is an X-linked dominant trait.

3.5. Phenotype Definition: Genetic and Allelic Heterogeneity

It is known that CRC can result from mutations in several different genes including Adenomatous Polyposis Coli (APC) and any of the mismatch repair genes. This means that, in any collection of CRC cases, genetic susceptibility is heterogeneous. Allelic heterogeneity describes the situation in which all affected individuals have mutations in a single gene, but there are many distinct mutations within that gene. A loss of power will result if, when analyzing all affected individuals (CRC and/or adenomatous polyps) together, genetic and allelic heterogeneity is ignored (3, 14).

There are several steps that may be taken to reduce the heterogeneity present in the sample:

1. Screen cases for known genetic variants. Although screening may be time-consuming and expensive, it is a necessary step because the exclusion of cases and families that link to known susceptibility loci will increase the analytical power of the study to detect new susceptibility loci.
2. Use clinical information and family history to identify cases and families with similar phenotypes (phenotypic homogeneity). This can result in genetic homogeneity, increasing the power of the genome-wide scan (3).
3. After completing the initial analysis, remove families or cases that link to the top hits and then redo the analysis.
4. When conducting a linkage genome-wide scan, a heterogeneity LOD (HLOD) score can be computed. The HLOD accounts for the fact that in any given collection of family samples there may be more than one susceptibility gene segregating in the collection. The HLOD does not account for heterogeneity within a family.

3.6. Population Stratification

When a genome-wide scan using a case-control or association approach is under consideration, the concept of population stratification and its effects on the design and analysis of a genome-wide scan must be understood in order that appropriate measures be taken to address this issue in the analysis. Population stratification occurs when there is hidden substructure in a population or there are systematic ancestry differences between the cases and controls, and there are allele frequency differences between the populations (63). Population stratification may lead to nonrandom rejection of markers from a genome-wide scan, thus resulting in a study bias (64). There are two main methods used to detect and control population stratification, namely genomic control and principal components.

1. *Genomic control* (*GC*): This concept was first introduced by Devlin and Roeder (65), who noted that the chi-squared distribution of test statistics, when confounded by population stratification, were more "spread out" than they should be, thereby resulting in higher median values and in a uniform inflation of the distribution. They termed the latter result the "inflation factor", denoted by the symbol, λ. To account for λ, they proposed taking the median of the distribution of the chi-square statistics observed over a set of "neutral" markers (or markers not being tested for association) and dividing this median value by the median of the corresponding (ideal) chi-square distribution, thus providing an estimate of λ. If $\lambda = 1$, there is no evidence for population stratification and no

correction is necessary. If $\lambda > 1$, then there is evidence for stratification and the correction factor is then applied by dividing the actual association test chi-square statistical results by λ. Two implementations of the method in wide use today are the following:

(a) Measure λ over a set of markers designed to identify population stratification, such as the ancestry informative markers (AIMS) for populations of European descent (66). These markers can then be used to estimate λ, with the correction being applied to the remaining markers (candidates to be tested for association). This approach is mainly used for candidate gene studies.

(b) Measure the inflation factor λ over all association tests conducted. Then, use the λ to correct all the chi-square results. This approach is recommended for genome-wide scans (see Note 3).

2. *Principal components*: This is a recently developed method in which all of the markers in a genome-wide association scan are used to infer the "axes of genetic variation" (52). The first two principal components have been demonstrated to have a high correlation with the northwest–southeast axes of the allele frequency distribution that is present in European populations (52, 66, 67). This approach has been incorporated into several freely available computer packages, EIGENSTRAT (52) and PLINK (68).

3.7. Data-Cleaning Steps

The purpose of the data-cleaning process is to remove data that may contain errors and that would reduce the power of a genome-wide scan. Data cleaning is one of the most important and most time-consuming tasks of any genome-wide scan. The numerous steps in the data-cleaning process are described below (see Notes 4 and 5).

3.7.1. Source and Type of Sample

DNA can be extracted from a variety of different biological sources (blood, saliva, spit, mouthwash, buccal swab, and cells) and extraction protocols and reagents, as well as the age of the samples (especially for longitudinal studies) may vary, thus creating variability that can affect the performance of the sample on the genotyping array. The following steps should be taken to reduce the effect of such factors:

1. Check for variability in the sample call rate by source, by age of the sample, and by study if there is a multicenter study design.

2. Include duplicate samples to search for errors in reproducibility. Compare the reproducibility error rates across sample source types.

3. Plot the distribution of sample call rates within each category.

4. Check the starting concentrations of samples with low call rates. One may decide to remove samples with low starting concentrations and/or volumes and then repeat the steps.

5. Determine a cut-off point for sample call rate. Generally, this will be between 95% and 98% (69). Samples that do not achieve this level would be discarded from the analysis (see Note 6).

6. Call whole-genome-amplified (WGA) DNA separately. If WGA DNA samples are used, these samples should be called separately from the genomic DNA and the QC steps done separately. One may form a further subset of the WGA samples according to the genomic source, as samples amplified from blood may perform better than samples amplified from cells. Additionally, one should consider the age of the source DNA sample, as older samples may be more degraded and/or have a higher likelihood of being contaminated. Genomic architecture, such as GC content or proximity to the telomeres, may also impact the performance rates (70, 71) of WGA samples.

7. Review gender errors. The genotyping center will provide a list of the samples showing gender inconsistencies (i.e., reported gender does not match X and Y chromosomes of the sample). One can choose to change the gender in the report or to discard the sample (see Note 7).

8. Check the Mendelian inheritance pattern in family studies. Families with inconsistencies that cannot be resolved should be removed.

9. Examine the identity by state sharing (IBS) for all samples (pair-wise). This can be done by using one of a variety of programs, such as GRR (72). This will not only identify duplicate samples (monozygotic twins or other unintentional duplicates), parent-offspring pairs, and siblings but will also confirm the putative relationships in family studies and identify unwanted related individuals for case-control studies.

10. Use multidimensional scaling plot (MDS) in case-control designs to confirm the ethnicity of individual samples. The algorithm plots the first two principal components (see Subheading 3.6 on population stratification for further details) on the x- and y-axes. HapMap samples (73) can be used as reference samples and can be color-coded by population (CEU, JPT, etc.); the study samples are then overlaid in a distinct color. This uses the genetic data to infer the ethnicity of the sample. The MDS algorithm is incorporated in the PLINK (68) software package.

3.8. QC Steps for Markers

The following steps may be used to evaluate the quality of the markers and to select the markers to be retained for analysis.

1. Use a high call rate. As there is a high correlation between call rate and accuracy, a call rate between 95% and 98% is recommended (69).
2. Remove monomorphic SNPs as they are not informative.
3. Evaluate Hardy Weinberg Equilibrium (HWE) for all SNPs. After poor quality SNPs and samples have been removed, test for HWE. Any SNP that fails HWE, as determined by a p-value less than 10^{-4} in the controls (74), should be excluded or flagged for further QC.
4. Compare the MAF in the sample to those obtained from HapMap. Allele frequencies will vary from population to population; however, if an allele is common in the HapMap population but rare in the sample, then this may reflect a problem with the genotype clusters. If appropriate, contact the genotyping center for support for removing these SNPs from the analysis or for flagging these SNPs for further QC.

3.9. Statistical Analyses

There are several layers to the statistical analysis of a genome-wide scan. Because of the computational burden and complexity, in most studies single-SNP associations will be investigated first, leaving the analyses of haplotype and of gene–gene and gene–environment interactions for later stages.

1. *Single-SNP associations*. As noted above, the first approach used in most genome-wide studies is that of single-marker tests of association. There are a variety of test statistics and programs that may be used, depending upon the study design and the trait under consideration. PLINK (68) is well suited to case-control designs; UNPHASED (75) uses a likelihood model that can be used for trio, case-control, or mixed designs (studies in which both families and cases and controls are used).
2. *Quantile–quantile (Q–Q) plots*. After completing single-SNP association tests, it is a good idea to check the distribution of the test statistic by using Q–Q plots for all SNPs that passed QC. The Q–Q plots allow comparison of the visual inspection of the observed distribution with the expected distribution of the test statistic (51). This step will identify SNPs that deviate from the expected distribution – such deviation may be due to population stratification (64, 76), genotyping error, or association (51) (see Note 8). Q–Q plots are constructed by rank ordering values from smallest to largest and plotting them against their expected values. It is also recommended to plot the 95% confidence interval bands (51).
3. *Haplotype tests*. These tests, generally performed after the single-SNP associations, are most informative when there are haplotype (cis and interaction) effects or when the disease allele is rare (0.05%) (77).

4. *Gene–gene and gene–environment interactions*: Evaluation of these interactions is generally reserved for the final stages of analyses. Although the importance of these interactions in the development of complex diseases is unquestioned, in practice the assessment of these interactions in a genome-wide scan poses significant challenges with respect to multiple comparisons and to the computational burden involved. The power to detect these interactions is generally considered to be poor (69, 78). It has been argued that if the genetic susceptibility is complex due to genetic and environmental interactions, then the only way to detect these interactions is by testing for them. If testing for interactions is planned, the reader may wish to refer to Cordell's excellent review on the topic, which includes a description of the current methods and software packages for investigating interactions (78).

3.10. Multiple Testing Issues

There are numerous, diverse approaches that may be taken into account for multiple testing. Because there is general debate about, and discussion of, these approaches (51, 69, 79), there is as yet no consensus as to which approach is the best; however, all the approaches have the common goal of maintaining an appropriate Type I error rate. To achieve this goal, it is necessary to account for the large number of statistical tests that are performed in genome-wide scans. A general overview of these methods is presented below. (The extensive mathematical details are provided in the original papers.)

1. *Bonferroni correction*: This method corrects for each SNP tested in the genome-wide scan. It is straightforward and easily implemented, but it assumes that each SNP is independent. This assumption is not valid; it is known from the LD structure present in the genome that there is dependence between SNPs. Therefore, it is widely accepted that the Bonferroni correction is an overly conservative approach for genome-wide scans.

2. *Permutation testing*: This is a traditional method, whereby the joint distribution of all the statistical tests being performed in the genome-wide study is repeatedly sampled (see Note 9). An empirical, or exact, *p*-value is then determined, based upon the number of times a *p*-value to the observed value is found.

3. *False Discovery Rate (FDR)*: The FDR, which aims to control the proportion of errors among the rejected hypothesis (80), has been incorporated into many statistical packages, including PLINK (68) and GoldenHelix (http://www.goldenhelix.com/).

4. *False Positive Report Probability (FPRP)*: The proponents of this approach cite the reliance upon *p*-values alone in the absence of prior probability as contributing to the plethora of

false-positive genetic associations reported in the literature. The FPRP uses factors, such as the prior probability for any SNP in the genome to be associated with the trait, the power of the study, and the significance threshold, to determine the probability that the null hypothesis (i.e., no association) is true, given a significant p-value (79). A related approach, which uses Bayes factors to account for the prior probability, was implemented by the Wellcome Trust Case Control Consortium in their analysis of seven common diseases (51).

3.11. Imputation

Imputation has been designed to extend the coverage of the genome-wide chips that currently interrogate between 500,000 and two million SNPs; imputation can increase this coverage up to four million SNPs. Statistical algorithms have been developed that can use information from the International HapMap project (73), from LD, and from SNPs that have been tested in a genome-wide association study (GWAS) to infer genotypes at SNPs that had not been directly genotyped in the GWAS, thereby allowing investigators to expand the coverage of a GWAS, or to combine studies in which different SNP panels were genotyped or distinct genotyping platforms were used (see Note 10). There are several imputation algorithms from which to choose, including Bim-Bam, Fast-PHASE, BEAGLE, MACH (available at http://www.sph.umich.edu/csg/abecasis/MACH/download/), PLINK, IMPUTE, and IMPUTE v2) (68, 81–85). Brief descriptions of the algorithms and the evaluation of their performance and power can be found in the article by Pei et al. (86).

3.12. Selection of Markers for Follow-up Studies

It is well accepted that results from genetic-association studies need validation and confirmation in independent samples. There are several options for the selection of the markers to carry forward for validation:

1. Set a threshold and carry forward those markers that have corrected p-values less than or equal to the threshold.
2. If FDR is used, select all markers that meet the specified alpha level.
3. Use Bayesian approaches that use prior information to weigh the evidence for linkage or association (69).

4. Notes

1. Two factors that strongly affect the power of an association study are the LD and the difference between the marker-allele frequency and the disease-allele frequency. If the LD parameter is not included in the model, then the user is making the

implicit assumption that the marker being tested is the actual disease allele; this assumption is unrealistic and artificially inflates the power. Similarly, for association studies, if the difference in allele frequencies between the marker and disease allele is not included, the implicit assumption is that they are of equal frequency. Again, this is an unrealistic assumption, as the power of the association study is highly dependent upon the frequency gap between marker and disease allele.

2. Mitochondrial inheritance patterns are not included in this section. The mitochondrial genome is distinct from the autosomes (chromosomes inherited from both parents) and the sex chromosomes (X and Y). Mitochondrial DNA, inherited from the mother and transmitted to both sexes, has been implicated in myopathic syndromes (OMIM 530000, 540000, 545000) and deafness (OMIM 520000). Investigators studying complex disease should be aware that mitochondrial inheritance is a possibility and that most of the current GWAS chips do not include mitochondrial markers. If interested, investigators should include plans for separate studies of the mitochondrial genome.

3. GC is optimally used with study design considerations that minimize population stratification, such as the matching of cases and controls by ethnicity (87). Additionally, if used in a genome-wide scan, one may wish to use the GCF (87) method.

4. The order of performing the data-cleaning steps can vary, as can the steps themselves, depending upon the type of genome-wide scan and the study design being used. Additionally, it should be noted that it may be necessary to repeat many of the steps.

5. It has been argued that data cleaning introduces bias into the analysis. An alternative to the data-cleaning steps outlined would be the use of error models (88).

6. An alternative approach may be to infer the missing values; however, this is computationally intensive and will inflate the type I error if not done correctly.

7. As gender is a relatively straightforward variable, errors are likely to reflect errors in charting or in database entry. As such, the gender-error rate may provide an estimate for the overall error rate in a study.

8. There are methods to determine whether an observed deviation is due to association, genotyping error, or stratification. If the number of markers that deviate from the expected distribution is large and if the deviation starts early in the distribution as demonstrated by Clayton et al. (64), this more than likely represents population stratification and systematic genotyping error rather than association. To evaluate the

effectiveness of the QC measures, the researcher may wish to plot the test statistics for all SNPs versus those SNPs that passed QC (51). Deviation due to association is generally observed in the tails of the distribution (51).

9. For determining the number of permutations to be carried out, a good general rule of thumb is 10,000 permutations for every significant digit of the p-value; for example, for p-values = 0.05, 10,000 permutations only would be needed.

10. Imputation performs best in samples of European descent; therefore, caution should be used when applying these methods to other populations (89).

Acknowledgments

The author would like to thank Veronica Yakoleff for editing the manuscript.

References

1. Kemp, Z., Carvajal-Carmona, L., Spain, S., Barclay, E., Gorman, M., Martin, L., et al. (2006) Evidence for a colorectal cancer susceptibility locus on chromosome 3q21-q24 from a high-density SNP genome-wide linkage scan. *Hum. Mol. Genet.* **15**, 2903–2910.
2. Tomlinson, I. P., Webb, E.L., Carvajal-Carmona, P., Broderick, K., Howarth, A. Pittman, M., et al. (2008). A genome-wide association study identifies colorectal cancer susceptibility loci on chromosomes 10p14 and 8q23.3. *Nat. Genet.* **40**, 623–630.
3. Daley, D., Lewis, S., Platzer, P., MacMillen, M., Willis, J., Elston, R.C., et al. (2008). Identification of susceptibility genes for cancer in a genome-wide scan: results from the colon neoplasia sibling study. *Am. J. Hum. Genet.* **82**, 723–736.
4. Zanke, B.W., Greenwood, C.M., Rangrej, J., Kustra, R., Tenesa, A., Farrington, S.M., et al. (2007) Genome-wide association scan identifies a colorectal cancer susceptibility locus on chromosome 8q24. *Nat. Genet.* **39**, 989–994.
5. Tomlinson, I., Webb, E., Carvajal-Carmona, L., Broderick, P., Kemp, Z., Spain, S., et al. (2007) A genome-wide association scan of tag SNPs identifies a susceptibility variant for colorectal cancer at 8q24.21. *Nat. Genet.* **39**, 984–988.
6. Tenesa, A., Farrington, S.M., Prendergast, J.G., Porteous, M.E., Walker, M., Haq, N., et al. (2008) Genome-wide association scan identifies a colorectal cancer susceptibility locus on 11q23 and replicates risk loci at 8q24 and 18q21. *Nat. Genet.* **40**, 631–637.
7. Broderick, P., Carvajal-Carmona, L., Pittman, A.M., Webb, E., Howarth, K., Rowan, A., et al. (2007) A genome-wide association study shows that common alleles of SMAD7 influence colorectal cancer risk. *Nat. Genet.* **39**, 1315–1317.
8. Houlston, R.S., Webb, E., Broderick, P., Pittman, A.M., Di Bernardo, M.C., Lubbe, S., et al. (2008) Meta-analysis of genome-wide association data identifies four new susceptibility loci for colorectal cancer. *Nat. Genet.* **40**, 1426–1435.
9. Djureinovic, T., Skoglund, J., Vandrovcova, J., Zhou, X.L., Kalushkova, A., Iselius, L., et al. (2006) A genome wide linkage analysis in Swedish families with hereditary non-familial adenomatous polyposis/non-hereditary non-polyposis colorectal cancer. *Gut* **55**, 362–366.
10. Wiesner, G.L., Daley, D., Lewis, S., Ticknor, C., Platzer, P., Lutterbaugh, J., et al. (2003) A subset of familial colorectal neoplasia kindreds linked to chromosome 9q22.2-31.2. *Proc. Natl. Acad. Sci. U.S.A.* **100**, 12961–12965.
11. Papaemmanuil, E., Carvajal-Carmona, L., Sellick, G.S., Kemp, Z., Webb, E., Spain, S., et al. (2008) Deciphering the genetics of hereditary non-syndromic colorectal cancer. *Eur. J. Hum. Genet.* **16**, 1477–1486.

12. Aaltonen, L., Johns, L., Jarvinen, H., Mecklin, J.P., and Houlston, R. (2007) Explaining the familial colorectal cancer risk associated with mismatch repair (MMR)-deficient and MMR-stable tumors. *Clin. Cancer Res.* **13**, 356–361.

13. Haines, J.L., and Pericak-Vance, M.A. (2006) *Genetic analysis of complex diseases.* Wiley-Liss, Hoboken, N.J.

14. Thomas, D.C. (2004) *Statistical methods in genetic epidemiology.* Oxford University Press, Oxford, New York.

15. Ziegler, A., and König, I.R. (2006) *A statistical approach to genetic epidemiology: concepts and applications.* Wiley-VCH, Weinheim.

16. Khoury, M.J., Beaty, T.H., and Cohen, B.H. (1993). *Fundamentals of genetic epidemiology.* Oxford University Press, New York.

17. Lipton, L.R., Johnson, V., Cummings, C., Fisher, S., Risby, P., Eftekhar Sadat, A.T., et al. (2004) Refining the Amsterdam Criteria and Bethesda Guidelines: testing algorithms for the prediction of mismatch repair mutation status in the familial cancer clinic. *J. Clin. Oncol.* **22**, 4934–4943.

18. Risch, N. (1990) Linkage strategies for genetically complex traits. II. The power of affected relative pairs. *Am. J. Hum. Genet.* **46**, 229–241.

19. Arcos-Burgos, M., and Muenke, M. (2002) Genetics of population isolates. *Clin. Genet.* **61**, 233–247.

20. Heutink, P., and Oostra, B.A. (2002) Gene finding in genetically isolated populations. *Hum. Mol. Genet.* **11**, 2507–2515.

21. Shifman, S., and Darvasi, A. (2001) The value of isolated populations. *Nat. Genet.* **28**, 309–310.

22. Roa, B.B., Boyd, A.A., Volcik, K., and Richards, C.S. (1996). Ashkenazi Jewish population frequencies for common mutations in BRCA1 and BRCA2. *Nat. Genet.* **14**, 185–187.

23. Laken, S., Petersen, G., Gruber, S., Oddoux, C., Ostrer, H., Giardiello, F., et al. (1997) Familial colorectal cancer in Askenazim due to a hypermutable tract in APC. *Nat. Genet.* **17**, 79–83.

24. Yuan, Z. Q., Wong, N. Foulkes, W. D. Alpert, L. Manganaro, F. Andreutti-Zaugg, C., et al. (1999) A missense mutation in both hMSH2 and APC in an Ashkenazi Jewish HNPCC kindred: implications for clinical screening. *J. Med. Genet.* **36**, 790–793.

25. Foulkes, W. D., Thiffault, I., Gruber, S., Horwitz, B.M., Hamel, N., Lee, C., et al. (2002) The founder mutation MSH2*1906G→C is an important cause of hereditary nonpolyposis colorectal cancer in the Ashkenazi Jewish population. *Am. J. Hum. Genet.* **71**, 1395–1412.

26. Toledano, H., Goldberg, Y., Kedar-Barnes, I., Baris, H., Porat, R.M., Shochat, C., et al. (2008) Homozygosity of MSH2 c.1906G→C germline mutation is associated with childhood colon cancer, astrocytoma and signs of Neurofibromatosis type I. *Fam. Cancer* **8**, 187–194.

27. Jaeger, E.E., Woodford-Richens, K.L. Lockett, M., Rowan, A.J., Sawyer, E.J., Heinimann, K., et al. (2003) An ancestral Ashkenazi haplotype at the HMPS/CRAC1 locus on 15q13-q14 is associated with hereditary mixed polyposis syndrome. *Am. J. Hum. Genet.* **72**, 1261–1267.

28. Tomlinson, I., Rahman, N., Frayling, I., Mangion, J., Barfoot, R., Hamoudi, R., et al. (1999) Inherited susceptibility to colorectal adenomas and carcinomas: evidence for a new predisposition gene on 15q14-q22. *Gastroenterology* **116**, 789–795.

29. Jaeger, E., Webb, E., Howarth, K., Carvajal-Carmona, L., Rowan, A., Broderick, P., et al. (2008) Common genetic variants at the CRAC1 (HMPS) locus on chromosome 15q13.3 influence colorectal cancer risk. *Nat. Genet.* **40**, 26–28.

30. Ott, J. (1999) *Analysis of human genetic linkage.* Johns Hopkins University Press, Baltimore.

31. Elston, R.C., Buxbaum, S., Jacobs, K. B., and Olson, J. M. (2000) Haseman and Elston revisited. *Genet. Epidemiol.* **19**, 1–17.

32. Kerber, R.A., Amos, C.I., Yeap, B.Y., Finkelstein, D.M., and Thomas, D.C. (2008) Design considerations in a sib-pair study of linkage for susceptibility loci in cancer. *BMC Med. Genet.* **9**, 64.

33. Zhao, H., Zhang, H., and Rotter, J.I. (1997) Cost-effective sib-pair designs in the mapping of quantitative-trait loci. *Am. J. Hum. Genet.* **60**, 1211–1221.

34. Elston, R.C., Song, D., and Iyengar, S.K. (2005) Mathematical assumptions versus biological reality: myths in affected sib pair linkage analysis. *Am. J. Hum. Genet.* **76**, 152–156.

35. Edwards, J.H. (2003) Sib-pairs in multifactorial disorders: the sib-similarity problem. *Clin. Genet.* **63**, 1–9.

36. Zollner, S., Wen, X., Hanchard, N.A., Herbert, M.A., Ober, C., and Pritchard, J.K. (2004) Evidence for extensive transmission distortion in the human genome. *Am. J. Hum. Genet.* **74**, 62–72.

37. Risch, N., and Zhang, H. (1995) Extreme discordant sib pairs for mapping quantitative trait loci in humans. *Science* **268**, 1584–1589.
38. Spielman, R.S., McGinnis R.E., and Ewens. W.J. (1993) Transmission test for linkage disequilibrium: the insulin gene region and insulin-dependent diabetes mellitus (IDDM). *Am. J. Hum. Genet.* **52**, 506–516.
39. Rabinowitz, D., and Laird, N. (2000) A unified approach to adjusting association tests for population admixture with arbitrary pedigree structure and arbitrary missing marker information. *Hum. Hered.* **50**, 211–223.
40. Lange, C., and Laird, N.M. (2002) Power calculations for a general class of family-based association tests: dichotomous traits. *Am. J. Hum. Genet.* **71**, 575–584.
41. Lange, C., and Laird, N.M. (2002) On a general class of conditional tests for family-based association studies in genetics: the asymptotic distribution, the conditional power, and optimality considerations. *Genet. Epidemiol.* **23**, 165–180.
42. Lange, C., DeMeo, D.L., and Laird, N.M. (2002) Power and design considerations for a general class of family-based association tests: quantitative traits. *Am. J. Hum. Genet.* **71**, 1330–1341.
43. Lange, C., DeMeo, D. Silverman, E.K. Weiss, S.T., and Laird, N.M. (2003) Using the non-informative families in family-based association tests: a powerful new testing strategy. *Am. J. Hum. Genet.* **73**, 801–811.
44. Lange, C., Lyon, H., DeMeo, D., Raby, B., Silverman, E.K., and Weiss, S.T. (2003) A new powerful non-parametric two-stage approach for testing multiple phenotypes in family-based association studies. *Hum. Hered.* **56**, 10–17.
45. Lange, C., Silverman, E.K., Xu, X., Weiss, S.T., and Laird, N.M. 2003. A multivariate family-based association test using generalized estimating equations: FBAT-GEE. *Biostatistics* **4**, 195–206.
46. Lange, C., DeMeo, D., Silverman, E.K., Weiss, S.T., and Laird, N.M. (2004) PBAT: tools for family-based association studies. *Am. J. Hum. Genet.* **74**, 367–369.
47. Laird, N.M., Horvath, S., and Xu, X. (2000) Implementing a unified approach to family-based tests of association. *Genet. Epidemiol.* **19**, Suppl 1: S36–S42.
48. Horvath, S., Xu, X., Lake, S.L., Silverman, E.K., Weiss, S.T., and Laird, N.M. (2004) Family-based tests for associating haplotypes with general phenotype data: application to asthma genetics. *Genet. Epidemiol.* **26**, 61–69.
49. Spielman, R.S., and Ewens, W.J. (1998) A sibship test for linkage in the presence of association: the sib transmission/disequilibrium test. *Am. J. Hum. Genet.* **62**, 450–458.
50. Risch, N., and Merikangas, K. (1996) The future of genetic studies of complex human diseases. *Science* **273**, 1516–1517.
51. Burton, P.R., Clayton, D.G., Cardon, L.R., Craddock, N., Deloukas, P., Duncanson, A., et al. 2007. Genome-wide association study of 14,000 cases of seven common diseases and 3,000 shared controls. *Nature* **447**, 661–678.
52. Price, A.L., Patterson, N.J., Plenge, R.M., Weinblatt, M.E., Shadick, N.A., and Reich, D. (2006) Principal components analysis corrects for stratification in genome-wide association studies. *Nat. Genet.* **38**, 904–909.
53. Purcell, S., Cherny, S.S., and Sham, P.C. (2003) Genetic Power Calculator: design of linkage and association genetic mapping studies of complex traits. *Bioinformatics* **19**, 149–150.
54. Menashe, I., Rosenberg, P.S., and Chen, B.E. (2008) PGA: power calculator for case-control genetic association analyses. *BMC Genet.* **9**, 36.
55. Ploughman, L.M., and Boehnke, M. 1989. Estimating the power of a proposed linkage study for a complex genetic trait. *Am. J. Hum. Genet.* **44**, 543–551.
56. Boehnke, M. (1986) Estimating the power of a proposed linkage study: a practical computer simulation approach. *Am. J. Hum. Genet.* **39**, 513–527.
57. Terwilliger, J.D., and Ott, J. (1994) *Handbook of human genetic linkage.* Johns Hopkins University Press, Baltimore.
58. (2009) S.A.G.E. Statistical Analysis for Genetic Epidemiology.
59. Whittaker, J.C., and Lewis, C.M. (1999) Power comparisons of the transmission/disequilibrium test and sib-transmission/disequilibrium-test statistics. *Am. J. Hum. Genet.* **65**, 578–580.
60. Knapp, M. (1999) A note on power approximations for the transmission/disequilibrium test. *Am. J. Hum. Genet.* **64**, 1177–1185.
61. Knapp, M. (1999) The transmission/disequilibrium test and parental-genotype reconstruction: the reconstruction-combined transmission/disequilibrium test. *Am. J. Hum. Genet.* **64**, 861–870.
62. Passarge, E. (2002) Dissecting Hirschsprung disease. *Nat. Genet.* **31**, 11–12.

63. Knowler, W.C., Williams, R.C., Pettitt, D.J., and Steinberg, A.G. (1988) Gm3;5,13,14 and type 2 diabetes mellitus: an association in American Indians with genetic admixture. *Am. J. Hum. Genet.* **43**, 520–526.
64. Clayton, D.G., Walker, N.M., Smyth, D.J., Pask, R., Cooper, J.D., Maier, L.M., et al. (2005) Population structure, differential bias and genomic control in a large-scale, case-control association study. *Nat. Genet.* **37**, 1243–1246.
65. Devlin, B., and Roeder, K. (1999) Genomic control for association studies. *Biometrics* **55**, 997–1004.
66. Price, A. L., Butler, J., Patterson, N., Capelli, C., Pascali, V.L., Scarnicci, F., et al. (2008) Discerning the ancestry of European Americans in genetic association studies. *PLoS Genet.* **4**, e236.
67. Nelis, M., Esko, T., Magi, R., Zimprich, F., Zimprich, A., Toncheva, D., et al. (2009). Genetic structure of Europeans: a view from the North-East. *PLoS One* **4**, e5472.
68. Purcell, S., Neale, B., Todd-Brown, K., Thomas, L., Ferreira, M.A., Bender, D., et al. (2007) PLINK: a tool set for whole-genome association and population-based linkage analyses. *Am. J. Hum. Genet.* **81**, 559–575.
69. Ziegler, A., Konig, I.R., and Thompson, J.R. (2008) Biostatistical aspects of genome-wide association studies. *Biom. J.* **50**, 8–28.
70. Cunningham, J.M., Sellers, T.A., Schildkraut, J.M., Fredericksen, Z.S., Vierkant, R.A., Kelemen, L.E., et al. (2008). Performance of amplified DNA in an Illumina GoldenGate BeadArray assay. *Cancer Epidemiol. Biomarkers Prev.* **17**, 1781–1789.
71. Berthier-Schaad, Y., Kao, W.H., Coresh, J., Zhang, L., Ingersoll, R.G., Stephens, R., et al. (2007) Reliability of high-throughput genotyping of whole genome amplified DNA in SNP genotyping studies. *Electrophoresis* **28**, 2812–2817.
72. Abecasis, G.R., Cherny, S.S., Cookson, W.O., and Cardon, L.R. (2001) GRR: graphical representation of relationship errors. *Bioinformatics* **17**, 742–743.
73. International HapMap Consortium. (2005) A haplotype map of the human genome. *Nature* **437**, 1299–1320.
74. Samani, N. J., Erdmann, J., Hall, A.S., Hengstenberg, C., Mangino, M., Mayer, B., et al. (2007) Genomewide association analysis of coronary artery disease. *N. Engl. J. Med.* **357**, 443–453.
75. Dudbridge, F. (2008) Likelihood-based association analysis for nuclear families and unrelated subjects with missing genotype data. *Hum. Hered.* **66**, 87–98.
76. Marchini, J., Cardon, L.R., Phillips, M.S., and Donnelly, P. (2004) The effects of human population structure on large genetic association studies. *Nat. Genet.* **36**, 512–517.
77. de Bakker, P.I., Yelensky, R., Pe'er, I., Gabriel, S.B., Daly, M.J., and Altshuler, D. (2005) Efficiency and power in genetic association studies. *Nat. Genet.* **37**, 1217–1223.
78. Cordell, H.J. (2009) Genome-wide association studies: detecting gene–gene interactions that underlie human diseases. *Nat. Rev. Genet.* **10**, 392–404.
79. Wacholder, S., Chanock, S., Garcia-Closas, M., El Ghormli, L., and Rothman, N. (2004) Assessing the probability that a positive report is false: an approach for molecular epidemiology studies. *J. Natl. Cancer Inst.* **96**, 434–442.
80. Hochberg, Y.B.A.Y. (1995) Controlling the false discovery rate: a practical and powerful approach to multiple testing. *J. Roy. Stat. Soc.* **57**, 289–300.
81. Howie, B.N., Donnelly, P., and Marchini, J. (2009) A flexible and accurate genotype imputation method for the next generation of genome-wide association studies. *PLoS Genet.* **5**, e1000529.
82. Aschard, H., Bouzigon, E., Corda, E., Ulgen, A., Dizier, M.H., Gormand, F., et al. (2009) Sex-specific effect of IL9 polymorphisms on lung function and polysensitization. *Genes Immun.* **10**, 559–565.
83. Browning, B.L., and Browning, S.R. (2009) A unified approach to genotype imputation and haplotype-phase inference for large data sets of trios and unrelated individuals. *Am. J. Hum. Genet.* **84**, 210–223.
84. Marchini, J., Howie, B., Myers, S., McVean, G., and Donnelly, P. (2007) A new multipoint method for genome-wide association studies by imputation of genotypes. *Nat. Genet.* **39**, 906–913.
85. Scheet, P., and Stephens, M. (2006) A fast and flexible statistical model for large-scale population genotype data: applications to inferring missing genotypes and haplotypic phase. *Am. J. Hum. Genet.* **78**, 629–644.
86. Pei, Y.F., Li, J., Zhang, L., Papasian, C.J., and Deng, H.W. (2008) Analyses and comparison of accuracy of different genotype imputation methods. *PLoS One* **3**, e3551.
87. Devlin, B., Bacanu, S.A., and Roeder, K. (2004) Genomic Control to the extreme. *Nat. Genet.* **36**, 1129–1130; author reply 1131.

88. Tintle, N.L., Gordon, D., McMahon F.J., and Finch, S.J. (2007) Using duplicate genotyped data in genetic analyses: testing association and estimating error rates. *Stat. Appl. Genet. Mol. Biol.* **6**, Article 4.

89. Huang, L., Li, Y., Singleton, A.B., Hardy, J.A., Abecasis, G., Rosenberg, N.A., et al. (2009) Genotype-imputation accuracy across worldwide human populations. *Am. J. Hum Genet.* **84**, 235–250.

Chapter 2

Prioritizing Candidate Genetic Modifiers of *BRCA1* and *BRCA2* Using a Combinatorial Analysis of Global Expression and Polymorphism Association Studies of Breast Cancer

Logan C. Walker and Amanda B. Spurdle

Abstract

Epidemiological evidence from different studies has shown that genes harboring sequence variations may modify breast cancer risk in *BRCA1* and *BRCA2* mutation carriers. Current attempts to identify genetic modifiers of *BRCA1* and *BRCA2* associated risk have focused on a candidate gene-based approach or the development of large genome-wide association studies. However, both methods have notable limitations. This chapter describes a novel approach for analyzing gene expression differences to prioritize candidate modifier genes for single nucleotide polymorphism association studies. The advantage that gives this strategy an edge over other candidate gene-based studies is its potential to identify candidate genes that interact with exogenous risk factors to cause or modify cancer, without detailed a priori knowledge of the molecular pathways involved.

Key words: Familial, Breast cancer, BRCA1, BRCA2, Genetic modifiers, Microarray, Irradiation, Genome wide association study, Lymphoblastoid cell lines

1. Introduction

Epidemiological evidence from family-based studies has indicated that genes harboring polymorphisms or mutations may modify breast cancer risk in *BRCA1* and *BRCA2* mutation carriers (1–3). As a result of this evidence, a number of studies have attempted to identify genetic modifiers of *BRCA1*- and *BRCA2*-associated risk by targeting candidate genes in breast cancer-related pathways, such as DNA repair and steroid hormone receptor signaling (4–10). To date, the identification of an SNP (rs1801320) in the 5′UTR of *RAD51* has provided the best evidence for a genetic modifier in *BRCA2* mutation carriers using the candidate gene approach (11).

Importantly, RAD51 is known to play an important role in the recombinational repair of radiation-induced double-strand DNA breaks (12), particularly through interaction with BRCA2 (13). Since ionizing radiation is known to be an environmental risk factor associated with breast cancer development in *BRCA1* and *BRCA2* mutation carriers (14), additional genes associated with irradiation response may also be candidates for potential risk modifiers. However, a major disadvantage of using the candidate gene (or candidate SNP) approach for identifying potential risk modifiers is the limited understanding of mechanisms and pathways that underlie breast cancer development in families carrying mutations in *BRCA1* or *BRCA2*. An alternative and powerful approach that can overcome such issues is the use of genome-wide association (GWA) studies to identify candidate SNPs. The analysis of breast cancer risk-associated SNPs identified by a large population-based GWA study (15) has shown that several of these SNPs also appear to modify risk in *BRCA1* and/or *BRCA2* carriers (16). However, only some of the breast cancer-associated SNPs assessed were shown to modify risk in carriers, and some of those associated with risk showed effects in *BRCA2* but not in *BRCA1* (16), suggesting that additional approaches are required to more comprehensively identify modifiers of *BRCA1* and *BRCA2*. While GWA studies specifically addressing risk among *BRCA1* and/or *BRCA2* carriers provide a more direct approach to identifying modifiers of these genes using an agnostic approach, GWA studies require large sample sizes to identify genetic modifiers with confidence. To address this issue, the Consortium of Investigators of Modifiers of *BRCA1* and *BRCA2* (CIMBA) was established in 2005 to link clinical and epidemiological data from about 30 groups from around the world (17). Collaborative CIMBA projects now have access to more than 10,000 *BRCA1* and 5,000 *BRCA2* mutation carriers, and the potential power of >80% at a threshold of $P<0.0001$ to detect polymorphisms in *BRCA1* carriers with minor allele frequencies >10% that confer risk ratios >1.2 (17). However, the GWA approach is still limited in that study designs involve predefined selection criteria for which SNPs identified from the initial whole genome scan are going to be analyzed in subsequent replication studies, a study design enforced by current genotyping costs. Due to insufficient power to detect low-risk SNPs, it is possible that cancer-associated SNPs that show no obvious correlation in the initial scan may be excluded from further study. Moreover, GWA studies are often limited in information about exogenous risk factors, such as environmental exposures, which confounds any effort to explore the effect of environmental factors in modifying gene–disease associations. Global gene expression analysis as a means to agnostically identify candidates has the potential to enhance the analysis of GWA studies.

We have previously explored the value of analyzing gene expression differences in irradiated lymphoblastoid cell lines from

BRCA1 or BRCA2 mutation carriers and mutation-negative controls to prioritize candidate modifier genes for polymorphism association studies (18). Genes that discriminated between BRCA1 or BRCA2 mutation carriers and mutation-negative controls were identified and filtered based on cellular function. We theorized that genes which modify BRCA1 and BRCA2 are likely also to contribute to increased risk of developing breast cancer, and so aligned these refined gene lists against data derived through the National Cancer Institute's Cancer Genetic Markers of Susceptibility (CGEMS) genome-wide association results for a large breast cancer case-control sample set (18). The intention was to identify genes whose expression is associated with BRCA1 and BRCA2 mutation status as a method for prioritizing candidate modifier genes for polymorphism association studies in large cohorts of BRCA1 and BRCA2 carriers. Assessing the effect of exogenous cellular stimulants by mRNA expression analysis was a way to target genes involved in biological pathways perturbed by such exogenous factors. We have used the example of irradiation to identify specific genetic risk factors that interact with this stimulant to cause or modify breast cancer in mutation carriers. However, similar array-based experiments could be designed that use exogenous stimulants to affect other biological pathways that appear to play a role in familial or population-based cancers, and so prioritize candidate genes for further study as potential genetic modifiers in the appropriate sample sets.

2. Materials

1. Epstein Barr virus-transformed lymphoblastoid cell lines derived from breast cancer-affected women in multicase families in which a BRCA1 or BRCA2 mutation had been identified. Samples used in the study were acquired as part of a research project approved by the familial breast cancer resource the Kathleen Cuningham Consortium for Breast Cancer (kConFab), Peter MacCallum Cancer Centre, Melbourne, Australia.
2. Epstein Barr virus-transformed lymphoblastoid cell lines derived from healthy female controls, recruited via the Australian Red Cross Blood Services for ethically approved genetic studies (Queensland Institute of Medical Research, Australia).
3. RPMI-1640 (Gibco Invitrogen) supplemented with 10% Serum Supreme (Lonza BioWhittaker) and 1% penicillin-streptomycin (Gibco Invitrogen).
4. Tissue culture flasks (25 cm^2) (Techno Plastic Products).

5. GammaCell 40 irradiator (Best Theratronics, formerly MDS Nordion).
6. 10 mL centrifuge tube (Sarstedt).
7. 50 mL centrifuge tube (Nunc).
8. RNeasy® Mini Kit (Qiagen).
9. 21-gauge × 38 mm needle (Terumo).
10. 1 mL Syringe (Terumo).
11. Agilent RNA 6000 Nano Chip kit.
12. Agilent 2100 Bioanalyzer.
13. NanoDrop™ 1000 Spectrophotometer (Thermo Scientific).
14. Illumina® TotalPrep RNA Amplification Kit (Ambion).
15. 0.2 mL thin-walled PCR tubes.
16. PCR-Cooler 0.2 mL (Eppendorf).
17. 0.6 mL microfuge tubes.
18. Sentrix® BeadChip Array for Gene Expression (Illumina®).
19. Illumina® Gene Expression System.
20. Streptavidin-Cy3 solution: Resuspend 1 mg of streptividin-Cy3 dye (Amersham) in 1 mL of ddH$_2$O and store in single use aliquots at −20°C.
21. Illumina® Hybridization Oven.
22. Illumina® BeadArray Reader.

3. Methods

The methodology describes the use of aligning gene expression data with genome-wide association data from a population-based breast cancer case-control study to identify candidate modifier genes of *BRCA1* and *BRCA2*. This protocol utilizes the Human-6 version 1 BeadChips along with the Illumina Gene Expression System and Illumina BeadStation. Other array platforms (e.g. Affymetrix, Roche NimbleGen, Agilent, spotted cDNA arrays) may be adapted with appropriate probe annotation. An overview of the steps used in the methodology is presented in Fig. 1.

3.1. Cell Culture and Irradiation

1. Culture LCLs in a 25 cm² flask containing supplemented RPMI 1640 medium (20 mL) and passage when approaching confluence (see Note 1).
2. Twenty four hours prior to irradiation treatment, normalize cells to a concentration of 10×10^6 cells per 20 mL of medium. This is carried out by calculating the total cell number using a hematocytometer and discarding excess cells. For example,

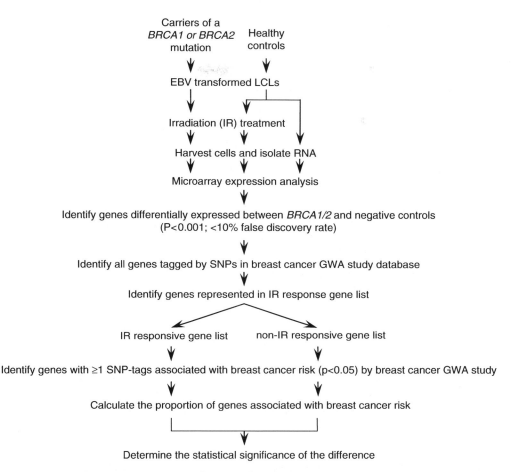

Fig. 1. An overview of the steps involved in identifying candidate modifiers of high-risk susceptibility genes in carriers of a *BRCA1* or *BRCA2* deleterious mutation.

in a 20 mL cell culture that contained a total of 16×10^6 cells, 7.5 mL of cell suspension would be discarded to leave 10×10^6 cells in 12.5 mL of medium. Transfer these cells to a 50 mL tube and pellet by centrifugation at $300 \times g$ for 5 min. Remove the supernatant by aspiration and resuspend cells in 20 mL of fresh supplemented RPMI 1640 medium by gently pipetting. Transfer the cell suspension to a new 25 cm² flask and culture cells for a further 24 h.

3. Immediately prior to irradiation treatment, mix cells and transfer 10 mL of cell suspension to a 10 mL centrifuge tube. Centrifuge the cells at $300 \times g$ for 5 min and remove the supernatant by aspiration. Transfer the tubes containing the cell pellet into dry ice for 10–15 min to maintain the integrity of the cellular RNA (see Note 2). Cells can be stored at −80°C until required for RNA isolation. These cells are the untreated LCLs.

4. Irradiate the remaining 5×10^6 cells within the culture flask at 10 Gy with a GammaCell 40 irradiator that uses a calibrated Cesium-137 source (e.g. 1 Gy/min would deliver 10 Gy in 10 min). Remove the cells from the irradiator and incubate at 37°C for a further 30 min (see Note 3).

5. Pellet the treated LCLs in a 10 mL centrifuge tube and store at −80°C using methods identical to those used for the untreated LCLs in step 3.

3.2. RNA Isolation

1. To lyse cells, add 350 µL of RNeasy Buffer RLT and proceed immediately to the next step. Do not thaw frozen cells without first adding Buffer RLT.

2. Homogenize the lysate by passing 5–10 times through an 18-gauge needle using a sterile 1 mL syringe. Once homogenized, use the syringe to transfer the lysate to a 1.5 mL microcentrifuge tube.

3. Isolate and purify total RNA using the RNeasy Mini Kit. We made no modifications to the protocol for the purification of total RNA from animal cells using spin technology. Elute the RNA from the RNeasy spin column using 30 µL of RNase-free H_2O.

4. Assess the quality of RNA. We used the Agilent RNA 6000 Nano Chip kit and the Agilent 2100 Bioanalyzer. An RNA integrity number (RIN) greater than nine would be expected after purifying RNA from cell lines (see Note 4).

5. Quantify the RNA using a NanoDrop™ 1000 Spectrophotometer.

3.3. RNA Amplification

The Illumina TotalPrep RNA Amplification Kit is used to amplify and biotinylate the LCL derived RNA. The protocol for this procedure is well described in the instruction manual. Samples are most efficiently processed in batches but this approach can cause nonbiological variation or "batch effects" as evidenced by downstream microarray data analysis (see Note 5). Although statistical methods have been proposed that reduce "batch effects" (19), such effects are minimized if samples are processed in random order to prevent batches being overrepresented by samples belonging to a single biological class (e.g. *BRCA1* or *BRCA2* mutation status). It is also important that the incubation time used for the in vitro transcription step is the same for all samples.

3.4. Microarray Analysis

We have used Sentrix® Human-6 version 1.0 BeadChips that allow the simultaneous assessment of expression profiles of >46,000 transcripts (including >23,000 RefSeq fully annotated genes) for six RNA samples in parallel. Illumina have since superseded this version BeadChip (currently version 3.0) by redesigning probe sequences derived from successive updates of NCBI RefSeq and UniGene databases. To reduce costs of microarray analysis, 8- or 12-sample Illumina BeadChips could be used in place of the 6-sample BeadChip.

3.4.1. cRNA Hybridization, Washing, and Signal Detection

Hybridize the cRNA samples to the BeadChip following the protocol that accompanies the Illumina Gene Expression System. Each step is adequately detailed from hybridization through to scanning and needs no modification (see Note 6). The protocol will differ slightly according to whether the 6-, 8-, or 12-sample BeadChip is being used.

3.4.2. Data Extraction and Preanalysis Processing

After the BeadChips are dried by centrifugation, scan each array by loading up to three BeadChips in the BeadArray Reader special tray (Illumina has since superseded this scanner with their new iScan System). Ensure that only the Cy3 channel is enabled and each scan uses the following settings: Gain = 2, PMT = 545 and Filter = 100%. Once all the slides have been scanned, import the data into BeadStudio (currently version 3.4) to form a single project containing all samples. Export the Sample Probe Profile to a *.txt file (see Note 7) ensuring the average signal intensity (AVG_Signal) and Detection_Score corresponding to each probe is included for each sample. Import the data into GeneSpring GX (Agilent Technologies; currently version 10.0) and normalize using the option of per chip normalization to the 50th percentile and per gene normalization to the median. Other normalization methods, such as quantile normalization, may also be considered at this stage. Filter the probes by excluding all that have an Illumina detection score of <0.99 in at least one sample. This will yield a subset of probes to use in downstream analyses.

3.5. Identify BRCA1- and BRCA2-Associated Genes

Identify genes that are differentially expressed between irradiated LCLs of mutation-negative controls and of the *BRCA1* and *BRCA2* classes. For this analysis, we import the normalized data into BRB-ArrayTools (http://linus.nci.nih.gov/BRB-ArrayTools.html) to utilize the multivariate permutation test that controls for false discoveries. The proportion of false discoveries allowed in the analysis can be selected by the user. We typically perform the test to provide 90% confidence that the number of false discoveries does not exceed 10%. To limit the analysis to the most differentially expressed genes, a stringent α-level threshold (i.e. ≤ 0.001) is also applied to each two-sample *T*-test performed.

3.6. Identify Irradiation Response Genes

Irradiation response genes are defined as those genes whose expression levels change as a result of LCL exposure to irradiation. There are two methods which could be used to identify irradiation response genes:

Option 1: Compare microarray expression profiles of the treated (irradiated) and untreated normal LCL pairs using the paired *T*-test option. As in the previous section, restrict the number of false discoveries to 10% and set a α-level threshold of 0.001. This gene list contains the irradiation responsive genes.

Option 2: In our study (18), we had expression data from irradiated LCLs derived from healthy controls, but we did not have expression data from the same LCLs prior to treatment. We were therefore unable to generate a list of irradiation responsive genes and so we utilized a gene list from a published study (20) (see Note 8). In this situation, where data is compared across two different arrays, it is necessary to exclude all genes that are not represented on both arrays.

3.7. Identify All Genes Tagged by SNPs in the CGEMS Database

1. Use gene symbols approved by the Human Genome Organization (HUGO) Gene Nomenclature Committee (www.genenames.org) to link the *BRCA1*-, *BRCA2*- and irradiation-associated gene lists with the CGEMS Breast Cancer GWA (currently Phase 1) dataset.

2. Where gene lists contain aliases for some gene symbols, convert each alias to an official symbol. Use the "Batch Lookup" tool in MatchMiner (21) or an equivalent annotation tool to translate the gene symbols and standardize the gene lists.

3. To identify all *BRCA1*-, *BRCA2*- and irradiation-associated genes tagged by SNPs in the CGEMS database, separately enter the HUGO gene symbol lists into the CGEMS Association Finding dataset. Select the Covariate Adjustment to return a *p*-value ($P \leq 0.05$) for an adjusted score test (see Note 9). The output table from CGEMS will contain a column with SNP-associated (tagged) gene symbols.

4. In many cases, the HUGO gene symbol will be listed alongside one or more aliases. Therefore, separate the terms so that the official symbol can be used as a search term. One way to do this is to import the output table as a *.txt file into Excel and separate each symbol using an "|" as a delimiter. This process will likely identify a high proportion of genes that are tagged with one or more SNPs. These SNP-tagged genes are to be retained for further analysis.

3.8. Alignment of GWA Study Association Results with BRCA1- and BRCA2- Associated Genes Categorized by Irradiation

1. Classify irradiation responsive genes in the *BRCA1*- and *BRCA2*-associated gene lists by aligning data against the irradiation gene list.

2. For each irradiation responsive and nonirradiation responsive gene list, identify those genes with ≥1 SNP-tags (i.e. genes reported by CGEMS to be associated with breast cancer risk ($P < 0.05$)) and calculate the proportion of these genes in their respective gene lists.

3. Apply the chi-squared statistic to test the null hypothesis that irradiation responsive genes whose expression correlated with *BRCA1* and/or *BRCA2* mutation status are no more likely to be tagged by risk-associated SNPs in the CGEMS dataset.
4. To exclude potential bias as a result of gene size, obtain the transcriptional start and stop sites for each gene in their respective gene lists using the annotation tool MatchMiner and determine whether the average gene sizes differ significantly between the irradiation and nonirradiation response groups.

If genes defined by gene expression analysis to play an important role in irradiation response are potential breast cancer risk modifiers, we would predict that breast cancer associated SNPs would be more likely to be linked to these genes. These genes (and the breast cancer associated SNPs in them) would be suitable for prioritization as potential modifiers of *BRCA1* and *BRCA2* in large sample sets of *BRCA1* and *BRCA2* carriers.

4. Notes

1. We suggest that LCLs grown from frozen stocks be cultured over a period of at least 2 weeks to ensure that the cells no longer exhibit growth irregularities as a result of being cryogenically stored in DMSO.
2. Batching LCLs for treatment is an efficient way of carrying out the experiment; however, it is important to either freeze or homogenize the treated (or nontreated) cells in Buffer RLT immediately after centrifugation. Allowing cells to sit at room temperature increases the possibility of RNA degradation and may also allow gene expression levels to change so that treated LCLs may no longer reflect an irradiation induced profile.
3. A relatively early time-point of 30 min post irradiation was chosen to target early transcriptional response and to minimize possible downstream compensation effects. It has previously been shown that 10 Gy irradiation treatment of normal LCLs has an effect on the transcriptional response, with greatest change in mRNA levels for most genes within 1 h posttreatment (20). Interestingly, a study of mouse brain gene expression after whole-body low-dose irradiation also showed that expression changes in a large number of irradiation response genes can be measured at the 30 min time point (22).
4. RIN < 9 indicates partial RNA degradation. To avoid this, see Note 2.

5. We have observed expression profile differences between RNA amplification sample batches but not between array hybridization batches. These experimentally induced differences are likely to be enhanced when the biological difference between the samples with respect to gene expression magnitude is relatively small, which is the case with LCLs.

6. According to the protocol, the hybridization step can be between 16 and 20 h. We believe that to minimize batch bias, it is important that the incubation time used for the hybridization step is kept consistent for each BeadChip. We adhered strictly to an incubation time of 19 h and always found a high correlation ($r > 0.98$) for duplicate arrays.

7. Data can also be exported as a "Sample Gene Profile". The "Sample Gene Profile" format takes the average value of all probes that target a specific gene regardless of whether the probe sequences differ. Therefore, probes that target specific mRNA isoforms for a particular gene may be combined with a probe that makes no such discrimination. For this reason, we have chosen to work with probe-based profiles.

8. A disadvantage with this method is that it might be difficult to find a study that has employed the similar treatment/posttreatment conditions (e.g. dose, posttreatment incubation period).

9. The rationale for choosing a nominal P-value cut-off of 0.05 was based on the following: (1) Comparing data from the breast cancer genome-wide association study of Easton et al. (15) with those from CGEMS revealed that two of the five top-ranking SNPs in named genes (TNRC9, LSP1) from Easton et al. had P-values greater than 0.05 in CGEMS, suggesting that a more stringent cut-off may exclude potential candidate risk associated SNPs; (2) Approximately 15,000–20,000 of the top-ranking SNPs from CGEMS Phase I will be selected for the Phase II replication study (http://cgems.cancer.gov/about/executive_summary.asp), and will therefore carry a P-value less than 0.04.

Acknowledgments

We thank Nic Waddell, Anette Ten Haaf, Georgia Chenevix-Trench, Denis Moss and kConFab for their contribution in developing the protocols described here. We also thank Nic Waddell for critical reading of the manuscript. This work was supported by the Susan G. Komen Breast Cancer Foundation and the NHMRC.

References

1. Antoniou, A., Pharoah, P. D., Narod, S., Risch, H. A., Eyfjord, J. E., Hopper, J. L., et al. (2003) Average risks of breast and ovarian cancer associated with BRCA1 or BRCA2 mutations detected in case Series unselected for family history: a combined analysis of 22 studies. *Am. J. Hum. Genet.* 72, 1117–1130.

2. Simchoni, S., Friedman, E., Kaufman, B., Gershoni-Baruch, R., Orr-Urtreger, A., Kedar-Barnes, I., et al. (2006) Familial clustering of site-specific cancer risks associated with BRCA1 and BRCA2 mutations in the Ashkenazi Jewish population. *Proc. Natl. Acad. Sci. U.S.A.* 103, 3770–3774.

3. Smith, A., Moran, A., Boyd, M. C., Bulman, M., Shenton, A., Smith, L., et al. (2007) Phenocopies in BRCA1 and BRCA2 families: evidence for modifier genes and implications for screening. *J. Med. Genet.* 44, 10–15.

4. Dagan, E., Friedman, E., Paperna, T., Carmi, N., and Gershoni-Baruch, R. (2002) Androgen receptor CAG repeat length in Jewish Israeli women who are BRCA1/2 mutation carriers: association with breast/ovarian cancer phenotype. *Eur. J. Hum. Genet.* 10, 724–728.

5. Hughes, D. J., Ginolhac, S. M., Coupier, I., Barjhoux, L., Gaborieau, V., Bressac-de-Paillerets, B., et al. (2005) Breast cancer risk in BRCA1 and BRCA2 mutation carriers and polyglutamine repeat length in the AIB1 gene. *Int. J. Cancer* 117, 230–233.

6. Kadouri, L., Easton, D. F., Edwards, S., Hubert, A., Kote-Jarai, Z., Glaser, B., et al. (2001) CAG and GGC repeat polymorphisms in the androgen receptor gene and breast cancer susceptibility in BRCA1/2 carriers and non-carriers. *Br. J. Cancer* 85, 36–40.

7. Kadouri, L., Kote-Jarai, Z., Easton, D. F., Hubert, A., Hamoudi, R., Glaser, B., et al. (2004) Polyglutamine repeat length in the AIB1 gene modifies breast cancer susceptibility in BRCA1 carriers. *Int. J. Cancer* 108, 399–403.

8. Kadouri, L., Kote-Jarai, Z., Hubert, A., Durocher, F., Abeliovich, D., Glaser, B., et al. (2004) A single-nucleotide polymorphism in the RAD51 gene modifies breast cancer risk in BRCA2 carriers, but not in BRCA1 carriers or noncarriers. *Br. J. Cancer* 90, 2002–2005.

9. Levy-Lahad, E., Lahad, A., Eisenberg, S., Dagan, E., Paperna, T., Kasinetz, L., et al. (2001) A single nucleotide polymorphism in the RAD51 gene modifies cancer risk in BRCA2 but not BRCA1 carriers. *Proc. Natl. Acad. Sci. U.S.A.* 98, 3232–3236.

10. Wang, W. W., Spurdle, A. B., Kolachana, P., Bove, B., Modan, B., Ebbers, S. M., et al. (2001) A single nucleotide polymorphism in the 5' untranslated region of RAD51 and risk of cancer among BRCA1/2 mutation carriers. *Cancer Epidemiol. Biomarkers Prev.* 10, 955–960.

11. Antoniou, A. C., Sinilnikova, O. M., Simard, J., Leone, M., Dumont, M., Neuhausen, S. L., et al. (2007) RAD51 135G→C modifies breast cancer risk among BRCA2 mutation carriers: results from a combined analysis of 19 studies. *Am. J. Hum. Genet.* 81, 1186–1200.

12. Karran, P. (2000) DNA double strand break repair in mammalian cells. *Curr. Opin. Genet. Dev.* 10, 144–150.

13. Shivji, M. K., Davies, O. R., Savill, J. M., Bates, D. L., Pellegrini, L., and Venkitaraman, A. R. (2006) A region of human BRCA2 containing multiple BRC repeats promotes RAD51-mediated strand exchange. *Nucleic Acids Res.* 34, 4000–4011.

14. Broeks, A., Braaf, L. M., Huseinovic, A., Nooijen, A., Urbanus, J., Hogervorst, F. B., et al. (2007) Identification of women with an increased risk of developing radiation-induced breast cancer: a case only study. *Breast Cancer Res.* 9, R26.

15. Easton, D. F., Pooley, K. A., Dunning, A. M., Pharoah, P. D., Thompson, D., Ballinger, D. G., et al. (2007) Genome-wide association study identifies novel breast cancer susceptibility loci. *Nature* 447, 1087–1093.

16. Antoniou, A. C., Spurdle, A. B., Sinilnikova, O. M., Healey, S., Pooley, K. A., Schmutzler, R. K., et al. (2008) Common breast cancer-predisposition alleles are associated with breast cancer risk in BRCA1 and BRCA2 mutation carriers. *Am. J. Hum. Genet.* 82, 937–948.

17. Chenevix-Trench, G., Milne, R. L., Antoniou, A. C., Couch, F. J., Easton, D. F., and Goldgar, D. E. (2007) An international initiative to identify genetic modifiers of cancer risk in BRCA1 and BRCA2 mutation carriers: the Consortium of Investigators of Modifiers of BRCA1 and BRCA2 (CIMBA). *Breast Cancer Res.* 9, 104.

18. Walker, L. C., Waddell, N., Ten Haaf, A., Grimmond, S., and Spurdle, A. B. (2008) Use of expression data and the CGEMS genome-wide breast cancer association study to identify genes that may modify risk in BRCA1/2 mutation carriers. *Breast Cancer Res. Treat.* 112, 229–236.

19. Johnson, W. E., Li, C., and Rabinovic, A. (2007) Adjusting batch effects in microarray

expression data using empirical Bayes methods. *Biostatistics* **8**, 118–127.

20. Jen, K. Y., and Cheung, V. G. (2003) Transcriptional response of lymphoblastoid cells to ionizing radiation. *Genome Res.* **13**, 2092–2100.

21. Bussey, K. J., Kane, D., Sunshine, M., Narasimhan, S., Nishizuka, S., Reinhold, W. C., et al. (2003) MatchMiner: a tool for batch navigation among gene and gene product identifiers. *Genome Biol.* **4**, R27.

22. Yin, E., Nelson, D. O., Coleman, M. A., Peterson, L. E., and Wyrobek, A. J. (2003) Gene expression changes in mouse brain after exposure to low-dose ionizing radiation. *Int. J. Radiat. Biol.* **79**, 759–775.

Chapter 3

Microarray-Based Comparative Genomic Hybridization (Array-CGH) as a Useful Tool for Identifying Genes Involved in Glioblastoma (GB)

Yolanda Ruano, Manuela Mollejo, Angel Rodríguez de Lope, José Luis Hernández-Moneo, Pedro Martínez, and Bárbara Meléndez

Abstract

Alterations in the genome that lead to changes in DNA sequence copy number are a characteristic of Glioblastomas (GBs). Microarray-based comparative genomic hybridization (array-CGH) is a high-throughput technology that allows the hybridization of genomic DNA onto conventional cDNA microarrays, normally used in expression profiling, to analyze genomic copy number imbalances. In this way, thousands of genes can be reviewed in a high resolution analysis to define amplicons and to identify? candidate genes showing recurrent genomic copy number changes in GB tumors.

Key words: GB, cDNA microarray, Array-CGH, Amplification, Copy number changes, Genomic DNA, Hybridization

1. Introduction

Comparative genomic hybridization (CGH), a technique that detects and maps genomic copy number variations, has been widely used for the analysis of various tumor types (1). However, the low resolution of the method, due to it being restricted to the chromosome level, makes the identification of candidate genes difficult. The development and application of microarray-based formats for CGH has been a major step in improving genomic profiling. The main advantages over the use of chromosome CGH are: higher resolution and dynamic range, direct mapping aberrations to the genome sequence, and higher throughput. In contrast, a limitation of this technique is the clone spacing of the constructed array (2).

A number of different array platforms have been used for CGH measurements of tumor genomes. The various approaches have employed large insert genomic clones, such as bacterial artificial chromosomes (BACs), cDNA clones, and oligonucleotides for array spots. In addition, the analyses of tumor genomes by microarray CGH have used arrays focused on a particular region of the genome (3, 4), selected regions known to be frequently altered in tumors (5) or genome-wide arrays (6).

The application of cDNA microarrays as a platform for CGH makes it possible to integrate information on gene copy numbers and expression levels. The cDNA microarrays were initially produced to measure gene expression and frequently contain a large number of clones. The hybridization of the same cDNA microarrays for expression and genomic analysis has permitted assessment of the relationship of mRNA expression levels to DNA copy number variations across the genome. This can be used to directly identify genes that are activated or silenced due to the underlying unbalanced genomic alterations (7–10).

2. Materials

2.1. Genomic DNA Extraction

1. Saline solution: 0,9 % (w/v) sodium chloride (NaCl), (B. Braun). Store at room temperature.
2. Blood lysis buffer: 2 M Tris-HCl, pH 7.5, 1 M magnesium-chloride (Cl$_2$Mg). Store at 4°C.
3. Protein digestion buffer: 5 M NaCl, 250 mM ethylenediamine tetraacetic acid (EDTA), pH 8.0, and 10 % (w/v) sodium dodecyl sulfate (SDS). Filter the solution with a Syringe Driven Filter Unit (MF Membrane for Clarification of Aqueous Solution; Millipore, Billerica, MA). Store at room temperature.
4. Proteinase K, recombinant (Roche, Basilea, Switzerland) is dissolved at 10 mg/ml in distilled water and stored in aliquots at −20°C.
5. Phenol/chloroform/isoamyl alcohol (25:24:1) (Applichem, Darmstadt, Germany). Store at 4°C.
6. Chloroform/Isoamyl alcohol (24:1). Prepare in an opaque glass bottle; shake overnight and store at 4°C.
7. 5 M NaCl solution. Store at 4°C.
8. Ethanol, absolute and 70%. Store at −20°C.
9. Tris-EDTA buffer (TE), pH 8.0: 1 mM Tris-HCl, 0.1 mM EDTA. Store at room temperature.

2.2. DNA Digestion

1. Digestion enzymes (Life Technologies, Inc., Rockville, MD): 25 units of 100 units/µL RsaI and 25 units of 10 units/µL AluI.

2.3. Clean-up of Digested DNA

1. Purification kit (Qiagen, Hilden, Germany)
2. TE buffer, pH 8.0: 1 mM Tris-HCl, 0.1 mM EDTA. Store at room temperature.
3. Phenol/chloroform/isoamyl alcohol (25:24:1) (Applichem). Store at 4°C.
4. Chloroform/Isoamyl alcohol (24:1). Prepare as detailed above and store at 4°C.
5. 3 M sodium acetate. Store at 4°C.
6. Ethanol, absolute and 70%. Store at −20°C.

2.4. Genomic DNA Labeling

1. 2.5× Random Primers Solution from the BioPrime DNA Labeling System kit (Life Technologies, Inc): 125 mM Tris-HCl, pH 6.8, 12.5 mM $MgCl_2$, 25 mM 2-mercaptoethanol, 750 µg/mL random octamers. Store at −20°C.
2. 10× dNTP mixture: 1.2 mM dATP, 1.2 mM dGTP, 1.2 mM dCTP and 0.6 mM dTTP dissolved in Tris-EDTA buffer, pH 8.0. Store at −20°C (see Note 1).
3. 25 nmol Cy3- and Cy5-dUTP (Amersham Biosciences, Piscataway, NJ). Store in the dark, in single-use aliquots at −20°C (see Note 2).
4. 40 units/µL Klenow Fragment (Large Fragment of DNA Polymerase I) from the BioPrime DNA Labeling System kit (Life Technologies, Inc). Store at −20°C.
5. Stop buffer: 0.5 M EDTA, pH 8.0. Store at room temperature.

2.5. Purification of Labeled DNA

1. T.E. buffer, pH 7.4: 1 mM Tris-HCl, 0.1 mM EDTA. Store at room temperature.
2. Microcon 30 filter (YM-30) (Amicon/Millipore, Billerica, MA).

2.6. Precipitation and Hybridization of Labeled DNA

1. Human Cot-1 DNA (Roche, 1 mg/mL stocks). Store at −20°C.
2. Yeast tRNA (Life Technologies, Inc). Prepare a 10 mg/mL stock solution with distilled water and store in single-use aliquots at −20°C.
3. Poly (dA)-(dT) (Sigma, St. Louis, MO). Prepare a 5 mg/mL stock solution with distilled water and store in single aliquots at −20°C.
4. T.E. buffer, pH 7.4: 1 mM Tris-HCl, 0.1 mM EDTA. Store at room temperature.
5. Microcon 30 filter (YM-30, Amicon/Millipore).
6. Hybridization solution (3.4× SSC, 0.3% (w/v) SDS): 20× SSC, 10% (w/v) SDS. Store at room temperature.

7. CMT-Hybridization chambers for use with 2×75 mm slides (Corning Incorporated, Corning, NY). Humidify the hybridization chambers with 3× SSC.

8. Cover slips (24×60 mm) (Corning Incorporated, Corning, NY).

2.7. Washing the Slides

1. Wash solution 1: 2× SSC/0.03% (w/v) SDS. Store at room temperature.
2. Wash solution 2: 1× SSC. Store at room temperature.
3. Wash solution 3: 0.2× SSC. Store at room temperature.

2.8. Analysis

1. Confocal scanner Axon GenePix 4100A (Axon Instruments Inc., Union City, CA).
2. GenePix Pro 6.0 software (Axon Instruments Inc.).
3. Gene Expression Preprocessing Analysis Suite (GEPAS) website tool (http://gepas.bioinfo.cipf.es/) (11).

3. Methods

The analysis of genomic copy number variations (amplifications, gains, and losses of genetic material) in GB tumors was performed by using cDNA microarrays containing 27,454 cDNA clones, including 9,900 known genes and uncharacterized expression sequence tags (ESTs) related to tumorigenesis (Oncochip v2.0). DNA from a GB tumor (test DNA) and genomic DNA from a pool of normal individuals (reference DNA) are differentially labeled with fluorochromes (Cy5- and Cy3-dUTP), and cohybridized onto the cDNA microarray.

The copy number ratios between the test and reference DNA are determined for each clone, and self versus self hybridizations of reference DNA allowed to define the cut-off points to determine the copy number variations in the test DNA (9, 10, 12).

The hybridization of DNA on cDNA microarrays provides sufficient fluorescece signal to detect large copy number changes (amplifications) with high resolution. However, the detection of lower copy number changes requires calculating the running average of multiple and consecutive clones, typically five to ten clones along the genome, because the gains and losses of genetic material do not provide adequate signals to detect them. The results obtained from this technique can be represented by using the available genome sequence alignment data. In particular, the clones can be mapped to their genomic basepair positions and the clone-derived ratios plotted as a function of position along the genome (6–8) (see example figures later).

3.1. Preparation of Samples to Identify Candidate Cancer Genes in GB by CGH on cDNA Microarrays

1. Collect fresh or frozen tissue material (7–10 μm sections) from human GB tumors in epperdorf tubes (see Note 3). As reference DNA, normal human lymphocytes from 5 mL whole blood (EDTA, heparin, citrate) of at least five healthy individuals are collected in 50 mL tubes. Tissue samples and whole blood are washed with 0.9% saline solution and centrifuged at maximum speed. After the removal of the supernatant (see Note 4), 30–40 mL blood lysis buffer is added to the whole blood pellet (if necessary, 1 mL blood lysis buffer should be added to the tumor tissue pellet) and centrifuged at $1,800 \times g$ for 15 min at 4°C. Remove the supernatant and repeat this step until the blood is completely lysed. At this point, the pellets are resuspended in protein digestion buffer with 10 μL proteinase K (10 mg/mL) for 1 mL protein digestion buffer added. The samples must be shaked gently, and incubated overnight at 40°C in a waterbath (see Note 5).

2. The genomic DNA is extracted following standard phenol/chloroform purification protocols:

    a. Add a volume of phenol/chloroform/isoamyl alcohol (25:24:1) to the sample, shake by hand for a couple of minutes, and centrifuge at $1,800 \times g$ for 15 min at 4 C (in case of 15–50 mL tubes) or $15,000 \times g$ for 3 min at 4°C (if using eppendorf tubes).

    b. Remove aqueose layer (top layer) to a new tube and repeat the phenol/chloroform/isoamyl step described above.

    c. Add a volume of chloroform/Isoamyl alcohol (24:1) to the sample, shake by hand for some minutes, and centrifuge.

    d. Transfer the aqueose layer (top layer) to a new tube and precipitate by adding two volumes of absolute ethanol and 80 μl of 5 M NaCl solution by millilitre of DNA extracted. Shake gently until the DNA is precipitated (see Note 6).

    e. The precipitated DNA is washed in 70% ethanol and dissolved in 0.1–1 mL TE buffer, pH 8.0 overnight on a rotating shaker (see Note 7).

3. The quality and quantity of the DNA extracted is checked in a spectrophotometer (NanoDrop Technologies, LLC, Wilmington, Delaware). The DNAs can be stored at 4°C or −20°C.

3.2. DNA Digestion

1. A total of 20 μg of genomic DNA is digested with 2.5 μL (25 units) of AluI, 2.5 μL (25 units) of RsaI, and 10 μL of 10× React1 Buffer supplied with the enzymes. Distilled water is added to make a final volume of 100 μL. The digestion mixture is incubated overnight at 37°C.

3.3. Clean-up of Digested DNA

1. Add 400 μL of TE, pH 8.0 to 100 μL of digestion and mix. The digestion mixture can be cleaned-up by using a Qiagen purification kit or following standard phenol-chloroform purification protocol described above in Subheading 3.1. In this case, the purification is carried out in eppendorf tubes.
2. The precipitation of the genomic DNA is performed with 1 mL of absolute ethanol and 60 μL of 3 M sodium acetate. The samples are incubated at −80°C for 15–30 min, and centrifuged at 15,000×g for 10 min at 4°C. Then, the pellet is washed with 70% ethanol, centrifuged again for 10 min and allowed to dry for 5 min or until almost dry. Redissolve the digested DNA in 35 μL of distilled water and measure the concentration by A260 absortion.

3.4. Genomic DNA Labeling

1. Add 2 μg of test DNA to three 0.5 mL tubes for Cy3 labeling, and 2 μg of control DNA to three 0.5 ml tubes for Cy5 labeling. Thus, a total of 6 μg of test DNA and 6 μg of control DNA is labeled for each hybridization. To each tube, add distilled water or T.E., pH 8.0 to bring the total volume to 21 μL, and 20 μL of 2.5× random primer/reaction buffer mix. Then, the tubes are boiled for 5 min and placed on ice.
2. Prepare a mix for Cy3 tubes and Cy5 tubes containing 5 μL 10× dNTP mix, 3 μL Cy3-dUTP or 3 μL Cy5-dUTP, and 1 μL Klenow Fragment for each reaction (see Note 1). While the tubes are on ice, add 9 μL of the mix to each tube and incubate at 37°C in a termocycler for 2 h. Then, stop the labeling reaction by adding 5 μL 0.5 M EDTA.

3.5. Purification of Labeled DNA

1. Purify each labeling reaction separately by using microcon 30 filter (Amicon/Millipore): add 450 μL TE 7.4 to the stopped labeling reaction and lay onto microcon 30 filter. Centrifuge ~10 min at 9,000×g. Invert and spin 1 min at 9,000×g to recover 20–40 μL of the purified probe in a new tube (see Note 8).

3.6. Precipitation and Hybridization of Labeled DNA

1. For two-color array hybridizations, combine one Cy3 purified probe with one Cy5 purified probe in a new eppendorf tube. Then, add to each of the three tubes: 50 μg of human Cot-1 DNA (blocks the hybridization to repetitive DNAs if present on array), 100 μg yeast tRNA (blocks nonspecific DNA hybridization), 20 μg Poly (dA)-(dT) (blocks hybridization to polyA tails of cDNA array elements) and 450 μL TE 7.4.
2. Concentrate each probe mixture with a microcon 30 filter as above (9,000×g for ~12 min) to recover a volume of 16 μL or less (see Note 8).
3. Combine the three purified probe mixtures and adjust the volume to 48 μL with distilled water. Then, pipette 10.2 μL

20× SSC (for a final concentration of 3.4×) and 1.8 μL 10% SDS (for a final concentration of 0.3%) to two different tubes. Add half of the probe to the tube with 20× SSC and the other half of the probe to the tube with 10% SDS. Mix well and combine the two tubes.

4. Denature the hybridization mixture at 100°C for 1.5 min, and incubate at 37°C for 30 min to allow Cot-1 preannealing. Then centrifuge at 15,000 ×g for 5 min to bring down precipitated material. Remove carefully all the supernatant to another tube except 2–3 μL at the bottom. Repeat centrifugation again to recover the probe solution left without any precipitate (see Note 9).

5. Hybridize the mixture to the microarray applying the probe solution to the coverslip. Invert array and place on top of coverslip (see Note 10). Hybridize for 16–24 h at 65°C in a sealed and humidified chamber with 40 μL of 3× SSC.

3.7. Wash of the Slides

1. Remove the coverslip in a 50 mL falcon tube with wash solution 1 at 60°C. Then wash the slide with this solution at 60°C for 5 min (see Note 11).

2. Wash the slide with wash solution 2 at room temperature for 5 min.

3. Was the slide twice with wash solution 3 at room temperature for 5 min.

4. To dry the slides, centrifuge immediately at 900 ×g for 3 min at room temperature.

3.8. Analysis

1. After the hybridization, the slides are scanned using an Axon GenePix 4100A confocal scanner. Then the images are analyzed using GenePix Pro 6.0 software. An example result is shown in Fig. 1.

2. The mean log2-transformed ratios derived from the self versus self experiments of normal genomic DNA in control hybridizations made it possible to establish the cut-off points for defining gains and losses of genetic material in the test hybridizations. A value of the mean ratio ± two standard deviations in control hybridizations showed a normal range of variation corresponding to log2-transformed values of −0.42 to 0.42. In order to ensure a fluorescence ratio of gain or loss, log2 ratios ≥ 0.5 were considered gene gains, log2 ratios ≤ −0.5 were considered gene losses, and log2 fluorescent ratios ≥ 2 were considered gene amplifications.

3. Finally, data is processed using bioinformatic tools such as Gene Expression Preproccessing Analysis Suite (GEPAS). Examples of the copy number variations and the amplicons detected in GB tumors are shown in Figs. 2 and 3.

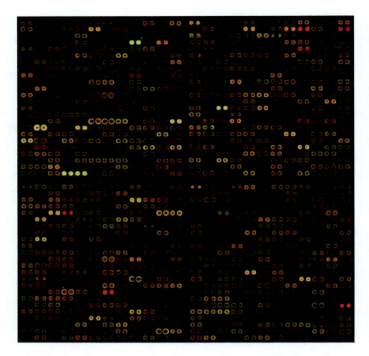

Fig. 1. Hybridization of genomic DNA from GB onto a cDNA microarray (Oncochip v2.0). The cDNA microarray includes 12 × 4 subgrids, and each subgrid contains 24 × 24 spots, which represent a total of 27,454 cDNA clones. Tumor DNA was labeled in *red* (Cy5-dUTP) and reference DNA was labeled in *green* (Cy3-dUTP). The cohybridization of GB and reference DNA showed three main color pattern signals: *yellow signals*, when gene dosage is similar in test and reference DNA, *red signals*, when gene dosage is higher in test DNA than in reference DNA, and *green signals*, when gene dosage is lower in test DNA than in reference DNA.

4. Notes

1. Do not use the dNTP mix provided in the BioPrime DNA Labeling System kit. This mixture includes 1 mM biotin-14-dCTP to produce sensitive biotinylated-DNA probes. In this experiment, however, it is not necessary because the labeling of DNA probes is performed with Cy3- and Cy5-dUTP. Use the Bioprime labeling kit for random primer, reaction buffer, and high concentration klenow.
2. The Cyanine dyes are fluorescence products sensitive to environmental conditions (ozone or ambient light). All exposures to light must be minimal and restricted to the time taken to complete a required operation. As far as possible, carry out experimental procedures in low light conditions.

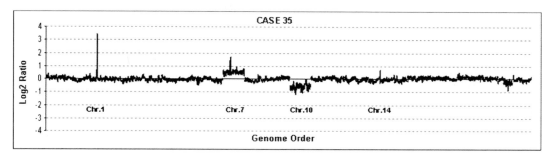
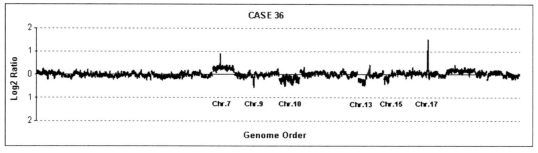

Fig. 2. Whole genome array-CGH copy number profiles in two different GB tumors (case 35 and 36). The average log$_2$ genomic ratios over five neighboring genes are plotted according to their map positions on the EnsEMBL database for each chromosome in order from 1p to Xqter. Chromosome 7 gain, chromosome 10 loss, and 7p amplification are observed in both tumors. In particular, amplifications at chromosomes 1 and 14 together with chromosome 22 loss are observed in case 35, while an amplification at chromosome 17, and loss of chromosomes 13 and 15 are observed in case 36.

3. In order to verify tumor viability, samples should be reviewed by means of tissue sections stained with hematoxylin and eosin (H&E).

4. After washing the pellets with saline solution and removing the supernatant, it is possible to store them at −80°C until the DNA extraction.

5. The protein digestion buffer should cover the pellet and the consistency should be viscous. If there are still some tissue pieces visible after the incubation at 40°C, add protein digestion buffer and proteinase K again, shake gently and incubate until the pellet is completely disaggregated.

6. To better remove the phenol/chloroform solutions from the DNA extracted, the aqueous layer can be centrifuged alone in a new tube before precipitation. In case the DNA does not precipitate after shaking by hand, the aqueous layer can be incubated at −20°C overnight and precipitated by centrifugation at maximum speed. Then, the pellet is washed with 70% ethanol and resuspended in TE buffer, pH 8.0.

7. The volume of TE depends on the amount of precipitated DNA, and initially should be less than necessary. In case the DNA is not dissolved completely, add more TE and leave it longer on the rotating shaker.

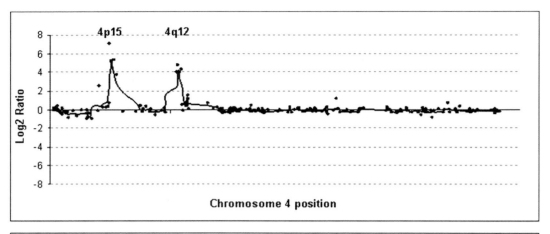
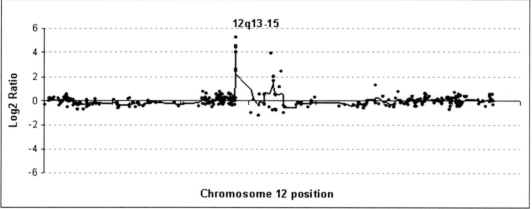

Fig. 3. Detection of amplicons at chromosomes 4 and 12. The average log$_2$ genomic values over five neighboring genes for chromosomes 4 and 12 are plotted with respect to their map position (EnsEMBL database). Two amplicons at 4p15 and 4q12 in GBM case 39, and two amplicons at 12q13-15 in case 33 were detected.

8. If the volume of the purified probe is more than 40 µL, then layer again onto the microcon column and check the volume every 1 min until appropriate.

9. Since the mixture of 20× SSC and 10% SDS produces extra small precipitates, it is very important to remove them so as to avoid artefacts in the image analysis.

10. The application of the probe could generate undesirable air bubbles, which would impede a homogeneous hybridization. Therefore, the application of the probe should be slow and careful. If the bubbles persist, then use a needle to lift the cover-slip and eliminate them.

11. The first washing step should be performed at 60°C to significantly increase the specific hybridization signal. In addition, it is important to perform all the wash steps in a rotating shaker or shaking by hand to reduce the background.

Acknowledgments

The author would like to thank Elena Gómez from the Virgen de la Salud Hospital for her technical assistance. This work was partially supported by grants FIS CA07/00119, FIS 03/0727, FIS PI070662 and INT 07/028 from the Fondo de Investigaciones Sanitarias; and FISCAM PI-2006/29 from the Consejeria de Sanidad de la Junta de Comunidades de Castilla-La Mancha.

References

1. Kallioniemi, A., Kallioniemi, O. P., Sudar, D., Rutovitz, D., Gray, J.W., Waldman, F. et al. (1992) Comparative genomic hybridization for molecular cytogenetic analysis of solid tumors. *Science* **258**, 818-821.
2. Albertson, D.G., and Pinkel, D. (2003) Genomic microarrays in human genetic disease and cancer. *Hum. Mol. Genet.* **12**, R145–R152.
3. Blesa, D., Mollejo, M., Ruano, Y., de Lope, A. R., Fiano, C., Ribalta, T. et al. (2009) Novel genomic alterations and mechanisms associated with tumor progression in oligodendroglioma and mixed oligoastrocytoma. *J. Neuropathol. Exp. Neurol.* **68**, 274–285.
4. Monni, O., Barlund, M., Mousses, S., Kononen, J., Sauter, G., Heiskanen, M. et al. (2001) Comprehensive copy number and gene expression profiling of the 17q23 amplicon in human breast cancer. *Proc. Natl. Acad. Sci. U.S.A.* **98**, 5711–5716.
5. Zhao, J., Roth, J., Bode-Lesniewska, B., Pfaltz, M., Heitz, P.U., and Komminoth, P. (2002) Combined comparative genomic hybridization and genomic microarray for detection of gene amplifications in pulmonary artery intimal sarcomas and adrenocortical tumors. *Genes Chromosomes Cancer* **34**, 48–57.
6. Pollack, J.R., Sorlie, T., Perou, C.M., Rees, C.A., Jeffrey, S.S., Lonning, P.E. et al. (2002) Microarray analysis reveals a major direct role of DNA copy number alteration in the transcriptional program of human breast tumors. *Proc. Natl. Acad. Sci. U.S.A.* **99**, 12963–12968.
7. Hyman, E., Kauraniemi, P., Hautaniemi, S., Wolf, M., Mousses, S., Rozenblum, E. et al. (2002) Impact of DNA amplification on gene expression patterns in breast cancer. *Cancer Res.* **62**, 6240–6245.
8. Pollack, J. R., Perou, C.M., Alizadeh, A. A., Eisen, M.B., Pergamenschikov, A., Williams, C.F. et al. (1999) Genome-wide analysis of DNA copy-number changes using cDNA microarrays. *Nat. Genet.* **23**, 41–46.
9. Ruano, Y., Mollejo, M., Ribalta, T., Fiano, C., Camacho, F.I., Gomez, E. et al. (2006) Identification of novel candidate target genes in amplicons of Glioblastoma multiforme tumors detected by expression and CGH microarray profiling. *Mol. Cancer* **5**, 39.
10. Wolf, M., Mousses, S., Hautaniemi, S., Karhu, R., Huusko, P., Allinen, M. et al. (2004) High-resolution analysis of gene copy number alterations in human prostate cancer using CGH on cDNA microarrays: impact of copy number on gene expression. *Neoplasia* **6**, 240–247.
11. Herrero, J., Diaz-Uriarte, R., and Dopazo, J. (2003) Gene expression data preprocessing. *Bioinformatics* **19**, 655–656.
12. Jiang, F., Yin, Z., Caraway, N.P., Li, R., and Katz, R.L. (2004) Genomic profiles in stage I primary non small cell lung cancer using comparative genomic hybridization analysis of cDNA microarrays. *Neoplasia* **6**, 623–635.

Chapter 4

Multiplex Amplifiable Probe Hybridization (MAPH) Methodology as an Alternative to Comparative Genomic Hybridization (CGH)

Ludmila Kousoulidou, Carolina Sismani, and Philippos C. Patsalis

Abstract

Genomic imbalances in locus copy-number are highly significant for the diagnosis and prognosis of cancer. Rapidly progressing DNA microarray technologies detect such pathogenic copy-number changes in the genome with high throughput, efficiency, and resolution. A variety of different microarray-based approaches have emerged, with array comparative genomic hybridization (array-CGH) being the method of choice in current clinical practice. Here we describe an alternative microarray-based technique called array-MAPH, derived from conventional Multiplex Amplifiable Probe Hybridization (MAPH).

The main novelty of array-MAPH is the directed reduction of test DNA complexity prior to hybridization, yielding a mixture of specific probes, identical to target sequences on the microarray and thus increasing hybridization specificity. Unique amplifiable 400–600 bp fragments can be designed for any genomic region of interest, PCR-amplified, and spotted onto arrays as targets. The same sequences are combined into a probe mixture and hybridized to genomic DNA immobilized on a membrane. Bound probes are recovered by quantitative PCR and hybridized to the array. Array-MAPH can be used for the detection of small-scale copy-number changes, thereby providing new insights into the genetic basis of several diseases, including cancer.

Key words: Array-MAPH, Array-CGH, DNA microarrays, Subtle genomic imbalances, Copy-number detection

1. Introduction

Cancer research has made considerable progress since the introduction of genome-wide screening techniques for subtle genomic imbalances (1). High-resolution DNA microarrays have further contributed to the investigation of cancer aetiology and manifestation with array-based comparative genomic hynbridization (array-CGH) applied as the main method of choice (2–4).

Despite the progress in the optimization of microarray probe size and genomic coverage, some technical issues, such as the need for multiple analyses of normal samples and the presence of redundant sequences in both sample and target due to the complexity of human genomic DNA, still remain unresolved. Here we describe an alternative microarray-based technique for the detection of small-scale copy-number changes throughout the human genome, named array-MAPH (5–7), derived from gel-based Multiplex Amplifiable Probe Hybridization (MAPH) (8). This new microarray platform should limit the need for normal sample analysis, provide the required flexibility in terms of resolution and locus selection and exclude the interference of redundant sequences from hybridization procedure (9–12). Moreover, array-MAPH provides an excellent tool for specifically reducing the complexity of human genomic DNA, thereby increasing the signal to noise ratio, which is critical for obtaining reliable data (13, 14).

The basis for the development of array-MAPH was Multiplex Amplifiable Probe Hybridization (MAPH) – a gel-based technique for the detection of changes in DNA copy-number with a resolution up to 100 base pairs (bp) within a defined region of interest (8). The principle of this method is that a number of specific probes can be recovered and quantitatively amplified after hybridization to genomic DNA immobilized on a solid matrix. The amount of product obtained for each probe represents the copy number of the corresponding sequence in a patient's genome. Several MAPH assays have been developed to identify anomalies in locations with known function (gene exons) or unknown function, such as losses or gains of subtle chromosomal segments in subtelomeric or subcentromeric regions and interstitial submicroscopic abnormalities (12). However, gel-based detection places a limit on the multiplicity of MAPH – a maximum of 100 probes spaced at minimum 5 bp can be analyzed simultaneously in one experiment (12).

To overcome this limitation, DNA microarrays were employed to replace the final quantification step of MAPH. In the first pilot study, which was based on a PamGene 3-Dimensional Flow-Through microarray platform (15), the authors demonstrated successful copy-number assessment of six different probes from PMP22 gene. More recently, we introduced a microarray platform (array-MAPH) similar to that used for array-CGH. In contrast to the PamGene approach (15), there is no need to obtain specialized equipment, as any laboratory with a microarray facility for CGH, can successfully apply array-MAPH without additional modifications to the existing infrastructure. Although both microarray MAPH methodologies aim for high multiplicity, it is only with array-MAPH that a large number of probes (about 700) have been simultaneously analyzed (5). The new array-MAPH method has enabled an accurate determination of copy-number changes on chromosome X (6, 9–11) and can be adjusted to virtually any targeted locus of complex genomes. The procedure consists of three major steps (outlined in Fig. 1): (a) Probe selection and preparation, (b) Microarray preparation and (c) Array-MAPH hybridization and data analysis.

Array-MAPH can be useful for several applications, including the detection of microdeletions or microduplications in cancer, high-resolution screening of patients with abnormal phenotype and no genetic findings, and screening of new possible disease-causative CNVs.

A more extensive discussion of array-MAPH methodology is given in ref. (7).

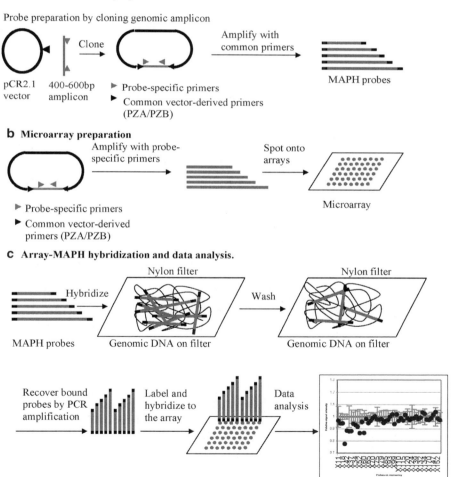

Fig. 1. Array-MAPH methodology. (a) Probes (genomic amplicons) are cloned into pCR2.1 vector and recovered by amplification with common vector-derived primers (b) cloned amplicons are amplified from clone library using probe-specific primers and spotted onto arrays (c) probes are hybridized to genomic DNA on filters, recovered by amplification with common primers, labeled, and hybridized to the arrays for quantification. The figure is reproduced with the permission of the authors (5).

2. Materials

2.1. Probe Selection and Preparation

1. Genomic DNA, isolated from normal individuals and patients.
2. Primers, designed according to the probes required (metabion International AG, Martinsried, Germany).
3. dNTP set, 100 mM each (MBI Fermentas, Vilnius, Lithuania).
4. Taq DNA polymerase (MBI Fermentas).
5. 10× PCR buffer with $(NH_4)_2SO_4$ (MBI Fermentas).
6. 25 mM $MgCl_2$ (MBI Fermentas).
7. 100 bp ladder (New England Biolabs).
8. Low-Range DNA Mass Ruler (MBI Fermentas).
9. PZA primer: 5'AGTAACGGCCGCCAGTGTGCTG3', common vector-derived forward primer for the simultaneous amplification of all probes from bacterial cultures and for the recovery of bound probes after hybridization to genomic DNA. It is also added to hybridization mixture to prevent probe cross-hybridization by blocking homologous sequences.
10. PZB primer: 5'CGAGCGGCCGCCAGTGTGATG3', common vector-derived reverse primer for simultaneous amplification of all probes from bacterial cultures and for recovery of bound probes after hybridization to genomic DNA. It is also added to hybridization mixture to prevent probe cross-hybridization by blocking homologous sequences.
11. TOPO TA cloning kit with TOP 10 chemically competent cells, version R (Invitrogen Co, Carlsbad, CA, USA).
12. Thermal cycler, programmed with the desired amplification protocol.
13. Vacuum concentrator.
14. Vacuum pump.
15. The DUST program (source code is available from ftp://ftp.ncbi.nlm.nih.gov/pub/tatusov/dust/).
16. GenomeMasker and GenomeTester programs (binaries are available from http://bioinfo.ut.ee/download/).
17. Primer3 (source code is available from http://fokker.wi.mit.edu/primer3/).
18. MegaBlast (binaries are available from http://blast.ncbi.nlm.nih.gov/Blast.cgi).
19. SSAHA (binaries are available from http://www.sanger.ac.uk/Software/analysis/SSAHA/).

20. "MAPHDesigner software": This software allows flexible design of probes and PCR primers for array-MAPH and array-CGH microarrays. With MAPHDesigner, the user can design hybridization probes for the whole genome, specified chromosome, specified target regions or cytogenetic bands in the human genome. Also, if interested in a specific target gene, it is possible to insert the ID of the gene of interest. At present, ENSEMBL, RefSeq, and Vega annotations can be used. Additionally, the user can specify the number of desired hybridization probes and different PCR primer/hybridization probe related parameters such as primer/probe length and melting temperature. A fully functional version of the MAPHDesigner is freely available (http://bioinfo.ut.ee/maphdesigner/) for all academic users as a web-based service and does not require any prior registration.

2.2. Microarray Preparation

1. UNI3 oligonucleotide 5'GAATTCGCCCTT3', vector-derived sequence flanking each probe, added to hybridization mixture along with PZA and PZB to prevent probe cross-hybridization by blocking homologous sequences.
2. UNI5 oligonucleotide 5'GATATCTGCAGAATTCGC-CCT3', vector-derived sequence flanking each probe, added to hybridization mixture along with PZA and PZB to prevent probe cross-hybridization by blocking homologous sequences.
3. Genorama™ SAL-1 microarray slides (Asper Biotech Ltd., Tartu, Estonia).
4. Microarray spotter (VersArray ChipWriter Pro; BioRad Laboratories, Hercules, CA, USA).

2.3. Array-MAPH Hybridization and Data Analysis

1. MAPH prehybridization buffer (mix the reagents to achieve the following final concentrations: 0.5 M Na_2HPO_4/NaH_2PO_4 (pH 7.2), 7% (v/v) SDS, 1 mM EDTA; denature the required amount of herring sperm DNA by heating at 95°C for 3 min and add to the solution at a final concentration of 10 mg/mL).
2. Wash solution 1: 1× SSC, 1% SDS.
3. Wash solution 2: 0.1× SSC, 0.1% SDS.
4. 10× Nick-translation buffer with dNTPs (prepare Nick-translation buffer by mixing reagents to achieve the following final concentrations: 500 mM Tris-HCl (pH 7.8); 50 mM $MgCl_2$; 100 mM mercaptoethanol. Add dNTP mix to the prepared Nick-translation buffer to the following final concentrations: 200 μM dATP; 200 μM dCTP; 200 μM dGTP). *CAUTION!* Mercaptoethanol is toxic by inhalation, ingestion, and through skin contact and may cause severe eye irritation. Handle in hood.

5. Array hybridization buffer degassed (mix the reagents to achieve the following final concentrations: 50% formamide, 6× SSC, 0.5% (v/v) SDS, 5× Denhardt's solution. Degas indicated solutions by sonicating for 5 min at room temperature (20–25°C) in an ultrasonic bath while applying a vacuum. The degassing of the hybridization solution will help to prevent the appearance of bubbles in the hybridization chamber). *CAUTION!* Formamide is embryotoxic, and may cause reproductive damage, and eye and skin irritation. Handle in hood and avoid breathing in.
6. Cot-1 human DNA (Roche Diagnostics Corporation, Indianapolis, IN, USA).
7. Cy™3 Monoreactive dye (GE Healthcare UK Ltd, Little Chalfont Buckinghamshire), one tube diluted in 45 µL 100% DMSO.
8. 0.1 M Na_2CO_3.
9. 5-(3-Aminoallyl)-2′-deoxyuridine-5′-triphosphate (aa-dUTP) (Sigma-Aldrich Co, St. Louis, MO, USA).
10. Bovine Serum Albumine (BSA) (Promega, Madison, WI, USA).
11. Shrimp Alkaline Phosphatase (USB Corporation, Cleveland, OH, USA).
12. Exonuclease I (MBI Fermentas, cat#EN0581).
13. Hydroxylamine (Sigma-Aldrich Chemie GmbH, Steinheim, Germany).
14. DNA Polymerase/DNAse mix (Invitrogen).
15. HYBOND-N+ filter (GE Healthcare, formerly Amersham Pharmacia Biotech, Little Chalfont Buckinghamshire, UK).
16. UltraClean PCR Clean-up DNA Purification Kit (Mo Bio Laboratories Inc., Solana Beach, CA, USA).
17. 100 mM NaOAcetate.
18. Array prewash solution: 6× SSC, 0.5% SDS. Degas before use as described above. Also, SDS tends to precipitate at low temperatures and high ionic strength, but can be easily redissolved by warming the solution to 37°C or higher.
19. Array wash solution 1: 2× SSC, 0.03% SDS. Degas before use as above.
20. Array wash solution 2: 1× SSC. Degas before use as above.
21. Array wash solution 3: 0.2× SSC. Degas before use as above.
22. Spectrophotometer (we used ND-1000, NanoDrop Technologies Inc., Wilmington, DE, USA).
23. Hybridization oven.
24. Automated hybridization station Tecan HS-400 (Tecan AG, Zurich, Switzerland).

MAPH Methodology 53

25. Microarray scanner (we used Affymetrix 428 microarray scanner, Affymetrix Inc., Santa Clara, CA, USA).
26. Software: Image ProPlus™ (Media Cybernetics, Silver Spring, MD, USA); Genorama™Genotyping Software 4.2 Package (Asper Biotech Ltd.); MAPHStat (available upon request for academic use).

3. Methods

3.1. Probe Selection and Preparation

1. Select the region of interest from the genome and the number of probes required. The main factors that should be taken into account when deciding the number of probes are the length of the region to be investigated and the desired spacing between probes. For example, to screen the whole 154 Mb chromosome X with a median spacing of 300 kb, a total of approximately 500 probes should be used.
2. Download the genomic sequence of the region of interest to allow the selection of candidate probes and PCR primers. Steps 3–7 can be performed automatically using web-based software called MAPHDesigner at http://bioinfo.ut.ee/maphdesigner/ (see Note 1).
3. Mask repetitive elements in the downloaded sequences with the GenomeMasker program from the GenomeMasker package (16) (freely available for academic users from http://bioinfo.ut.ee/download). Low-complexity repetitive regions can be masked with the DUST program (17).
4. Use the Primer3 program (18) to design PCR primers for amplifying candidate sequences, using the following parameters:
PRIMER_PRODUCT_SIZE_RANGE=200-600
PRIMER_PRODUCT_OPT_SIZE=400
PRIMER_OPT_SIZE=24
PRIMER_MIN_SIZE=22
PRIMER_MAX_SIZE=26
PRIMER_OPT_TM=62
PRIMER_MIN_TM=59
PRIMER_MAX_TM=65
PRIMER_MAX_DIFF_TM=4
PRIMER_OPT_GC_PERCENT=35
PRIMER_MIN_GC=20
PRIMER_MAX_GC=50
PRIMER_SALT_CONC=20

PRIMER_FILE_FLAG=0
PRIMER_EXPLAIN_FLAG=1
PRIMER_MAX_POLY_X=4
PRIMER_NUM_RETURN=1
PRIMER_PRODUCT_MIN_TM=60
PRIMER_PRODUCT_MAX_TM=70

5. Test all designed primers for their uniqueness in the human genome and their ability to form PCR products, using the GenomeTester program from the GenomeMasker package (16). Detach a substring of 16 nucleotides from the 3 end of each primer and count the number of occurrences in chromosomes as potential binding sites. Discard primers that have more than 10 putative binding sites in the genome and primer pairs that can generate more than one PCR product. Predict a product if two primers bind to opposite strands within 1,000 bp from each other.

6. Test candidate probes (PCR products) for their uniqueness by comparing them against each other with the MegaBLAST program (19). Reject probes that contain regions longer than 50 bp with more than 75% identity to other probes.

7. Test the remaining probes for their uniqueness in the human genome as follows: apply the SSAHA program (20) to reject probes that have stretches of identity longer than 30 bp to regions other than their own correct binding site in the human chromosomes. Additionally, perform a more comprehensive test of all probes against human chromosome sequences using the MegaBLAST program. The DUST filter within the MegaBLAST is switched off with the –F F option, otherwise some repeated regions in the human genome could remain unnoticed. Remove probes that show identity higher than 75% in regions longer than 50 bp within sequences other than their own correct binding site.

8. Amplify probe sequences from a normal 46,XY source of genomic DNA (see Note 2). For each sequence to be amplified, set up the following reaction in 200 µL PCR tubes:

Component	Amount per reaction	Final
Genomic DNA	50 ng	2.5 ng/µL
10× PCR buffer	2 µL	1×
25 mM MgCl$_2$	1 µL	1.25 mM
12.5 mM each dNTP mix	0.5 µL	0.3 mM each
10 µM Forward probe-specific primer	1 µL	10 pmoles

(continued)

(continued)

Component	Amount per reaction	Final
10 µM Reverse probe-specific primer	1 µL	10 pmoles
5 U/µL Taq DNA polymerase (see Note 3)	0.2 µL	1 U
ddH$_2$O	to 20 µL	

9. Amplify the reactions according to the following program:

Cycle number	Denaturation	Annealing	Polymerization
1	5 min at 94°C		
2–26	1 min at 94°C	1 min at 67°C	1 min at 72°C
27			30 min at 72°C (see Note 4)

10. Analyze PCR efficiency and specificity by loading 5 µL of each reaction on a 2% (wt/vol) agarose gel for electrophoresis (see Note 5). A single band of the expected size should be clearly visible on the gel, without any signs of unspecific amplification (additional bands) or low efficiency (faint band).

Archiving Probes into a Library

11. Clone amplicons into pCR2.1 vector using the TOPO TA cloning kit (see Note 6).

12. Analyze transformants by direct amplification from bacterial colonies, without plasmid extraction. For each colony to be analyzed, set up the following reaction in 200 µL PCR tubes:

Component	Amount per reaction	Final
10× PCR buffer	2 µL	1×
25 mM MgCl$_2$	1 µL	1.25 mM
12.5 mM each dNTP mix	0.5 µL	0.3 mM each
10 µM PZA primer	1 µL	10 pmoles
10 µM PZB primer	1 µL	10 pmoles
5 U/µL Taq DNA polymerase	0.2 µL	1 U
ddH$_2$O	to 20 µL	

13. Pick three or four single colonies per probe and resuspend them individually in 20 µL of the above PCR reaction mix. Amplify the reaction according to the following program:

Cycle number	Denaturation	Annealing	Polymerization
1	10 min at 94°C		
2–26	1 min at 94°C	1 min at 60°C	1 min at 72°C

Restreak and grow each selected colony on selective plates for further use (see step 15).

14. Visualize the PCR products by agarose gel electrophoresis. Positive clones will give a single clear band of the expected size (keep in mind that PZA-PZB primers add 77 bp to probe length).

15. Select positive clones, transfer to 96 well plates containing liquid culture with 10% glycerol and freeze at −80°C after growing at 37°C, as described in TOPO TA cloning instruction manual, version R.

16. Verify clone identity by direct amplification from bacterial glycerol cultures (see Note 7). For each colony to be analyzed, set up the following reaction in 200 μL PCR tubes:

Component	Amount per reaction	Final
10× PCR buffer	2 μL	1×
25 mM MgCl$_2$	1 μL	1.25 mM
12.5 mM each dNTP mix	0.5 μL	0.3 mM each
10 μM Forward probe-specific primer	1 μL	10 pmoles
10 μM Reverse probe-specific primer	1 μL	10 pmoles
5 U/μL Taq DNA polymerase	0.2 μL	1 U
ddH$_2$O	to 19.5 μL	

17. Add 0.5 μL of glycerol stock of the corresponding clone. Amplify the reaction according to the following program:

Cycle number	Denaturation	Annealing	Polymerization
1	10 min at 94°C		
2–26	1 min at 94°C	1 min at 67°C	1 min at 72°C

18. Load 5 μL of each PCR reaction to a 2% (wt/vol) agarose gel for electrophoresis. A single band of the expected size should be clearly visible on the gel. The absence of visible PCR product indicates that the identity of the insert is incorrect. In such a case, discard the clone and repeat cloning or, alternatively, resequence the insert in order to identify the inserted sequence.

19. Archive clone library and create a database with all information about probes, locations, sizes and amplification protocols.

3.2. Microarray Preparation

1. Amplify array-MAPH target sequences from glycerol stocks. For each target sequence, prepare two of the following reactions in 200 µL PCR tubes:

Component	Amount per reaction	Final
10× PCR buffer	5 µL	1×
25 mM MgCl$_2$	3 µL	1.5 mM
12.5 mM each dNTP mix	2.5 µL	0.6 mM each
10 µM Forward probe-specific primer	1 µL	10 pmoles
10 µM Reverse probe-specific primer	1 µL	10 pmoles
5 U/µL Taq DNA Polymerase	0.3 µL	1.5 U
ddH$_2$O	to 49.5 µL	

Add 0.5 µL of glycerol culture of the corresponding clone. Amplify the reaction according to the following program (see Note 8).

Cycle number	Denaturation	Annealing	Polymerization
1	10 min at 94°C		
2–26	1 min at 94°C	1 min at 67°C	1 min at 72°C

2. Combine products from duplicate reactions. Purify and concentrate amplified sequences by ethanol precipitation and dissolve in 20 µL of water (21). Estimate individual concentrations and quality by electrophoresis on 1.5% (wt/vol) agarose gel using Low Range DNA Mass Ruler and quantification software (e.g. Image ProPlus). The concentration of PCR products has to be in the range of 50–200 ng/µL. Alternatively, use your method of choice for quantification.

3. Dissolve array target sequences in 25% DMSO to a final concentration of 30 ng/µL and spot onto Genorama™ SAL-1 Ultra microarray slides, in at least duplicates, with a microarray spotter. Instructions for the particular spotter should be followed (see Note 9).

3.3. Array-MAPH Hybridization and Data Analysis

3.3.1. Preparation of MAPH Hybridization Probes

1. Amplify MAPH hybridization probes from the corresponding glycerol cultures, using the common PZA-PZB primer set. For each probe, prepare the following reaction in 200 µL PCR tubes:

Component	Amount per reaction	Final
10× PCR buffer	2 µL	1×
25 mM MgCl$_2$	1 µL	1.25 mM
12.5 mM each dNTP mix	0.5 µL	0.3 mM each
10 µM PZA primer	1 µL	10 pmoles
10 µM PZB primer	1 µL	10 pmoles
5 U/µL Taq DNA Polymerase	0.2 µL	1 U
ddH$_2$O	to 19.5 µL	

2. Add 0.5 µl of glycerol culture of the corresponding clone. Amplify the reaction according to the following program:

Cycle number	Denaturation	Annealing	Polymerization
1	10 min at 94°C		
2–26	1 min at 94°C	1 min at 60°C	1 min at 72°C

3. Estimate individual concentrations and quality by electrophoresis on 1.5% (wt/vol) agarose gel using Low Range DNA Mass Ruler and Image ProPlus software. The concentration of PCR products has to be in the range of 50 ng/µL. Alternatively, use your method of choice for quantification.

4. Mix all probes together in equal quantities. The final volume can vary depending on the probe concentrations (see Note 10). The probe mixture(s) will be concentrated by vacuum concentration using SpeedVac and dissolved in ddH$_2$O so that the final concentration of each probe in the mixture will be 1 ng/µL.

MAPH Hybridization

5. Measure the concentrations of DNA samples to be tested, using your quantification method of choice. Select samples with a concentration higher than 200 ng/µl or adjust the DNA concentration using ethanol precipitation or vacuum concentration. Prepare at least five phenotypically normal male and female DNA samples. These samples will be used in control experiments to create male and female reference panels. Mix 2 µg of genomic DNA (see Note 11) with 1.5 µL of 1 M NaOH and immobilize on a small piece (2 × 3 mm) of Hybond-N + filter, by applying 1 µL at a time, allowing to dry before the next application.

Prepare filters in a DNA-free environment. If possible use a hood or a separate room. Take all necessary steps to prevent contamination. To detect any possible contamination on the filters, include two controls: one filter with NaOH only (to detect contamination of the NaOH) and one blank to detect other sources of contamination during preparation procedure (air, instruments etc.). The time needed for filters to dry depends on temperature and humidity (see Note 12).

6. Transfer filters to a screw-top 1.5 mL tube containing 1 mL MAPH prehybridization buffer and prehybridize in a water bath or heat block at 65°C for at least 2 h (see Note 13).

7. Denature 3 μg of human Cot-1 DNA at 95°C for 2 min, cool on ice, and mix with 300 μL fresh prehybridization buffer.

8. Remove prehybridization buffer from the tubes and quickly replace with 300 μL of the solution prepared in step 7. Incubate at 65°C for 30–60 min.

9. Prepare hybridization probe mixture. Mix per filter (see Notes 14–16):

Component	Amount per reaction	Final
Probe mixture, as prepared in step 4	Up to 10 μL	2 ng each probe
Human Cot-1 DNA	1 μL	1 μg
10 μM PZA primer	1 μL	10 pmoles
10 μM PZB primer	1 μL	10 pmoles
10 μM UNI3 oligonucleotide	1 μL	10 pmoles
10 μM UNI5 oligonucleotide	1 μL	10 pmoles
1 M NaOH	4.5 μL	0.45 M

10. Denature at 37°C for 1 min.

11. Place denatured mixture on ice and neutralize with 7 μL of 1 M Na_2HPO_4/NaH_2PO_4 per filter. Add to the tube from step 8, containing the prehybridized filter in 300 μL of solution. Hybridize overnight at 65°C (see Note 17).

12. Wash away unbound probes from filters as follows (see also http://www.nottingham.ac.uk/~pdzjala/maph/maph.html). Pipette off the hybridization mix, and replace with 1 mL prehybridization solution: mix and remove.

13. Use 1 mL of wash solution 1 to rinse the filters out into a 50 mL centrifuge tube.

14. Wash at 65°C in wash solution 1, prewarmed to 65°C. Leave the tube to rotate on the carousel of the hybridization oven. Replace the wash solution frequently so that 500 mL of wash solution 1 is used within 15–20 min.

15. Wash in 500 mL of solution 2 (0.1× SSC, 0.1% SDS, 65°C). When all the wash solution is used up (should take 35–45 min), tip out the filters into a Petri dish.

16. Recover bound probes by PCR amplification with PZA-PZB primers. For each filter, prepare the following reaction in 200 µL PCR tubes:

Component	Amount per reaction	Final
10× PCR buffer	5 µL	1×
25 mM $MgCl_2$	2 µL	1 mM
2 mM each dNTP mix	5 µL	0.2 mM each
10 µM PZA primer	1.5 µL	15 pmoles
10 µM PZB primer	1.5 µL	15 pmoles
5 U/µl Taq DNA Polymerase	0.5 µL	2.5 U
ddH_2O	to 50 µL	

17. Place one filter in each tube. Amplify the reaction according to the following program:

Cycle number	Denaturation	Annealing and polymerization
1	2 min at 94°C	
2–5	1 min at 94°C	1 min at 70°C

Include a control sample of PCR solution without filter to detect possible contamination in PCR reagents (see Note 18).

18. Amplify recovered probes with PZA-PZB primers. For each filter and blank control, prepare the following reaction in 200 µL PCR tubes:

Component	Amount per reaction	Final
Amplification product from step 17	2 µL	
10× PCR buffer	2 µL	1×
25 mM $MgCl_2$	1.5 µL	1.8 mM
2 mM each dNTP mix	2 µL	0.2 mM each
50 µM PZA primer	1.4 µL	70 pmoles
50 µM PZB primer	1.4 µL	70 pmoles
5 U/µL Taq DNA polymerase	0.2 µL	1 U
ddH_2O	to 20 µL	

19. Amplify each reaction according to the following program:

Cycle number	Denaturation	Annealing and polymerization
1	5 min at 94°C	
2–20	1 min at 94°C	1 min at 70°C
21		20 min at 70°C

Amplify each sample twice. Apply one of the reactions on gel and save the remainder for further application (see Note 19).

20. Visualize the PCR reaction by agarose gel electrophoresis. Expect to see a smear of bands at the expected probe length. Control samples should contain no DNA bands (see Note 20).

Microarray Hybridization and Analysis

21. Treat amplified probes from step 19 with shrimp alkaline phosphatase (SAP) and exonuclease I (ExoI) (see Note 21). Mix in 200 µL PCR tube:

Component	Amount per reaction	Final
Amplified product from step 19	20 µL	
ExoI 10 U/µL	0.15 µL	1.5 U
SAP 1 U/µL	1.35 µL	1.35 U

22. Incubate in the thermal cycler at 37°C for 30 min, stop reaction by heating at 80°C for 15 min.
23. Purify the reactions using MoBio PCR product cleaning kit, according to the manufacturer's protocol.
24. Dry the samples in a vacuum concentrator and dissolve in 38.5 µL of water.
25. Label samples by nick-translation including aa-dUTP, which facilitates labeling with monoreactive Cy™3 dye. Mix on ice in 200 µL PCR tubes:

Component	Amount per reaction	Final
Purified sample	38.5 µL	
10× Nick-translation buffer with dNTPs (see REAGENT SETUP)	5 µL	1×
0.1 µg/µL BSA	0.5 µL	1 ng/µL
1 mM aa-dUTP	1 µL	20 µM
DNA polymerase/DNase (0.5 U/µL; 0.4 mU/µL) mixture	5 µL	2.5 U polymerase; 2 mU DNase

26. Incubate in a thermal cycler at 15°C for 90 min, stop the reaction at 80°C for 15 min and incubate at room temperature (20–25°C) for 20 min (see Note 22).
27. Purify reactions using MoBio PCR product cleaning kit, according to the manufacturer's protocol.
28. Dry samples in a vacuum concentrator (see Note 23).
29. Label samples with Cy™3 as follows (see Note 24): resuspend pellets in 4.5 µL of 0.1 M Na_2CO_3 (pH 9.0) (made freshly and heated to 60°C for 15 min to inactivate possible contamination of DNase). Add 4.5 µL of diluted Cy™3 monoreactive dye. Incubate at room temperature in the dark for 1 h.
30. Inactivate excess dye by adding 3.5 µL of 4 M hydroxylamine and incubate in the absence of light at room temperature for 15 min.
31. Add 35 µL of 100 mM sodium acetate (pH 5.2 adjusted with acetic acid), mix, and purify using MoBio PCR product cleaning kit, according to the manufacturer's protocol. Dehydrate in vacuum concentrator.
32. Dissolve in 80 µl of degassed array hybridization buffer.
33. Label microarray slides with a permanent ink pen outside the hybridization area and place into the Hybridization Station.
34. Prepare wash solutions: prewash solution, solution 1, solution 2 and solution 3.
35. Hybridize the slides using the hybridization program shown below:

Step	Temperature	Time	Comments
Prewash	85°C	1 min	Soak time 30 s
Probe injection	60°C		
Denaturation	95°C	5 min	
Hybridization	42°C	8 h	Medium agitation mode
Wash 1	42°C	1.5 min	30 s soak time, 3 cycles
Wash 2	42°C	1.5 min	30 s soak time, 3 cycles
Wash 3	42°C	1.5 min	30 s soak time, 3 cycles
Drying	30°C	1.5 min	

36. Remove slides from hybridization station and scan with a microarray scanner.
37. Extract raw signal intensities with BaseCaller module of Genorama™ Genotyping Software 4.2 Package. Any other

basecalling software can be used to extract the raw signal intensities, followed by conversion to a format suitable for analysis. Since on our platform each target sequence is present in duplicate, we use the mean fluorescence intensity for further analysis (see Note 25).

38. Normalize and analyze results using a suitable data analysis software. See Note 26 for important considerations on aspects of data manipulation. Data presented in this paper was analyzed by specifically designed analysis software called MAPHStat. This software with sample data is available for academic use from the authors upon request. A detailed description of the data analysis can be found elsewhere (5).

    For normalizing data from different experiments use median signal intensities of internal control probes. Compare normalized signal values of the analyzed samples to 90% tolerance interval (TI 90%) of the respective signal intensities for each target sequence from the control experiments. Signal intensity values of at least two adjacent targets falling to the same side above or below TI 90% are indicative for putative copy-number change in the corresponding region.

    Signal intensities are extracted and analyzed as described in steps 37–38, resulting in array-MAPH profiles (Figs. 2–4). If all relative signal intensity values remain within the reference panel's tolerance intervals (TI 90%), this is indicative of no copy-number variation. If data points should occur above or below the reference panel's TI 90%, this indicates a duplication or deletion, respectively.

39. Confirm detected copy-number changes with your method of choice (see Note 27). The confirmation strategy depends upon the nature of detected abnormalities. Use Fluorescence in situ hybridization (FISH) for confirmation of relatively large (more than 2 Mb) duplications or deletions. For smaller copy-number changes, use real-time PCR (22). For homozygous deletions or deletions on the X chromosome of male patients, a standard PCR followed by agarose gel detection is sufficient. In locus-specific PCR-based procedures, the primers for target-specific amplification in step 8 can be used or, to further refine the breakpoints, design new primers following the strategy described in steps 1–7. Primers for real-time PCR can be designed from the existing 500 bp probe region. For FISH, search for available clones in genomic libraries (www.sanger.ac.uk or http://bacpac.chori.org/) and follow the recommended procedure of culturing and extraction. Label and hybridize using a FISH protocol of choice, for example, the one provided by Abbott Molecular (www.abbott.com).

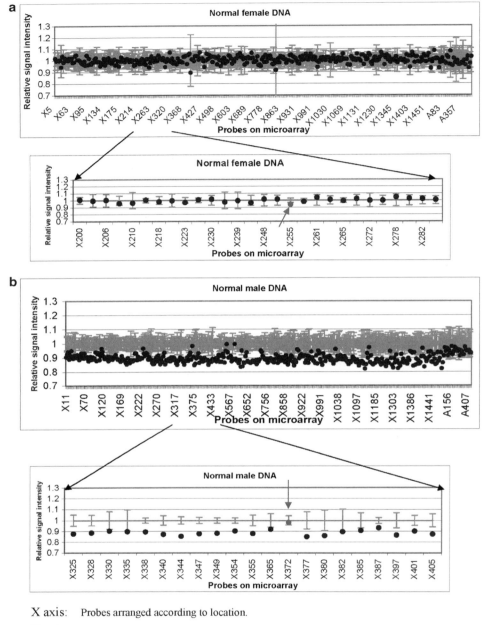

Fig. 2. Examples of chromosome X array-MAPH profiles for normal DNA samples. *Arrows* indicate probes that deviate from expected values. (**a**) Array-MAPH chromosome X profile of normal female, analyzed against female reference panel. Probes lie within TI90% as there is no copy-number change on chromosome X. (**b**) Array-MAPH chromosome X profile of normal male DNA sample, analyzed against female reference panel. Probes lie below TI 90% as males have only one chromosome X. The figure is reproduced with the permission of the authors (7).

MAPH Methodology 65

Patient A-2879

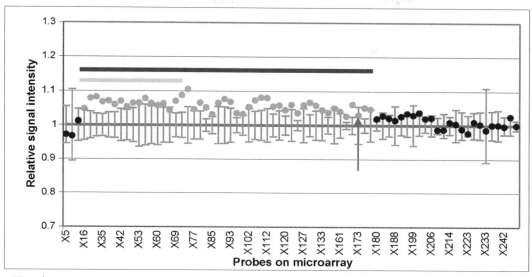

X axis: Probes arranged according to location.
Y axis: Relative signal intensity.

———— Normalized median value of the signal intensities of probes on the reference panel.

● ● Normalized values of fluorescence intensities in the test DNA.

I Tolerance Intervals (*TI90%*) of the reference panel for each probe.

———— Duplicated region, detected by initial FISH analysis.

———— Duplicated region, detected by Array-MAPH and confirmed by FISH analysis.

Fig. 3. Array-MAPH profile of patient A-2879 carrying a known duplication of Xp22.32-p22.31. Array-MAPH data showed that the duplicated region, indicated by probes with a ratio higher than the TI90%, extends to Xp22.12. The figure is reproduced with the permission of the authors (5).

4. Notes

1. Alternatively, other probe development tools can also be used to design gene- or region-specific hybridization probes (23, 24). Include internal control probes; for example, if chromosome X is to be analyzed, include a number (5–10% of studied probes) of autosomal control sequences.

2. It is important to use 46, XY DNA so that all chromosomes are represented in the template. This will help in the detection of primers with more than one binding site, in case it was missed in previous steps. DNA should represent an individual with normal phenotype and karyotype to ensure the presence of all primer-binding sites.

3. The use of Taq Polymerase is essential for creating A-overhangs on the 3′ end of the PCR product. These overhangs have a

Patient A045

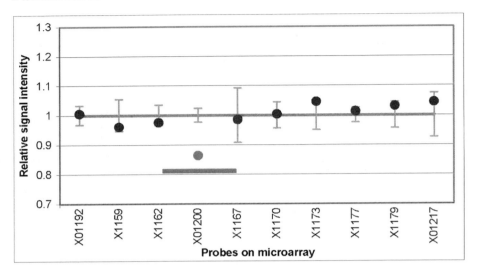

X axis: Probes arranged according to location.
Y axis: Relative signal intensity.

───── Normalized median value of the signal intensities of probes on the reference panel.

● ● Normalized values of fluorescence intensities in the test DNA.

I   Tolerance Intervals (*TI 90%*) of the reference panel for each probe.

───── Deleted region detected by array-MAPH.

Fig. 4. Array-MAPH profile of patient A045 resulted in the detection of a deletion on Xq25, based on a single-probe deviation. The figure is reproduced with the permission of the authors (5).

key role in the cloning procedure that will follow. For further details and alternative strategies, see TOPO TA cloning Instruction manual, version R (www.invitrogen.com).

4. A final 30 min polymerization step is required for Taq Polymerase to create A-overhangs and facilitate the subsequent cloning procedure. For further details, see TOPO TA cloning Instruction manual, version R (www.invitrogen.com).

5. If primers are designed correctly, the same PCR conditions should work for all probes. Use common PCR troubleshooting procedures only in case of very weak bands or low levels of specificity. If a primer gives more than one clear band, remove the corresponding probe from analysis, without proceeding with troubleshooting. Only highly specific PCR products are suitable for copy-number assessment.

6. The TOPO TA cloning system is ideal for cloning Taq polymerase-amplified PCR products of 100–1,000 bp in size.

Moreover, the cloning site is flanked by a common set of primers, facilitating cloning efficiency checks by rapid amplification from bacterial cultures. Subsequently, the products of this amplification carry a common flanking primer-binding sequence, as required for MAPH and can easily be used as hybridization probes. The PZA and PZB common primers are preferential instead of M13 primers provided with the kit, as they are located closer to the cloning site, adding only 77 bp to the size of PCR product, which does not significantly affect the probe's hybridization properties. For troubleshooting, see TOPO TA cloning Instruction manual, version R, www.invitrogen.com.

7. Amplification with common primers involves the risk of artefacts caused by mispriming or contaminated template. Moreover, probes cannot be identified by size so, even though a distinct PZA-PZB PCR product is produced, there is no guarantee that the cloned sequence is the expected one. A quick way to verify clone identity is direct amplification from bacterial cultures using probe-specific primers for each clone. As all primers are designed to have only one binding site in human genome, they will give a product only if the specific probe sequence is inserted in the cloning site.

8. Each target sequence is amplified twice in a volume of 50 µl to produce a greater concentration of the product for spotting.

9. For best results, keep freshly spotted slides at 4°C for 5–7 days before use. Spotted slides can be kept at 4°C for a maximum period of 1 year.

10. Probe concentrations in the mixture should be equal to avoid preferential hybridization of probes present in higher concentrations. Keep in mind that a minimum of 2 ng of each probe is required for one sample. Details and calculations concerning DNA and probe concentrations, as well as hybridization kinetics can be found at http://www.nottingham.ac.uk/~pdzjala/maph/maph.html. Probe mixture can be stored at –20°C for maximum 6 months.

11. The amount of DNA used for array-MAPH is twice the amount required for classical gel-based MAPH because of the increased number of simultaneously hybridized probes and the increased demands for probe outcome after hybridization.

12. Prolonged exposure to air increases the contamination risk. After cross-linking, filters can be kept at 4°C for a maximum period of 1 year.

13. For maximum efficiency, each tube should contain a maximum of four filters; use extra tubes to increase the number of simultaneously analyzed samples. Filters can be kept overnight in prehybridization buffer at 65°C.

14. The volume of probe mixture should not exceed 10 μL; otherwise, NaOH concentration will be affected, reducing denaturation efficiency. In addition, it might affect the concentration equilibrium in hybridization buffer. To decrease volume, take the required amount of probe mixture and concentrate on a vacuum concentrator. Proceed with adding all the other ingredients.

15. Quantities differ from those recommended for the classical MAPH protocol (8) because of the significantly increased probe number. The current array-MAPH protocol is adjusted to work with approximately 700 probes, but further optimization may allow an increase of this number.

16. Even if there is only one sample to analyze, at least 3 filters are required if the correct controls are included. Therefore, the above quantities should be adjusted accordingly.

17. Locus copy number can be correctly estimated only if hybridization is driven to completion and each probe anneals to all homologous sequences present in the DNA. To achieve this, it is important to have an excess of probes (see steps 9 and 10) and allow a minimum of 16 h for hybridization (see also http://www.nottingham.ac.uk/~pdzjala/maph/maph.html).

18. Filters can be kept in PCR mixture at 4°C for maximum 1 year.

19. Two-step amplification for 5 and 20 cycles remains within the quantitative phase of the PCR and at the same time gives a satisfactory product yield.

20. If traces of DNA appear in controls, discard all samples and repeat procedure from step 5 to step 20. If only the "filter with NaOH" control is contaminated, replace the NaOH solution used for DNA denaturation. If traces of DNA are present in all controls, including "no filter" control, replace all PCR reagents. If "filter with NaOH" and "empty filter" are contaminated, then the source of contamination could be air, instruments, or other factors of filter application procedure. Repeat with extra anticontamination measures (e.g. in a separate DNA-free environment, sterilize tubes, instruments, and bench with DNA contamination removing reagents or UV; avoid contact with potentially contaminating agents, etc).

21. SAP and ExoI treatment is performed to remove contaminating PCR components, such as dNTPs and primers that could interfere with the labeling process.

22. Do not use the heated lid on the thermal cycler or keep the lid open. The high temperature of the heated lid can affect the efficiency of labeling, which is set at relatively low temperature.

23. Dry pellets can be stored at −20°C for a maximum period of 2 weeks.
24. Cy™3 is the dye of choice, as it is more stable than Cy™5.
25. Array-MAPH hybridization outcome depends mostly upon the efficiency and reproducibility of spotting, labeling, and hybridization steps. Poor quality images may occur as a result of failure to maintain optimal reaction conditions during manual array hybridization, spotting artefacts or unsuccessful labeling reaction due to poor DNA quality, enzyme inactivation, or dye bleaching. It is much easier to obtain an informative image, using an automated hybridization system. Only high-quality hybridization results should be further analyzed to produce array-MAPH profiles.
26. Considerations for data normalization and analysis:
    (a) Microarray normalization: Normalize raw signal intensities to minimize technical and spatial defects of the array.
    (b) Between-slide normalization: In order to compare results from different experiments, use between-slide normalization for microarrays. Rescale signal intensities from different microarrays with respect to the median signal intensities of internal control probes.
    (c) Data transformation: In order to adjust the data to the normal distribution, which is required for correct calculation of tolerance intervals, convert signal intensity values to logarithmic scale with base of two.
    (d) Calculation of tolerance intervals: For each probe i, calculate the average ($AVERAGE_i$) and 90% tolerance interval values using data from the reference panel containing signals from several experiments carried out with control individuals.
    (e) Data transformation prior to sample analysis: Convert intensity values from studied DNA as follows: $CONVERTED\_VALUE_i = SIGNAL\_INTENSITY_i / AVERAGE_i$. Convert tolerance interval values for each probe by using the same principle.
27. For confirmation, there is no need to order and culture BAC, PAC or other clones, as all probe-specific primers are available to carry out PCR-based confirmation procedures for any detected copy-number alteration. Moreover, there is a well-established methodology for the rapid selection of additional primers from any genomic region. Homozygous deletions and deletions in chromosome X in males require a standard PCR reaction, followed by agarose gel detection, while quantitative real-time PCR can be used for duplications or hererozygous deletions.

Acknowledgments

The above work was funded by the grants 30/2001 from the Cyprus RPF, QLRT-2001-01810 from the EURO-MRX EU, 5467 from the Estonian Science Foundation, by 0182649s04 and PBGMR06907 from the Estonian Ministry of Education and Research, and by 070191/Z/03/Z from the Wellcome Trust International Senior Research Grant. We would also like to thank D. Andreou, C. Tryfonos, E. Hadjiyanni, C. Pitta, C. Antoniades, S. Bashiardes, and G. Slavin for their contribution.

References

1. Lucito, R., Nakimura, M., West, J.A., Han, Y., Chin, K., Jensen, K., et al. (1998) Genetic analysis using genomic representations. *Proc. Natl. Acad. Sci. U.S.A.* **95**, 4487–4492.
2. Solinas-Toldo, S., Lampel, S., Stilgenbauer, S., Nickolenko, J., Benner, A., Döhner, H., et al. (1997) Matrix-based comparative genomic hybridization: biochips to screen for genomic imbalances. *Genes Chromosomes Cancer* **20**, 399–407.
3. Wagenstaller, J., Spranger, S., Lorenz-Depiereux, B., Kazmierczak, B., Nathrath, M., Wahl, D., et al. (2007) Copy-number variations measured by single-nucleotide-polymorphism oligonucleotide arrays in patients with mental retardation. *Am. J. Hum. Genet.* **81**, 768–779.
4. Bignell, G.R., Huang, J., Greshock, J., Watt, S., Butler, A., West, S., et al. (2004) High-resolution analysis of DNA copy number using oligonucleotide microarrays. *Genome Res.* **14**, 287–295.
5. Patsalis, P.C., Kousoulidou, L., Männik, K., Sismani, C., Zilina, O., Parkel, S., et al. (2007) Detection of small genomic imbalances using microarray-based multiplex amplifiable probe hybridization. *Eur. J. Hum. Genet.* **15**, 162–172.
6. Sismani, C., Kousoulidou, L., and Patsalis, P.C. (2008) Multiplex Amplifiable Probe Hybridization, Molecular Biomethods Handbook, 2nd edition, (eds. Walker, J.M. and Rapley, R.), Chapter 13, Humana Press, USA, ISBN: 978-1-60327-374-9.
7. Kousoulidou, L.K., Männik, K., Sismani, C., Zilina, O., Parkel, S., Puusepp, H., et al. (2008) Array-MAPH: a methodology for the detection of locus copy-number changes in complex genomes. *Nat. Protoc.* **3**, 849–865.
8. Armour, J.A., Sismani, C., Patsalis, P.C., Cross, G., et al. (2000) Measurement of locus copy number by hybridisation with amplifiable probes. *Nucleic Acids Res.* **28**, 605–609.
9. Kousoulidou, L., Parkel, S., Zilina, O., Palta, P., Puusepp, H., Remm, M., et al. (2007) Screening of 20 patients from XLMR families for X-chromosomal subtle copy number alterations, using chromosome X-specific array-MAPH platform. *Eur. J. Med. Genet.* **50**, 399–410.
10. Kousoulidou, L., Männik, K., Zilina, O., Parkel, S., Palta, P., Remm, M., et al. (2008) Application of two different microarray-based copy-number detection methodologies – array-CGH and array-MAPH – with identical amplifiable target sequences. *Clin. Chem. Lab. Med.* **46**, 722–724.
11. Puusepp, H., Zordania, R., Paal, M., Bartsch, O., Ounap, K., et al. (2008) A girl with partial Turner syndrome and absence epilepsy. *Pediatr. Neurol.* **38**, 289–292.
12. Patsalis, P.C., Kousoulidou, L., Sismani, C., Männik, K., Kurg, A., et al. (2005) MAPH: from gels to microarrays. *Eur. J. Med. Genet.* **48**, 241–249.
13. Kennedy, G.C., Matsuzaki, H., Dong, S., Liu, W.M., Huang, J., Liu, G., et al. (2003) Large-scale genotyping of complex DNA. *Nat. Biotechnol.* **21**, 1233–1237.
14. Lucito, R., West, J., Reiner, A., Alexander, J., Esposito, D., Mishra, B., et al. (2000) Detecting gene copy number fluctuations in tumor cells by microarray analysis of genomic representations. *Genome Res.* **10**, 1726–1736.
15. Gibbons, B., Datta, P., Wu, Y., Chan, A., and Armour, J. (2006) Microarray MAPH: accurate array-based detection of relative copy number in genomic DNA. *BMC Genomics* **7**, 163.

16. Andreson, R., Reppo, E., Kaplinski, L., and Remm, M. (2006) GENOMEMASKER package for designing unique genomic PCR primers. *BMC Bioinformatics* **7**, 172.

17. Morgulis, A., Gertz, E.M., Schäffer, A.A., and Agarwala, R. (2006) WindowMasker: window-based masker for sequenced genomes. *Bioinformatics* **22**, 134–141.

18. Rozen, S., and Skaletsky, H. (2000) Primer3 on the WWW for general users and for biologist programmers. *Methods Mol. Biol.* **132**, 365–386.

19. Zhang, Z., Schwartz, S., Wagner, L., and Miller, W. (2000) A greedy algorithm for aligning DNA sequences. *J. Comput. Biol.* **7**, 203–214.

20. Ning, Z., Cox, A.J., and Mullikin, J.C. (2001) SSAHA: a fast search method for large DNA databases. *Genome Res.* **11**, 1725–1729.

21. Sambrook, J., and Russell, D.W. (2001) Molecular Cloning: A Laboratory Manual, Vol. 3, 3rd edition, (eds. Sambrook, J and Russell, D.W.) A8.9–A8.24, Cold Spring Harbour Laboratry Press, Cold Spring Harbor, New York, USA.

22. Kulka, J., Tôkés, A.M., Kaposi-Novák, P., Udvarhelyi, N., Keller, A., and Schaff, Z. (2006) Detection of HER-2/neu gene amplification in breast carcinomas using quantitative real-time PCR – a comparison with immunohistochemical and FISH results. *Pathol. Oncol. Res.* **12**, 197–204.

23. Mantripragada, K.K., Buckley, P.G., Jarbo, C., Menzel, U., and Dumanski, J.P. (2003) Development of NF2 gene specific, strictly sequence defined diagnostic microarray for deletion detection. *J. Mol. Med.* **81**, 443–451.

24. Mantripragada, K.K., Tapia-Páez, I., Blennow, E., Nilsson, P., Wedell, A., and Dumanski, J.P. (2004) DNA copy-number analysis of the 22q11 deletion-syndrome region using array-CGH with genomic and PCR-based targets. *Int. J. Mol. Med.* **13**, 273–279.

Chapter 5

Utilizing *Saccharomyces Cerevisiae* to Identify Aneuploidy and Cancer Susceptibility Genes

Erin D. Strome and Sharon E. Plon

Abstract

Cancers are commonly characterized as having an abnormal number of chromosomes, termed aneuploidy, which arise due to genomic instability. There is still debate over whether aneuploidy is a driving force of the disease or a resulting phenotype; however, the presence of aneuploidy can be used to grade the malignant potential of certain types of cancer. A simple hypothesis is that genome instability itself is tumorigenic in that it results in alterations in the number of chromosomes, which alters gene copy number and ultimately affects gene expression in cells.

Many gene disruptions that result in a propensity for cells to become aneuploid were first identified through mutagenesis screens designed to generate null or missense mutations in haploid strains of *Saccharomyces cerevisiae*. In contrast, the susceptibility to develop cancer can be transmitted as an autosomal dominant trait with affected individuals being heterozygous carriers of null mutations. In this chapter, we will describe a technique that can be used to identify heterozygous mutations in dosage-sensitive genes that mediate genomic stability by performing genome-wide screens in yeast.

Key words: *Saccharomyces cerevisiae*, Haploinsufficiency, Genome instability, Cancer susceptibility genes

1. Introduction

Current techniques for identifying mutations that convey small increased cancer risk are limited by the statistical power of epidemiologic studies, which require the screening of large populations or the use of candidate genes (1). Furthermore, due to the varying age of onset, type, and number of cancers developed, even among individuals carrying the same cancer susceptibility mutation, modifying factors have been explored to play a role in cancer development. These modifying factors include environmental factors such as carcinogen exposure, an individual's hormonal and reproductive status as well as genetic modifiers, defined as genetic changes occurring at a second locus, which result in the modification of cancer susceptibility (2–4).

Here we will outline a novel screening technique in *S. cerevisiae* to identify dosage-sensitive genes that mediate genomic stability as an alternative approach to identify genes, the orthologs of which may impact cancer susceptibility or modify cancer risk in carriers of high penetrant mutations. This comprehensive genome-wide screening method allows the identification of mutations, which confers a small increase in chromosome instability by utilizing two genome stability assays sensitive enough to detect the impact of heterozygous mutations.

S. cerevisiae has been frequently used as a model organism to identify genes that control genomic stability (5–10). Many of the genes that control the spindle, DNA replication, and DNA damage pathways are conserved between humans and *S. cerevisiae*, and were first identified through genetic screens, in this model organism, in studies focused on the control of genomic stability (11). Generally, these screens take one of two approaches – either looking at genomic instability itself as a read-out through the use of appropriately engineered strains, or identifying mutant strains with altered sensitivity or resistance to genotoxic stress agents (12–19). However, independent of the screening techniques utilized, the one main theme that previous screens have in common is the use of a haploid genetic background and therefore the cell retains no wild-type copies of the gene being studied (except in a few cases where the overexpression of genes and the resulting increase in ploidy are analyzed (20, 21)). In addition, it should be noted that mutant strains were normally identified due to large effects on genome stability, that is, several log differences in the degree of genomic instability or change in genotoxic sensitivity. Thus, screens to identify heterozygous mutations, which might model the impact of being heterozygous for a mutation in a cancer susceptibility gene in mammalian systems, have not been frequently undertaken.

2. Materials

2.1. Marker Systems and Strain Creation

1. *S. cerevisiae* diploid yeast strain: leu2-3/leu2-3, his3-Δ200/his3-Δ200, trp1Δ1/trp1Δ1, lys2-801/LYS2, ura3-52/ura3-52, can1-100/CAN1, ade2-101/ade2-101, 2× [CF:(ura3::TRP1, SUP11, CEN4, D8B)] (available upon request).

2. YPD (Yeast extract (VWR), Peptone (VWR), Dextrose (Fisher Scientific) – rich medium); Synthetic complete (Sc)-Arg⁻ CAN⁺; Sc-Trp⁻; Sc-His⁻ medium and plates poured in 100 cm dishes.

3. Low adenine (Sigma) containing (6 μg/mL) plates.

4. Plasmid carrying HIS3 gene. For example, pSH62 (22).
5. Primers to knockout your gene of interest with the HIS3 gene (22, 23).
6. Taq DNA Polymerase kit (Promega) supplied with 10× PCR buffer: 200 mM Tris–HCl, pH 8.4, 500 mM KCl; and 50 mM $MgCl_2$ and dNTPs.
7. 1% Agarose (ISC BioExpress) gel and TBE buffer: 89 mM Tris base (Roche Diagnostics Corporation), 89 mM Boric Acid, 2 mM EDTA.
8. 1 M and 100 mM Lithium Acetate (LiAc) (Sigma).
9. 50% PEG (Polyethyline glycol) (Sigma).
10. 2 mg/mL salmon sperm (Sigma).
11. Zymolase solution: 1.2 M Sorbitol (Sigma), 100 mM Na_2HPO_4, 2.5 mg/mL zymolase (Seikagaku America).
12. Sterile Toothpicks.
13. Agarose gel electrophoresis equipment.
14. 14 mL round-bottom Falcon tubes.
15. 30°C and 37°C incubator.
16. Rotating wheel in 30°C incubator.
17. Heatblock.

2.2. Insertional Mutagenesis

1. Transposon-mutagenized genomic library plasmid DNA (mTn-lacZ/LEU2-mutagenized library: available through http://ygac.med.yale.edu/mtn/insertion_libraries.stm).
2. Sc-LEU+ (Synthetic complete dropout medium deficient for HIS, TRP, and URA but proficient for LEU) (Amino acids from Sigma) medium and plates.
3. TE buffer: 10 mM Tris–HCl, 0.1 mM EDTA (Sigma), pH 8.0, sterile.
4. DH5α strain of *Escherichia coli*.
5. LB plates and medium supplemented with 40 μg/mL kanamycin and/or 50 μg/mL ampicillin (Antibiotics from Sigma).
6. LB medium: 10 g NaCl (Fisher), 10 g Tryptone (Fisher), 5 g Yeast Extract (VWR) per liter.
7. *Not*I restriction endonuclease and buffer (NEB).
8. 10 mg/mL denatured salmon sperm DNA (Sigma).
9. Water bath or incubator.

2.3. Fluctuation Analysis

1. Sterile water.
2. 96-well clear flat-bottom plates.
3. Vortex.

4. 30°C incubator with rotating platform.
5. 96-well plate absorbance capable plate reader.

2.4. Isolation of High Quality DNA from E. coli

1. 0.5 M EDTA (Sigma).
2. Beta-mercaptoethanol (Sigma).
3. TE Buffer: 10 mM Tris–HCl, 0.1 mM EDTA, pH 8.0, sterile.
4. 2 M Tris base.
5. 10% SDS (Sodium Dodecyl Sulfate) (Fisher).
6. 5 M Potassium Acetate.
7. Isopropanol (VWR).
8. Ethanol.
9. RNase A (Qiagen).
10. 5 M NaCl (Fisher).

2.5. Isolation of High Quality DNA from S. cerevisiae

1. 50 mL sorbitol/EDTA/zymolase solution: 22.5 mL 2 M Sorbitol, 10 mL 0.5 M EDTA, 100 µL β-mercaptoethanol, 3 mg 100 T zymolase (Seikagaku America), 17.4 mL sterile H_2O.
2. 4 mL EDTA/Tris/SDS solution: 2 mL 0.5 M EDTA, 1 mL 2 M Tris base, pH 7.5, 1 mL 10% SDS.

2.6. Vectorette PCR

1. Taq DNA Polymerase kit supplied with 10× PCR buffer 200 mM Tris–HCl, pH 8.4, 500 mM KCl; and 50 mM $MgCl_2$ and dNTPs.
2. *Rsa*I restriction endonuclease and buffer (NEB).
3. *Alu*I restriction endonuclease and buffer (NEB).
4. *Dra*I restriction endonuclease and buffer (NEB).
5. Anchor bubbles (see Note 1).
6. Qiagen QIAquick Gel Extraction Kit.

2.7. Inverse PCR

1. Taq DNA Polymerase kit supplied with 10× PCR buffer: 200 mM Tris–HCl, pH 8.4, 500 mM KCl, and 50 mM $MgCl_2$ and dNTPs.
2. *Hpa*II restriction endonuclease and buffer (NEB).
3. *Aci*I restriction endonuclease and buffer (NEB).
4. *Hae*II restriction endonuclease and buffer (NEB).
5. T4 DNA ligase and buffer (NEB).
6. ATP (USB).
7. Qiagen QIAquick PCR Purification Kit.

2.8. KAN-MX Knockouts

1. KAN-MX module plasmid.
2. Haploid deletion collection strains.
3. G418 Sulfate (EMD Biosciences) (VWR).

3. Methods

To focus on heterozygous mutations that increase chromosome loss, we developed a diploid parental strain, which includes the features required for a primary qualitative assay based on the spontaneous loss of a non-essential linear chromosome, referred to as a chromosome fragment (CF), and a secondary quantitative assay that determines the rate of loss or mitotic recombination of a natural endogenous chromosome (24).

We outline here the use of an insertional mutagenesis technique based on the Snyder mTn-lacZ/LEU2-mutagenized library (25) to create genome-wide heterozygous insertions potentially disrupting non-essential, essential and novel/uncharacterized genes as well as non-coding regions with potential function.

Our first screening technique is colorimetric based on loss of the CF; the second assay for genomic instability monitored the endogenous chromosome Vs, one containing the wild-type *CAN1* gene conferring sensitivity to canavanine and the second containing the *can1-100* recessive allele conferring resistance. The quantitative assessment of conversion to canavanine resistance assessed the combined effects of loss of the endogenous chromosome V containing the wild-type *CAN1* gene, mitotic recombination of the *CAN1* locus to *can1-100* or point mutation in the *CAN1* gene. However, spontaneous point mutations account for only 1–2% of the canavanine resistant mutants (26) and thus do not significantly contribute to this assay. In our published screen, we performed the experiment in a diploid strain background that was null for *RAD9* as a model for *BRCA1* null cells. This also facilitated the screen because it increased the CF loss rate. As described below, the screen can be performed in any specific null background by first deleting the gene of interest using the *HIS3* allele.

3.1. Strains and Assay Markers

1. Verify that the strain has all the required auxotrophies and markers by lack of growth after plating the strain on deficient medium plates and/or color observation.
2. Utilize short-flanking homology techniques to knock-out your gene of interest with a HIS3 cassette: design two primers (1) 40–45 bases homologous to the coding strand 5′ upstream of your gene of interest ORF and 18 bases homologous to the first 18 bps of the HIS3 gene (2) 40–45 bases

homologous to the non-coding strand 3′ downstream of your gene of interest ORF and 18 bases homologous to the last 18 bps of the HIS3 gene.

3. Set up the PCR to create a knockout cassette: standard PCR buffer, $MgCl_2$, dNTPs with primers (from step 2) and HIS3 containing plasmid template DNA; for example pSH62.

Step 1	94°C	4 min
Step 2	94°C	30 s
Step 3	Tm-5°C	30 s
Step 4	72°C	30 s/0.5 kb
Step 5	Go to step 2	29×
Step 6	72°C	10 min
Step 7	4°C	Hold

4. Screen for proper size construct by analysis in a 1% agarose TBE gel.

5. Transform yeast with knockout cassette using a modified lithium acetate protocol (27).

   (a) Grow 50 mL cultures of strains, to transform, to an OD of 0.6–0.9.
   (b) Spin 1 min at $2,500 \times g$.
   (c) Wash 1×100 mM LiAc.
   (d) Spin 1 min at $2,500 \times g$.
   (e) Resuspend at 2×10^9 cells in LiAc.
   (f) Transfer 50 µL of cells to 14 mL round-bottom Falcon tube.
   (g) Add in order: 240 µL 50% PEG, 36 µL 1 M LiAc, 50 µL 2 mg/mL salmon sperm, 5 µL knockout cassette from PCR reaction.
   (h) Let rest 1 h at 30°C.
   (i) Heat shock at 42°C for 45 min.
   (j) Add 5 mL YPD medium.
   (k) Incubate 3–4 h at 30°C on a rotating wheel.
   (l) Spin 1 min at $2,500 \times g$.
   (m) Remove supernatant, resuspend cells in 250 µL SC-his⁻ medium.
   (n) Plate at 50 and 200 µL dilutions on SC-his⁻ plates.
   (o) Incubate at 30°C for 3–4 days until single colonies appear.

6. Screen colonies that arise on SC-his⁻ plates by colony PCR with primer 1 homologous to the coding strand 5' upstream of your gene of interest (and upstream of the primer used to make the cassette and primer 2 homologous to the non-coding strand within the HIS3 gene (500–800 bps apart).

Step 1	94°C	4 min
Step 2	94°C	30 s
Step 3	Tm-5°C	30 s
Step 4	72°C	30 s/0.5 kb
Step 5	Go to step 2	29×
Step 6	72°C	10 min
Step 7	4°C	Hold

(a) Inoculate portion of yeast colony into 20 µL of zymolase solution.
(b) Incubate at 37°C for 15 min.
(c) Boil for 10 min; centrifuge briefly; add 40 µL of H_2O and vortex well; use 1–10 µL as template per PCR reaction.

7. Tetrad dissect strains that have been verified to have your GOI knocked out with HIS3. Plate for auxotrophies and drug resistance/sensitivity to determine genotype for all markers listed in strain description in Subheading 2.1. Mate two haploids of opposite mating type, each carrying a *goi*::HIS3 mutation and some portion of the appropriate markers listed in Subheading 2.1. Although not discussed in detail, you will need a haploid that has *goi*::HIS3 plus one distinct marker, therefore when you mate the two haploids you will have a diploid that can be selected for both markers (the specific details are not discussed because there are many possible combinations that can be used to select for the correct diploid strain). Confirm that a diploid was selected by the absence of mating to either MATa or MATalpha haploid tester strains and confirm genotype of the diploids.

3.2. Insertional Mutagenesis

Heterozygous mutations were created using the mTn-lacZ/LEU2-mutagenized library (25). Protocols for preparation and use of the library can be found at http://ygac.med.yale.edu/mtn/reagent/avail_reagents/lacZ_LEU2_lib_p.stm.

Briefly: Plasmid DNA is received as individual pools of the requested mTn-lacZ/LEU2-mutagenized library. DNA is resuspended, treated as individual pools, and transformed using standard procedures into the bacterial strain DH5α. Colonies resulting from the transformation are scraped from the surface of the plates and a large-scale DNA preparation is performed using standard techniques.

The insertion cassette is released from the plasmid by *Not*I digestion, which is then transformed into a *leu2⁻* yeast strain by the protocol listed above in Subheading 3.1 step 5 (see Note 2) to yield a large number of transformants which represent insertional mutants of the starting strain to be assayed for changes in genomic instability.

1. Streak Leu+ transformants onto 1/8 of a low-adenine concentration plate (6 μg/mL), to allow visualization of ~185 single colonies per insertionally mutagenized strain. This number of colonies assumes you are starting with a strain background that has a CF loss rate comparable to a *rad9* homozygous null background (see Note 2).

2. Grow for 3 days at 30°C, then incubate for 1 night at 4°C (for color development), and visually examine colonies for the appearance of pink/red sectors (see Note 3).

3. Determine the sectoring rate in your pre-mutagenized strains and set a statistically significant threshold level of sectoring for the insertionally mutagenized colonies (see Note 4).

4. All mutagenized strains that meet the threshold level of statistically significant sectoring should be restruck 3× to test the reproducibility of phenotype. Strains reproducibly achieving statistically significant sectoring (at least two of the additional three replicates) should be carried forward to fluctuation analysis.

3.3. Fluctuation Analysis: Estimation of Chromosome V Instability Rate via Modified Method of the Median

Chromosome V instability rate was measured as the conversion of a heterozygous can1-100/CAN1 strain to canavanine resistance using a modified median estimator that accounts for variations of the parallel culture population sizes N_t (24, 28).

1. Streak out mutants with increased CF loss, identified in Subheading 3.2, using a small innocula in order to maximize colonies, which arose from single cells. Allow plates to incubate for 3 days at 30°C.

2. Inoculate 24 separate colonies per strain by dispersal in 200 μL of water in a 96-well plate.

3. Measure absorbance using a 96-well plate reader, such as the Tecan Spectroflour Plus, at 620 nm. The goal is to identify 15 colonies of similar size using the optical density measurements. These colonies are carried forward.

4. The canavanine-resistant (k) and viable numbers of cells (N) in each of the 15 colonies are determined by plating the appropriate dilution on SC-Arg⁻ plus canavanine at 60 μg/mL and nonselective (YPD) plates, respectively (see Note 5).

5. Grow for 3 days at 30°C, and then count colonies on the canavanine and YPD plates (see Note 6).

6. Calculate Chromosome V instability rates using fluctuation analysis and a modification of the Lea and Coulson method of the median (29) (see Note 7).

3.4. Statistical Analysis of Chromosome V Instability Rates

Perform one-sided unequal Behrens–Fisher (30) variance t-tests for the estimated chromosome V instability rate of each strain (using the 15 estimated mutation rate data from all of the parallel cultures in each experiment) against the estimated parental (non-mutagenized) chromosome V instability rate to test if this rate was smaller.

3.5. Isolation of High Quality DNA from S. cerevisiae

DNA is prepared from the mutagenized strains with statistically significant increases in genomic instability.

1. Grow 10 mL cultures of mutagenized strains, in Sc-leu⁻, with increased genomic instability.
2. Spin cells, 5 min at 2,500 × g, pour off supernatant, resuspend cell pellet in residual medium and transfer to a microcentrifuge tube.
3. Add 600 µL sorbitol/EDTA/zymolase solution and incubate 1 h at 37°C.
4. Spin 3–7 s in tabletop centrifuge, pour off supernatant, resuspend in 600 µL TE Buffer.
5. Add 120 µL EDTA/Tris/SDS, mix by inversion, incubate 30 min at 65°C.
6. Add 200 µL 5 M Potassium Acetate, mix by inversion, put on ice for 1 h.
7. Spin at 4°C for 20 min at 13,000 × g, remove supernatant to a fresh microcentrifuge tube with 550 µL isopropanol, invert to mix, incubate on ice for 30 min.
8. Spin at 4°C for 15 min at 13,000 × g, pour off supernatant, wash with 1 mL 70% ethanol, invert to mix.
9. Spin at 4°C for 5 min at 13,000 × g, pour off supernatant, air dry pellets.
10. Resuspend dry pellets in 500 µL TE, add 3 µL RNase, incubate at 37°C for 30 min, vortex briefly, incubate at 37°C for an additional 30 min.
11. Spin at 4°C for 15 min at 13,000 × g, transfer the supernatant to a fresh microcentrifuge tube, add 20 µL 5 M NaCl, invert to mix, add 300 µL isopropanol, invert to mix.
12. Spin at 4°C for 15 min at 13,000 × g, remove the supernatant, wash with 1 mL 70% ethanol.
13. Spin at 4°C for 5 min at 13,000 × g, remove supernatant and air dry pellets.

14. Resuspend in 30 μL TE buffer, by gentle pipetting, and then allow to sit at RT at least 1 h.
15. Quantitate DNA.

3.6. Transposon Insertion Site Identification Utilizing Vectorette PCR

Vectorette PCR protocols were adapted from www.princeton.edu/genomics/botstein/protocols/vectorette.html.

Briefly: 3 μg of high quality genomic DNA is blunt end digested overnight with a frequent cutter such as *Rsa*I, *Alu*I, and *Dra*I. Digested fragments are ligated with anchor bubbles that are utilized as primer sites in subsequent PCRs. Unique bands from the PCR (compared to the products using non-mutagenized parental DNA as the template) are individually isolated, sequenced and aligned by BLAST to determine the site of transposon insertion.

3.7. Transposon Insertion Site Identification Utilizing Inverse PCR

Inverse PCR protocols were adapted from http://labs.fhcrc.org/gottschling/General%20Protocols/ipcr.html.

Briefly: Genomic DNA is digested with frequent cutters such as *Rsa*I, *Alu*I, *Dra*I, *Taq*I, *Hpa*II, *Aci*I, and *Hae*III. After digestion, the DNA is ligated at low concentration to favor intramolecular ligation, precipitated and then utilized in a PCR reaction with primers designed to amplify out from the transposon (primer sequences available on website above). PCR products are then sequenced and aligned by BLAST to identify the transposon insertion site.

3.8. Creation of Precise Heterozygous Mutations Utilizing the KAN-MX Cassette

This step allows you to create a heterozygous strain that contains a precise deletion of the coding region (or any sequence) in the *S. cerevisiae* genome. In this screen, it allows you to confirm that the phenotype (genome instability) identified by insertional mutagenesis is also seen found in the precise deletion.

1. Precise heterozygous deletions were created for a subset of the genes utilizing the KAN-MX cassette homologous recombination switch-out method (31).
2. KAN-MX module deletions for each gene were amplified using PCR on DNA isolated from individual strains from the haploid deletion collection (32) (for non-essential genes) or by flanking homology techniques (outlined above in Subheading 3.1).
3. For non-essential genes primers were designed 500–800 bp upstream and downstream of the KAN-MX cassette inserted in the ORF to create large areas of homology to facilitate recombination between the deletion cassette and the endogenous gene.
4. After amplification, the PCR generated products are transformed into the non-mutagenized parental strains (both with and without your gene of interest deleted).

5. Positive transformants are then selected on 200 μg/mL G418 plates and checked for proper integration via PCR with a forward primer upstream of the gene of interest and the PCR primer used to create the deletion cassette and a reverse primer within the KAN-MX cassette.

6. Fluctuation analysis assays as outlined in Subheadings 3.3 and 3.4 are then carried out on strains carrying precise deletions of the genes identified in the insertional mutagenesis as impacting genomic stability (see Notes 8–10).

4. Notes

1. A pair of oligonucleotides that hybridize at both the 3′ and 5′ ends but not-in in the middle, thereby when ligated together they form an oligonucleotide dimer with a bubble in the middle and therefore confer directionality to the PCR primers for amplification when ligated to the end of blunt-ended DNA molecules.

2. Fully pink or red colonies were not counted as sectored colonies.

3. For consistency, Leu+ transformed colonies should be screened by the same observer for the presence of sectors. Sectors arise due to loss of a CF, which harbors a SUP11 ochre-suppressing tRNA responsible for the suppression of the homozygous *ade2-101* ochre mutation that causes yeast to be red due to the build-up of adenine precursors. *S. cerevisiae* containing two copies of the CF are white, one copy is pink, and zero copies are red. The use of two CFs in the parental strain eases the identification of sectors due to the visualization of pink and red sectors on a white colony background.

4. Notes with the mutagenesis library indicate that screening 30,000 mutagenized colonies for their phenotype should yield 95% coverage of the genome; however, we recommend performing individual calculations of saturation as you screen to determine a stopping point.

5. Appropriate dilutions will be dependent on the mutation rate of your starting strains and the impact of the insertional mutant, therefore each mutagenized strain may need to be optimized for this assay. Ideally the dilution that gives 30–300 colonies per plate should be used.

6. Colony counting was expedited in our hands using the aCOLyte SuperCount colony counter.

7. To accommodate variations in N, chromosome V instability rate estimates were separately computed for the 15 colonies,

setting the initial cell count at $N_0 = 1$ and utilizing individual N and k values for each colony. A median of these estimates was accepted as a final estimate. The details of this method can be found in Wu et al. (28).

8. The comparison of mutation rates, calculated by fluctuation analysis, between strains deleted for screen-identified genes in GOI +/+ and GOI −/− strains yields information on the dependence of your mutant on the strain background.

9. It is useful to create profiles of the genes identified in the screen, for example, using gene ontologies or KEGG pathway characterizations, to determine if the genes identified cluster in certain genetic or biochemical pathways or networks. Gene Ontology (GO), a vocabulary of annotated gene assignments places genes into ontologies based on their known biological process, compartment location, or molecular function (33).

10. Homology searches to determine mammalian homologs of the genes identified in the screen that might mediate genomic instability in human cells and therefore a closer link to cancer susceptibility can be performed using multiple comparison tools of eukarYotic OrtholoGY (YOGY) available in the Comparison Resources section of www.yeastgenome.org.

Acknowledgments

The authors wish to express their thanks to Drs. Phil Heiter, Hannah Klein and Vicki Lundblad for donating strains to create their two genomic instability assay systems. We would also like to thank Dr. Marek Kimmel and Xiaowei Wu for their collaboration and for their help in the development of the statistical methods presented here.

References

1. Chenevix-Trench, G., Milne, R.L., Antoniou, A.C., Couch, F.J., Easton, D.F., and CIMBA. (2007) An international initiative to identify genetic modifiers of cancer risk in BRCA1 and BRCA2 mutation carriers: the Consortium of Investigators of Modifiers of BRCA1 and BRCA2. *Breast Cancer Res.* 9, 104

2. Mendiratta, P., and Febbo, P.G. (2007) Genomic signatures associated with the development, progression, and outcome of prostate cancer. *Mol. Diagn. Ther.* 11, 345–354

3. Hughes, D.J. (2008) Use of association studies to define genetic modifiers of breast cancer risk in BRCA1 and BRCA2 mutation carriers. *Fam. Cancer* 7, 233–244

4. Carneiro, F., Oliveria, C., Leite, M., and Seruca, R. (2008) Molecular targets and biological modifiers in gastric cancer. *Semin. Diagn. Pathol.* 25, 274–287

5. Hartwell, L.H. (1967) Macromolecule synthesis in temperature-sensitive mutants of yeast. *J. Bacteriol.* 93, 1662–1670

6. Hartwell, L.H., Culotti, J., and Reid, B. (1970) Genetic control of the cell-division cycle in yeast. I. Detection of mutants. *Proc. Natl. Acad. Sci. U. S. A.* 66, 352–359

7. Hartwell, L.H., Mortimer R.K., Culotti, J., and Culotti, M., (1973) Genetic control of the cell division cycle in yeast: V. Genetic analysis of cdc mutants. *Genetics* 74, 267–286

8. Hartwell, L.H., and Smith, D. (1985) Altered fidelity of mitotic chromosome transmission in cell cycle mutants of S. cerevisiae. *Genetics* **110**, 381–395

9. Spencer, F., Gerring, S.L., Conelly, C., and Hieter P. (1990) Mitotic chromosome transmission fidelity mutants in *Saccharomyces cerevisiae*. *Genetics* **124**, 237–249

10. Hoyt, M.A., Stearns T., and Botstein, D. (1990) Chromosome instability mutants of *Saccharomyces cerevisiae* that are defective in microtubule-mediated processes. *Mol. Cell Biol.* **10**, 223–234

11. Elledge, S.J. (1996) Cell cycle checkpoints: preventing an identity crisis. *Science* **274**, 1664–1672

12. Zhou, Z., and Elledge, S.J. (1993) DUN1 encodes a protein kinase that controls the DNA damage response in yeast. *Cell* **75**, 1119–1127

13. Osborn, A.J., and Elledge, S.J. (2003) Mrc1 is a replication fork component whose phosphorylation in response to DNA replication stress activates Rad53. *Genes Dev.* **17**, 1755–1767

14. Begley, T.J., Rosenbach, A.S., Ideker, T., and Samson, L.D. (2004) Hot spots for modulating toxicity identified by genomic phenotyping and localization mapping. *Mol. Cell* **16**, 117–125

15. Bennett, C.B., Lewis, L.K., Karthikeyan, G., Lobachev, K.S., Jin, Y.H., Sterling, J.F., et al. (2001) Genes required for ionizing radiation resistance in yeast. *Nat. Genet.* **29**, 426–434

16. Lee, M.S., and Spencer, F.A. (2004) Bipolar orientation of chromosomes in *Saccharomyces cerevisiae* is monitored by Mad1 and Mad2, but not by Mad3. *Proc. Natl. Acad. Sci. USA.* **101**, 10655–10660

17. Pan, X., Yuan, D.S., Diang, X., Wang, X., Sookhai-Mahadeo, S., Bader, J.S., et al. (2004) A robust toolkit for functional profiling of the yeast genome. *Mol. Cell* **16**, 487–496

18. Wheelan, S.J., Martinez-Murillo, F., Irazarry, R.A., and Boeke, J.D. (2006) Stacking the deck: double-tiled DNA microarrays. *Nat. Methods* **3**, 903–907

19. Pan, X., Yaun, D.S., Ooi, S.L., Wang, X., Sookhai-Mahadeo, S., Meluh, P., et al. (2007) dSLAM analysis of genome-wide genetic interactions in *Saccharomyces cerevisiae*. *Meth. Cell Cycle Res.* **41**, 206–221

20. Storchova, Z., Breneman, A., Cande, J., Dunn, J., Burbank, K., O'Toole, E., et al. (2006) Genome-wide genetic analysis of polyploidy in yeast. *Nature* **443**, 541–547

21. Ouspenski, I.I., Elledge, S.J., and Brinkley, B.R. (1999) New yeast genes important for chromosome integrity and segregation identified by dosage effects on genome stability. *Nucleic Acids Res.* **27**, 3001–3008

22. Guldener, U., Heinisch, J., Kohler, G.J., Voss, D., and Hegemann, J.H. (2002) A second set of loxP marker cassettes for cre-mediated multiple gene knock-outs in budding yeast. *Nucleic Acids Res.* **30**, e23

23. Wach, A. (1998) PCR-synthesis of marker cassettes with long flanking homology regions for gene disruptions in S. cerevisiae. *Yeast* **12**, 259–265

24. Strome, E.D., Wu, X., Kimmel, M., and Plon, S.E. (2008) Heterozygous screen in *Saccharomyces cerevisiae* identifies dosage-sensitive genes that affect chromosome stability. *Genetics* **178**, 1193–1207

25. Kumar, A., Vidan, S., and Synder, M. (2002) Insertional mutagenesis: transposon-insertion libraries as mutagens in yeast. *Methods Enzymol.* **350**, 219–229

26. Ohnishi, G., Endo, K., Doi, A., Fujita, A., Daigaku, Y., Nunoshiba, T., et al. (2004) Spontaneous mutagenesis in haploid and diploid *Saccharomyces cerevisiae*. *Biochem. Biophys. Res. Commun.* **325**, 928–933

27. Gietz, R.D., and Woods, R.A. (2002) Transformation of yeast by the LiAc/SS carrier DNA/PEG method. *Meth. Enzymol.* **350**, 87–96

28. Wu, X., Strome, E.D., Ming, Q., Hastings, P., Plon, S.E., and Kimmel M. (2009) A robust estimator of mutation rates. *Mutat. Res.* **661**, 1–2

29. Lea, D.E., and Coulson, C.A. (1949) The distribution of the numbers of mutants in bacterial populations. *J. Genet.* **49**, 264–285

30. Lix, L.M., Keselman, H.J., and Hinds, A.M. (2005) Robust tests for the multivariate Behrens-Fisher problem. *Comput. Methods Programs Biomed.* **77**, 129–139

31. Wach, A., Brachat, A., Pohlmann, R., and Philippsen, P. (1994) New heterologous modules for classical or PCR-based gene disruptions in *Saccharomyces cerevisiae*. *Yeast* **10**, 1793–1808

32. Winzeler, E.A., Shoemaker, D.D., Astromoff, A., Liang, H., Anderson, K., Andre, B., et al. (1999) Functional characterization of the *S. cerevisiae* genome by gene deletion and parallel analysis. *Science* **285**, 901–906

33. Ashburner, M., Ball, C.A., Blake, J.A., Botstein, D., Butler, H., Cherry, J.M., et al. (2000) Gene ontology: tool for the unification of biology. The Gene Ontology Consortium. *Nat. Genet.* **25**, 25–29

Chapter 6

Computational Identification of Cancer Susceptibility Loci

Marko Laakso, Sirkku Karinen, Rainer Lehtonen, and Sampsa Hautaniemi

Abstract

The identification of novel cancer susceptibility syndromes and genes from very limited numbers of study individuals has become feasible through the use of high-throughput genotype microarrays. With such an approach, highly sensitive genome-wide computational methods are needed to identify the regions of interest. We have developed novel methods to identify and compare homozygous and compound heterozygous regions between cases and controls, to facilitate the identification of recessively inherited cancer susceptibility loci. As our approach is optimized for sensitivity, it creates many hits that may be unrelated to the phenotype of interest. We compensate for this compromised specificity by the automated use of additional sources of biological information along with a ranking function to focus on the most relevant regions. The methods are demonstrated here by comparing colorectal cancer patients to controls.

Key words: Bioinformatics, Cancer genetics, Recessive inheritance, High-throughput data analysis, Data integration, Visualization, Homozygosity

1. Introduction

The development of microarray technology has significantly improved genetic analyses of human diseases and traits. The most up-to-date methods are capable of detecting hundreds of thousands or even up to a million genetic markers simultaneously in small and large cohort studies (1). This progress was made possible by the completion of the human genome sequence supplemented with accumulating knowledge of structure and variation in the human genome. Development of extensive and informative whole-genome genotyping platforms could not have been possible without information from the International HapMap project (2). The goal of the HapMap project is to develop a haplotype map of the human genome representing different populations and describing the common pattern of human DNA sequence variation. The knowledge that the genome is organized into discrete linkage disequilibrium (LD) blocks (3), a minimal set of single nucleotide polymorphisms (SNP) can be selected for SNP microarrays to tag most of the individual genetic variation (tagSNPs).

Modern SNP microarray technologies enable the detection of smaller regions and more uncommon variations contributing to human diseases than previously possible. The identification of Mendelian cancer susceptibility loci in seemingly isolated populations, such as Finns, has been successful. Finns can be divided into genetically differentiated sub-populations based on genome-wide SNP data. Especially North-Eastern Finns who represent the outcome of a classical bottleneck effect and they are additionally affected by a substantial amount of inbreeding caused by small sub-population size (4). This effect causes a higher probability of sharing substantially long genomic regions inherited from a common ancestor. Chromosomal regions inherited from a common ancestor are called identical by descent (IBD) opposite to a definition of identical by state (IBS) which represent identity by change. More information can be obtained when tracing data from haplotypes (sets of associated SNPs) rather than individual SNPs. The use of extended homozygous segments to find rare disease alleles, such as a Meckel syndrome has been utilized in Finland (5). This strategy could offer a way to localize even more common variants especially among young population isolates with substantial excess of extended runs of homozygosity (ROH) (6). For example, each individual from Eastern Finland may have on the average 20 ROH regions (homozygous segment over 1 Mb long).

Isolated populations with extensive and reliable genealogical records are ideal for genetic studies of hereditary diseases (7–9). In addition to Finland, especially the northern and eastern part of the country, suitable populations can be found, for example, from Quebec, Iceland, and Northern Sweden (8). The likelihood for consanguineous parents is increased in such populations, and thus recessively heritable phenotypes are seen more frequently. The genealogical records can be used to identify clusters of affected individuals with putative founder mutations if the affected people are close relatives and the records are available.

Mutation identification of recessive inherited phenotypes is based on the knowledge that a mutant allele is inherited from both parents so the genotype is either homozygous or compound heterozygous. Homozygous regions have identical alleles in both homologous chromosomes contrary to compound heterozygous regions which have two different mutated alleles. Extended homozygous or compound heterozygous regions shared by similarly affected individuals originating from the same population are candidate loci for causative mutations (9). A chromosomal region is called hemizygous if the genome contains only one copy of an allele and its homologies. Hemizygous cells might have lost a chromosome or its fragments.

The two chromosomal copies of an individual are approximately 99.5% identical (10). Thus, the remaining 0.5% containing the genetic variants is a very interesting fraction because that is what makes us different from each other. The similarity of the sequences is especially noted for genes and other evolutionary conserved parts of the genome. Even those loci that vary between individuals are likely to be homozygous as one of the alleles may be more common than the others. The distributions of two alleles can be estimated using the binomial distribution if a random mating is assumed within the (infinitely large) population as stated by the Hardy-Weinberg principle (11).

Here, we demonstrate the use of two rule-based approaches to identify loci that potentially harbor recessive mutations in colorectal cancer patients. The first approach is based on homozygosity detection and the other approach on haplotypes. We also present computational tools for interpreting genomic loci that were ranked high by the computational methods. We assume an isolated population in order to attain a reasonable chance of IBD while the number of required samples is kept in minimum.

1.1. SNP Microarrays

SNP-microarrays are small chips covered by an array of tiny droplets of short single-stranded DNA fragments called probes. These fragments of 25 to 50 nucleotides are complementary to sequences around the SNP loci. Fragmented and stained sample DNA is hybridized on an array. The single-stranded sample fragments binds to the probes with complementary sequences. The longer oligonucleotides are more sensitive and they work with lower DNA concentrations. On the other hand, shorter sequences are more specific in binding to their complements. To date, there is no consensus in selecting the optimal length for the oligonucleotides. The exact protocol used in the sample hybridization on an SNP-microarray depends on the platform. The sample fragments are hybridized with the matching complements attached to the microarray. The excess sample material is washed away and the microarray surface is scanned to a bitmap image.

Currently, Affymetrix and Illumina are the two major companies offering high-throughput SNP genotyping arrays for a variety of purposes and organisms. Here we focus on the Affymetrix technology though the discussed computational methods are applicable to other platforms as well. Affymetrix genome-wide SNP-microarrays for humans are currently available in formats of about $2 \times 50,000$, $2 \times 250,000$, and $2 \times 500,000$ SNPs. In the combination of two microarrays, the sample DNA is divided into two sets that are digested with different restriction enzymes producing fragments based on different splicing sequences for PCR amplification. The utilization of the restriction enzymes and the PCR amplification of the sequences up to 2,000 base pairs together produce copies of genomic regions that can be targeted by the microarrays (12).

Each SNP chosen to the microarray is targeted with 40 different probe sequences consisting of ten different probe quartets. A probe quartet consists of a mismatch (MM) and perfect match (PM) probes of both target alleles. PM probes match the sequence around the SNP loci and MM probes have one mismatching nucleotide in the middle of the probe. An illustration of a fictional probe quartet is shown in Fig. 1. The Affymetrix microarray architecture can detect only two alternative alleles for each SNP. The purpose of the MM probes is to measure the level of nonspecific hybridization that is considered as the background. The intensities of the PMs are determined based on their difference in the corresponding MM intensities.

The constitution of alleles in each SNP can be determined using a dynamic modeling algorithm that compares the likelihoods of models of homozygous (coded as AA or BB), heterozygous (AB) and missing data (NN) models (13). The algorithm makes no distinction between homozygous and hemizygous loci, so the most likely model is used as a genotype estimate. Genotype estimates of the studies using multiple SNP-microarrays can be done with the robust linear model that utilizes the information about

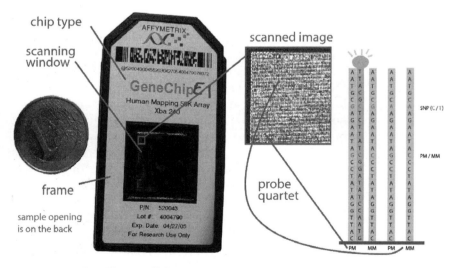

Fig. 1. Size and structure of an Affymetrix SNP-microarray. An example of a single probe quartet is shown on the *right*. The quartet consists of PM and MM probes of both alleles. The distinction between the PM and MM is always made in the *middle* of the sequence, whereas the SNP locus varies between the quartets. An example of a target sequence with a labeling dye residue has bound to the left-most probe, which represents the allele C. The other PM probe has not bound to its target and the sample can be considered as homozygous for the C allele.

the similarities between the probes and genotypes of different chips (14).

There are various causes for missing values in SNP genotypes, such as measurement errors and unexpected polymorphisms including unexpected alleles and copy number variants (15). The undetected alleles can be scored as missing values or hemizygous SNPs depending on whether they occur in one or both homologous chromosomes. Some of these undetected (null) alleles can be caused by a bi-allele deletion (16). The deletions can be of biological origin but they may also indicate sample degradation or other issues in the SNP experiment or array. The SNP-arrays with low overall SNP call rates (<95%) are likely to be defective according to the Affymetrix SNP-array manual. High missing value rate on a particular SNP often refers to technical problems. Some of the null alleles can be explained by another polymorphism that is so close to the SNP site that it interferes with the probes leading to a poor hybridization signal. Similar problems can be seen with multiallelic markers where some alleles are not supported by the arrays. Affymetrix arrays are built so that they are supposed to target only two known alleles, but the fact that there are four possibilities in reality may introduce bias to the measured alleles.

Technically, normalized probe signals for a sample are stored as a vector of genotypes. Genotype vectors can be combined into a data matrix where the rows and columns correspond to samples and markers, respectively. Such matrices can be formed for each chromosome, which reduces the computational complexity of the downstream analysis since the matrices require less memory and the algorithms do not need special handling of the chromosome boundaries.

2. Materials

1. The identification of recessive mutations using computational methods for SNP-arrays is illustrated with data obtained from a recessively inherited colorectal cancer (CRC) study (17). Samples of the CRC patients originated from Eastern Finland. A total of 49 patients were selected out of 1,044 prospectively collected CRC cases. The selection criteria were CRC in at least one sibling of a proband, and no evidence of dominant transmission. The cancers were microsatellite stable, and except for two samples, the common *MUTYH* gene mutations causing recessive CRC were excluded. The two samples having a different but homozygous *MUTYH* mutation were included in the data set to test whether the method is capable of identifying the *MUTYH* locus.

2. The microarray experiment is performed using an Affymetrix GeneChip Human Mapping 50K array (XbaI) according to the Affymetrix SNP-array standard protocol.

3. The DNA is extracted from normal fresh frozen colon tissue of the selected 49 patients and data from 51 control samples is available from different sources. The sample donors are not close relatives of each other. The samples were hybridized by Expression Analysis, Inc. (Durham, NC, US).

4. Samples with a mean call rate less than 95% (n = 8) are considered unsuccessful and excluded from the analysis as they would have introduced too many false positives in the homozygosity analysis. This phenomenon is caused by the higher odds of heterozygous genotype misclassification in low quality samples (18). A total of 41 patient samples are used in the downstream analyzes. The sample material is collected from healthy tissue surrounding the tumors. Therefore, the results are not biased due to large chromosomal aberrations that are common in CRCs.

3. Methods

Low statistical power caused by a small number of samples may become a limiting factor in finding chromosomal loci segregating with rare recessively inherited diseases. Furthermore, statistical tests estimate the likelihood for the case and control samples originating from the same distribution. Most cancer susceptibility gene cases are caused by somatic mutations and only a small fraction are due to an inherited mutation. Accordingly, the fraction of mutant carries is likely to be too small to be seen when the allele distributions are compared between the cases and the controls.

In order to overcome these challenges, biological databases are utilized to further classify genome regions into interesting and uninteresting segments. Two rule-based classifiers have been developed for genotype-derived features and their abundance in cases and controls. The main assumptions behind the first classifier are (i) an interesting region contains a long homozygous sequence that is shared by at least a certain fraction of case samples, and (ii) the region is detected in the control samples fewer times than a predetermined threshold. The second classifier extracts homozygous, heterozygous, and compound heterozygous haplotypes from genotype data, and similarly, evaluates the regions based on their abundance in cases and controls.

The identification of candidate regions compatible with the initial hypothesis can be obtained using an automated data analysis pipeline. In Fig. 2, a schematic diagram of such a pipeline is illustrated.

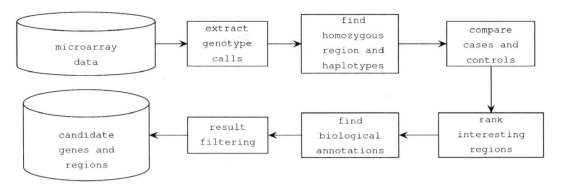

Fig. 2. Main steps of the computational analysis of SNP-data.

The original SNP array data were first normalized and converted into sample-specific genotype calls that are used for the identification of regional features, that is, multi-SNP structures that are either IBD homozygous regions or any combination of haplotypes. Samples are then divided into cases and controls and the overlap of the features calculated within and between the groups.

The overlaps that satisfied the enrichment criterion in cases are labeled as interesting and are ranked based on the scoring function. The regions that contained promising scores are selected for the functional annotation of the chromosome loci. The annotations consisted of known protein coding and non-coding, such as micro-RNA, genes, and transcription factor-binding sites or other regulatory elements. Finally, the most prominent regions and their biological constitutions are selected by combining them against the prior knowledge and the candidate genes.

3.1. Identification of Homozygous Regions

1. The major assumption behind efforts to identify recessive alleles is that a causal mutation for a recessive phenotype segregates within relatively long homozygous or compound heterozygous IBD haplotypes. Long continuous homozygous regions have been used to identify regions that are likely to be IBD (19) (see Note 1). No differences are made between homozygous and hemizygous regions, therefore genotypes A = {AA, A}, B = {BB, B}.

2. Homozygous regions in each sample are determined by using a sliding window to detect the continuous sequences of homozygous markers. A sliding window is used to consider long continuous homozygous sequences although a low number of heterozygous markers are accepted due to the possibility of genotyping errors. In this approach, the window length can be specified in base pairs or as a number of consecutive SNPs. As SNPs in commercial platforms are usually tagSNPs, they are not randomly or evenly distributed. Therefore, the

usage of a number of SNPs or the size of the region as a window parameter will result in different results in different genomic regions. In the next analysis step, chromosomal regions in which homozygosity was enriched are filtered out. Such regions represent common or uninformative IBD fragments and are therefore unlikely to carry rare founder mutations. Genomic loci containing more IBD fragments in cases than in controls are qualified as interesting candidate regions.

3. An example of identification of homozygous regions is shown in Fig. 3. The two samples containing a known *MUTYH* mutation in the shared homozygous region are easily and clearly detectable. The vertical axis represents the samples; the controls are at the top and the cases are below the black line. The effect of the uneven distribution of SNP markers can be seen in the middle of the horizontal axis as the homozygous regions of this centromere region are determined by its boundary sequences.

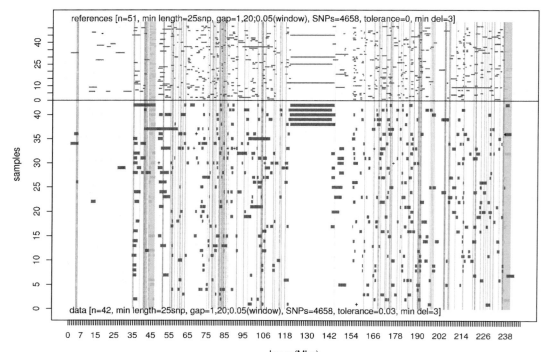

Fig. 3. Interesting regions found from the chromosome 1 are highlighted with *vertical bars*. *Orange bars* indicate allele-specific regions and *yellow bars* are allele-nonspecific regions. Homozygous regions of each sample are shown as *horizontal red* (common allele) and *blue* (rare allele) *lines*. *Gray lines* represent possible compound heterozygous regions for the homozygous regions of the interesting regions. *MUTYH* site has produced a wide *yellow bar* at 45.6 Mbp. Colored figure is available in (17).

3.2. Identification of Heterozygous and Compound Heterozygous Regions

1. The method described in Subheading 3.1 is designed exclusively to identify biologically relevant homozygous loci, as was shown with the *MUTYH* data. Thus, another approach can be developed to determine the number of compound heterozygous and heterozygous genotypes as well.
2. A heterozygous region has a different haplotype in both homologous chromosomes, and a homozygous region shares two identical haplotypes. The search of homozygous, heterozygous, or compound heterozygous chromosome regions is limited to a search of shared haplotypes in order to focus on the biological question, the detection of IBD fragments segregating with CRC.
3. In general, detecting homozygous genotypes is straightforward but heterozygous haplotypes cannot be observed from the data directly. To construct heterozygous haplotypes chromosome-specific haplotypes have to be estimated from the data.

3.2.1. Haplotype Estimation

1. As SNP marker data do not provide information about chromosome-specific sequences but only describe a genotype in each loci, the actual organization of alleles is estimated from the data. This procedure is called haplotype phasing and it aims at finding a plausible set of haplotypes that can be inferred from a given set of genotypes (20).
2. There are many methods to construct haplotypes from population data. HaploRec is the one of the most accurate and easily scalable of them (21). HaploRec uses Expectation-Maximization algorithm and assumes Hardy-Weinberg equilibrium in the population. With this method, common haplotypes in controls may hide the detection of rare haplotypes in cases. To avoid bias toward haplotypes in controls, haplotypes in cases and controls are inferred separately (see Note 2).

3.2.2. Evaluating Shared Haplotypes

1. After haplotype estimation, for each sample, two data rows that correspond to the alleles in both the copies of the chromosome are used. For generalization, both data rows from each sample are treated as individual samples and haplotypes that are shared between the two data rows of one sample are actually representing the homozygous region.
2. For each sample, all the haplotypes that it shares with the other samples are extracted. The search for shared haplotypes is performed separately for each locus along the chromosomes.
3. To find haplotypes that are likely to be IBD, the same sliding window technique that was used in the detection of homozygous genotypes is used. To avoid collecting shared IBS haplotypes

(shared just by chance), a probability value for each haplotype based on SNP allele frequencies is calculated. Only those haplotypes, whose probabilities are below a user-specified threshold, for instance, 0.05, are extracted from the data.

4. Finally, whether a haplotype is heterozygous, homozygous, or compound heterozygous is evaluated. A genome region is homozygous if both the haplotypes are the same, and heterozygous if they differ from each other. Compound heterozygous regions are more difficult to define because, by definition, in a compound heterozygous state, the two alleles carry a different recessive mutation. Obviously, which haplotypes carry the mutation cannot be determined. In this case, a region can be considered compound heterozygous if both the heterozygous haplotypes are also observed in homozygous conformations in the cases.

5. In our experiment, in addition to the two samples carrying the known *MUTYH* mutation, we added one artificial compound heterozygous sample to the data. This sample was a random combination of the actual mutation carriers. Figure 4 shows that using the rule-based classification we were able to discover the region including the haplotypes harboring the actual mutated *MUTYH* gene.

3.3. Scoring

1. The analysis of a genome-wide SNP data set may produce thousands of possibly interesting regions depending on the parameters and the number of samples. The complete manual validation of all discovered regions would need far too much time and resources. Thus, a scoring scheme is required to prioritize the biologically relevant interesting regions.

2. The scores are calculated to indicate the most promising candidates for the wet-lab validation. Quality values for the regions can be described in terms of the length, relative frequency of its features between the control and the case samples (19), and its biological content. Two scoring schemes to rank homozygous and compound heterozygous regions have been developed.

3.3.1. Scoring Homozygous Regions

1. A possibly interesting region consists of samples with homozygous alleles overlapping loci that are not present in control samples. The type of interesting region depends on the number of alleles that it covers. An interesting region may represent a feature of general homozygosity if there are not too many overlapping homozygous regions in controls. An interesting region may represent allele-specific features if it has an allele that is not homozygous in controls but the controls are homozygous for the other allele (see Note 3). An interesting region may also cover the entire extended homozygous region

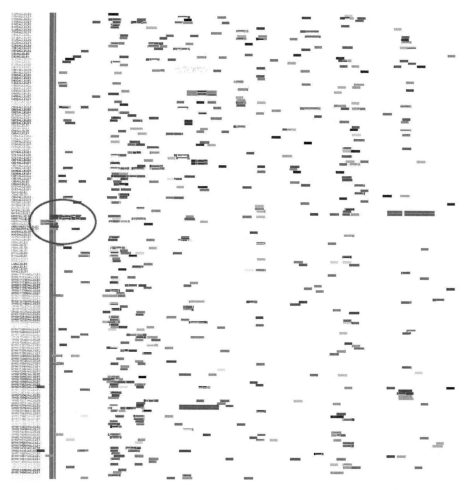

Fig. 4. Haplotypes found from each sample (ids on the *left*) from the chromosome 1 are drawn with *horizontal blocks*. *Vertical line* marks the interesting region, which is the chromosomal location of *MUTYH* mutations. Haplotype analysis discovered the two mutated homozygous alleles and one compound heterozygous allele and they are circulated in the picture. The number of markers was used as a unit of length; therefore, uneven distribution of markers along the chromosome is not seen.

in one sample but another sample may share only a fraction of the homozygous region. The scoring of the region is based on the length of the selected features and thus we are not calculating the actual length of the region itself but the total length of overlapping features.

2. Two different methods for scoring possibly interesting regions have been tested. First, a total score includes the length of the whole feature (such as a homozygous region or a fragment of an interesting allele) that made the region interesting. Second, a fraction score takes only the intersection of the feature and the region into account. Both scoring schemes have been tested in genome-wide analyses with the same parameters.

On the basis of the results, the fraction score method agrees better with the manual scoring given by an experienced cancer biologist. Long homozygous regions dominate the results of the total score method even if the interesting region is very short and shared by few individuals. Score values are most useful as sorting criteria. The interpretation of the meaningfulness of the value itself is quite hard since the range of possible scores is [0, k]. Getting the score of k would mean that all SNPs would differ in all samples between the data sets.

3.3.2. Scoring Haplotypes

1. A haplotype is given a score according to its length and the number of cases and controls sharing the haplotype. Each haplotype may be shared by different samples in each locus. Therefore, the number of cases and controls sharing the haplotype in each locus individually are calculated and then the individual scores from subsequent loci shared by the same cases and controls are summed up. This system highlights homozygous genotypes in which the same haplotype is seen twice because such genotypes get double scores.

2. Scoring based only on haplotypes does not give any insight into the interestingness of the overall chromosomal region. Thus, a score that describes all the haplotypes in the given region should also be used. This score is achieved by summing the scores from each haplotype that is present in each locus. The score can also be extended to a wider region by summing up the scores in neighboring SNPs that have the same score.

3.4. Interpreting Candidate Regions

1. Interesting chromosomal regions are easier to interpret if information about the biological functions can be linked to the identified, high-scoring regions. At the final stage in the analysis, annotations for genes and other functional elements in the identified chromosomal regions are searched for.

2. Many biological databases and electronic libraries are readily available, and integrating data from these sources may help prioritize chromosomal loci for validation. Interpretation and the functional analysis and filtering of the candidate regions require proper annotations about the biological functions of the regions. Databases containing information on gene, protein, micro-RNA (22), regulation elements (23) and Gene Ontology (GO) (24) for the regions are often beneficial.

3. We used the Ensembl database (22) to obtain the gene annotations for the best scoring genome regions. Regions with no gene annotations are of less interest as the interpretation of the functional role of possible genetic changes in these regions is challenging. Genes of the interesting regions are compared against CRC candidate genes obtained from the SNPs3D

database (25). The SNPs3D database can be queried for disease-associated genes. The Disease Candidate Gene module of the database provides an interface to a text-mining tool. This tool can be used to extract gene names based on keywords that are used in the abstracts of articles available in Medline. The set of keywords is constructed by selecting abstracts with the name of the disease. The words of these disease-related abstracts are compared against all abstracts to filter out common words that are not related to the disease. The most enriched terms are used as keywords. SNPs3D retrieves the gene names from the NCBI Gene database and compares them against the disease articles. The genes that are mentioned in articles are returned with an association score indicating how well the keywords and the gene name matched the abstracts.

4. In Table 1, we show how the comparison of the candidate regions against the CRC-associated genes can be used to emphasize the most prominent loci. Literature-based scoring works for the genes that are well known and it may explain the phenotypes of some case samples. This method is not suitable for the loci that are not associated with the phenotype of interest, and they may be ranked based on gene and GO annotations.

3.5. Summary

Statistical power in the analysis of rare recessive traits is often limited by the number of samples, and therefore rule-based methods are more suitable for such studies. The method described in this chapter was capable of identifying a site that was common for only two out of 41 case samples. In small sample sets, our haplotype-based approach supported by the formulation of rules for the classification of interesting loci is more powerful than commonly used statistical single SNP or haplotype-based association analysis methods. In our experiments, we were able to detect the known *MUTYH* mutation site in both settings, in the homozygous as well as in the artificial compound heterozygous haplotype states Our approach is not limited to recessively inherited phenotypes but is applicable to dominant and complex traits as well. Our method is not limited to population samples but can also be used in family studies. Basically, any experiment where haplotype information is available can substantially benefit from the methodologies described here.

An important aim of human genomics is to detect the entire spectrum of individual and population level variation and its impact on phenotypic differences, and more importantly on human diseases. Next-generation high-throughput sequencing technologies such as 1000Genomes(http://www.1000genomes.org/page.php, sequencing of the whole human genomes of over

Table 1
High scoring regions with colorectal cancer associated genes

Score	Region	Gene	Description
197287	9:33649571-35811797	VCP	Transitional endoplasmic reticulum ATPase (TER ATPase) (15S Mg(2+)-ATPase p97 subunit) (Valosin-containing protein) (VCP) [Source: UniProtKB/Swiss-Prot; Acc: P55072]
		C9orf127	Protein NGX6 (Nasopharyngeal carcinoma-associated gene 6 protein) (Protein NAG-5) [Source: UniProtKB/Swiss Prot; Acc: A6NDV4]
		UBAP1	Ubiquitin-associated protein 1 (UBAP) (Nasopharyngeal carcinoma-associated gene 20 protein) [Source: UniProtKB/Swiss-Prot; Acc: Q9NZO9]
197275	1:236777460-240462257	EXO1	Exonuclease 1 (hExo1) (EC 3.1) (Exonuclease I) (hExol) [Source: UniProtKB/Swiss-Prot; Acc: Q9UQ84]
195203	1:43494738-46829964	MUTYH	A/G-specific adenine DNA glycosylase (EC 3.2.2) (MutY homolog) (hMYH) [Source: UniProtKB/Swiss-Prot; Acc: Q9UIF7]
		RPS8	40S ribosomal protein S8 [Source UniProtKB/Swiss-Prot; Acc: P62241]
		CDC20	Cell division cycle protein 20 homolog (p55CDC) [Source: UniProtKB/Swiss-Prot; Acc Q12834]
		B4GALT2	Beta-1,4-galactosyltransferase 2 (Beta-1,4-GalTase 2) (Beta4Gal-T2) (b4Gal-T2) (EC 2.4.1) (UDP-galactose: beta-N acetylglucosamine beta-1,4-galactosyltransferase 2) (UDP-Gal beta-GlcNAc beta-1,4-galactosyltransferase 2) [Includes Lactose synthase A protein(EC 2.4.1.22); N-acetyllactosamine synthase (EC 2.4.1.90) (Nal synthetase); Beta N-acetylglucosaminylglycopeptide beta-1,4-galactosyltransferase (EC 2.4.1.38); Beta-N-acetylglucosaminyl-glycolipid beta-1,4-galactosyltransferase (EC 2.4.1)] [Source: UniProtKB/Swiss-Prot; Acc: O60909]
127989	22:40927203-43614979	ARHGAP8	Protor-1(Protein observed with Rictor-1) (Proline-rich protein 5) [Source: UniProtKB/Swiss-Prot; Acc: P85299]
		BIK	Bcl-2-interacting killer (Apoptosis inducer NBK) (BP4) (BIP1) [Source: UniProtKB/Swiss-Prot; Acc: Q13323]

(continued)

Table 1 (continued)

Score	Region	Gene	Description
		TSPO	Translocator protein (Peripheral-type benzodiazepine receptor) (PBR) (PKBS) (Mitochondrial benzodiazepine receptor) [Source: UniProtKB/Swiss-Prot; Acc: P30536]
114169	16:22705354-24217457	PLK1	Serine/threonine-protein kinase PLK1 (EC 2.7.11.21) (Polo-like kinase 1) (PLK-1) (Serine/threonine-protein kinase 13) (STPK13) [Source: UniProtKB/Swiss-Prot; Acc: P53350]

MUTYH mutation was found to be the third best scoring region

1,000 individuals) or the Cancer Genome Project (http://www.sanger.ac.uk/genetics/CGP/, including sequences of tens of entire cancer genomes), have made these plans affordable. Novel technologies will provide us with a huge amount of detailed genetic data calling for computational analysis methods to distinguish relevant mutations from random variation. For example, direct sequencing and the accurate detection of actual haplotypes is already possible (26) but the data needs efficient tools for haplotype comparisons. In addition to whole genome sequencing, targeted re-sequencing of the interesting cancer-associated locus has been recently carried through with the novel platforms (27). In addition to computational methods that are able to efficiently analyze massive amounts of genetic data, there is a high demand for more sophisticated visualization tools.

4. Notes

1. The determination of the shortest homozygous regions or haplotypes that should be considered IBD is a non-trivial task. The biological relevance of the findings is important; however, we should retain a high sensitivity for the recessive regions. Achieving a balance between these two exclusive objectives is challenging because the biological relevance cannot be determined without the actual identification of the predisposing mutation. Long regions are favored by our method as they are more likely to be IBD than IBS. Though computational methods for haplotype phasing are not comprehensive, the predictions are fairly robust for our purposes if enough SNP data from a homogenous population sample is available (21, 26). Only some estimates of the evolutional

background of the haplotypes can be estimated computationally since we do not know the pre-existed genomes or complete pedigrees. Some estimates about the sensitivity of the region selection can be obtained by comparing the probability of calling a region to a homozygous region between the real samples and the computationally generated random samples. These random samples can be constructed by sampling genotype calls for each marker from an observed distribution of genotypes independently of the other markers. Randomized samples will have an allele distribution equal to that of the real samples but the markers do not show any linkage dependencies.

2. Haplotype phasing from the population data is not straightforward and it is hardly ever completely accurate. The most obvious reasons that reduce the haplotype phasing accuracy are the number of samples, marker density, population heterogeneity, missing values, and bias toward typical haplotypes. Many of these cannot be controlled. In our case, we chose haplotype cases and controls separately to avoid bias toward common haplotypes in controls, potentially increasing the number of false negatives. This may introduce a new bias, as cases and control groups seemed more dissimilar than expected. Population differences led to an increase of false positive findings because more shared haplotypes are seen in cases that are not present in controls.

3. Balancing between biological relevance and sensitivity translates into tuning parameter values. In our experiments, it is evident that too stringent parameters lead to possible missdetection of interesting regions, while too loose settings increase the number of hits and the false positive rate. Selecting correct parameter values is a challenging task. Running the analysis iteratively with several alternative parameter values often provides a good solution. The best way to start is probably with the most stringent conditions and then, if the result set becomes too small, we move step by step to less stringent parameters.

References

1. Grant, S.F., and Hakonarson, H. (2008) Microarray technology and applications in the arena of genome-wide association. *Clin Chem.* **54**, 1116–1124
2. The International HapMap Consortium. (2003) The International HapMap Project. *Nature.* **426**, 789–796
3. Conrad, D.F., Jakobsson, M., Coop, G., Wen, X., Wall, J.D., Rosenberg, N.A. and Pritchard, J.K. (2006) A worldwide survey of haplotype variation and linkage disequilibrium in the human genome. *Nat. Genet.* **38**, 1251–1260
4. Salmela, E., Lappalainen, T., Fransson, I., Andersen, P.M., Dahlman-Wright, K., Fiebig, A., et al. (2008) Genome-wide analysis of single nucleotide polymorphisms uncovers population structure in Northern Europe. *PLoS ONE.* **3**, e3519
5. Tallila, J., Jakkula, E., Peltonen, L., Salonen, R. and Kestila, M. (2008) Identification of CC2D2A as a Meckel syndrome gene adds an

important piece to the ciliopathy puzzle. *Am J Hum Genet.* **82**, 1361–1367

6. Jakkula, E., Rehnstrom, K., Varilo, T., Pietilainen, O.P., Paunio, T., Pedersen, N.L., et al. (2008) The genome-wide patterns of variation expose significant substructure in a founder population. *Am J Hum Genet.* **83**, 787–794

7. Peltonen, L., Jalanko, A., and Varilo, T. (1999) Molecular genetics of the Finnish disease heritage. *Hum Mol Genet.* **8**, 1913–1923

8. Varilo, T., and Peltonen, L. (2004) Isolates and their potential use in complex gene mapping efforts. *Curr Opin Genet Dev.* **14**, 316–323

9. Mizrachi-Koren, M., Shemer, S., Morgan, M., Indelman, M., Khamaysi, Z., Petronius, D., et al. (2006) Homozygosity mapping as a screening tool for the molecular diagnosis of hereditary skin diseases in consanguineous populations. *J Am Acad Dermatol.* **55**, 393–401

10. Levy, S., Sutton, G., Ng, P.C., Feuk, L., Halpern, A.L., Walenz, B.P., et al. (2007) The diploid genome sequence of an individual human. *PLoS Biol.* **5**, e254

11. Stern, C. (1943) The Hardy-Weinberg Law. *Science.* **97**, 137–138

12. Syvanen, A.C. (2005) Toward genome-wide SNP genotyping. *Nat Genet.* **37** Suppl, S5–S10

13. Altshuler, D., Brooks, L.D., Chakravarti, A., Collins, F.S., Daly, M.J., and Donnelly, P. (2005) A haplotype map of the human genome. *Nature.* **437**, 1299–1320

14. Rabbee, N. and Speed, T.P. (2006) A genotype calling algorithm for affymetrix SNP arrays. *Bioinformatics.* **22**, 7–12

15. Carlson, C.S., Smith, J.D., Stanaway, I.B., Rieder, M.J. and Nickerson, D.A. (2006) Direct detection of null alleles in SNP genotyping data. *Hum Mol Genet.* **15**, 1931–1937

16. Conrad, D.F., Andrews, T.D., Carter, N.P., Hurles, M.E., and Pritchard, J.K. (2006) A high-resolution survey of deletion polymorphism in the human genome. *Nat Genet.* **38**, 75–81

17. Laakso, M., Tuupanen, S., Karhu, A., Lehtonen, R., Aaltonen, L.A., and Hautaniemi, S. (2007) Computational identification of candidate loci for recessively inherited mutation using high-throughput SNP arrays. *Bioinformatics.* **23**, 1952–1961

18. Xiao, Y., Segal, M.R., Yang, Y.H., and Yeh, R.F. (2007) A multi-array multi-SNP genotyping algorithm for Affymetrix SNP microarrays. *Bioinformatics.* **23**, 1459–1467

19. Woods, C.G., Valente, E.M., Bond, J., and Roberts, E. (2004) A new method for autozygosity mapping using single nucleotide polymorphisms (SNPs) and EXCLUDEAR. *J Med Genet.* **41**, e101

20. Halldórsson, B.V., Bafna, V., Edwards, N., Lippert, R., Yooseph, S., and Istrail, S. (2004), Lecture Notes in Computer Science. Springer Berlin/Heidelberg, Heidelberg, Vol. 2983/2004, pp. 613–614

21. Eronen, L., Geerts, F., and Toivonen, H. (2006) HaploRec: efficient and accurate large-scale reconstruction of haplotypes. *BMC Bioinformatics.* **7**, 542

22. Flicek, P., Aken, B.L., Beal, K., Ballester, B., Caccamo, M., Chen, Y., et al. (2008) Ensembl 2008. *Nucleic Acids Res.* **36**, D707–D714

23. Sandelin, A., Alkema, W., Engstrom, P., Wasserman, W.W., and Lenhard, B. (2004) JASPAR: an open-access database for eukaryotic transcription factor binding profiles. *Nucleic Acids Res.* **32**, D91–D94

24. Ashburner, M., Ball, C.A., Blake, J.A., Botstein, D., Butler, H., Cherry, J.M., D. et al. (2000) Gene ontology: tool for the unification of biology. The Gene Ontology Consortium. *Nat Genet* **25**, 25–29

25. Yue, P., Melamud, E., and Moult, J. (2006) SNPs3D: candidate gene and SNP selection for association studies. *BMC Bioinformatics.* **7**, 166

26. Kidd, J.M., Cheng, Z., Graves, T., Fulton, B., Wilson, R.K., and Eichler, E.E. (2008) Haplotype sorting using human fosmid clone end-sequence pairs. *Genome Res.* **18**, 2016–2023

27. Yeager, M., Xiao, N., Hayes, R.B., Bouffard, P., Desany, B., Burdett, L., et al. (2008) Comprehensive resequence analysis of a 136 kb region of human chromosome 8q24 associated with prostate and colon cancers. *Hum Genet.* **124**, 161–170

Chapter 7

Digital Candidate Gene Approach (DigiCGA) for Identification of Cancer Genes

Meng-Jin Zhu, Xiang Li, and Shu-Hong Zhao

Abstract

The candidate gene approach is one of the most commonly used methods for identifying genes underlying disease traits. Advances in genomics have greatly contributed to the development of this approach in the past decade. More recently, with the explosion of genomic resources accessible via the public Web, digital candidate gene approach (DigiCGA) has emerged as a new development in this field. DigiCGA, an approach still in its infancy, has already achieved some primary success in cancer gene discovery. However, a detailed discussion concerning the applications of DigiCGA in cancer gene identification has not been addressed. This chapter will focus on discussing DigiCGA in a generalized sense and its applications to the identification of cancer genes, including the cancer gene resources, application status, platform and tools, challenges, and prospects.

Key words: DigiCGA, Cancer gene, Cancer resource, Platform/tool, Prospect

1. Introduction

Cancer is one of the leading disease killers for people in many nations around the world. Topics relating to cancer biology, diagnostics, and therapeutics are of great interest not only to cancer specialists but also to the broader scientific community. There is also an increasing awareness of cancer among the general public. Although heavily involved in non-genetic factors such as environment and lifestyle (1), the revolution in cancer research has confirmed that cancer is, in essence, a genetic disease (2). Numerous studies have shown that cancer is a multiple-gene controlled disease rather than a single-gene one, and there are complex genetic and epigenetic events to participate in the molecular determinants of various carcinogenesis.

It is known that cancer is a consequence of the abnormal expressions of specific genes, which usually involve dynamic changes of the genome (3). Therefore, as the first step, gene discovery and identification are essential and preconditions for molecular genetic analyses and the mechanistic understanding of cancers. In the last decade, much effort has been devoted to unravel the mysteries of the molecular architecture of cancer. An increasingly large set of candidate genes or molecules underlying the genesis of various cancers have been discovered and the deregulation or dysregulation of pathways through which they act were also characterized (2). Much progress in this field has been achieved but there is still a long way to go. The identification of other potential causal/susceptibility genes responsible for cancers remains a priority.

Different strategies and approaches have been developed and are now established for identifying disease susceptibility genes. In this chapter, we will focus on the candidate gene approach (also named candidate gene identification approach), a popular method for cancer gene identification, and make a special emphasis on the recent advances of digital candidate gene approach (DigiCGA) and its related topics for identifying cancer-related genes.

2. Traditional Candidate Gene Approach

2.1. A Synoptic Description

One powerful and commonly used technique to dissect and identify genetic risk factors for cancer is the candidate gene approach. The rationale of candidate gene approach states that a major component of heritable variation of biological traits and diseases can be determined by a causal functional mutation of a putative gene (4), which, in a hypothesis-driven manner, detects the effective sizes of genetic variants of a potentially contributing gene through an association analysis. The major advantages of the candidate gene approach include quickness, simplicity, inexpensiveness, directness, high sensitivity for detecting the genes with small effect, and perfect plasticity in the practical application. The routine procedures of traditional candidate gene approach mainly involve:

1. Selecting a candidate gene according to the researcher's prior knowledge about the target trait;
2. Detecting a DNA polymorphism inside the candidate gene such as single nucleotide polymorphism (SNP);
3. Testing the already-conformed polymorphic site of the candidate gene on a large scale in specific populations or families

through convenient molecular biology techniques such as the PCR-based genotyping method;

4. Performing a statistical association analysis with phenotypic records of interest for genetic effect estimation;
5. Conducting further intensive validation experiments including transgenic or knockout animal models; in agricultural animals and crops, this usually involves a validation test in more future generations of the same population or other different populations, or the ultimately believable quantitative complementation test.

The candidate gene approach has been ubiquitously applied for gene disease research, genetic association studies, and biomarker and drug target selection in many organisms from animals to human beings (5). Candidate gene studies are better suited for detecting genes underlying common and more complex diseases where the risk associated with any given candidate gene is relatively small (6). Therefore, the candidate gene approach is not only useful in the single gene diseases/traits but also in the multiple-genic or polygenic diseases/traits to which cancer belongs (7). Unlike the genome-wide linkage analysis, the candidate gene approach is practically more efficient for direct gene discovery (8, 9), which has been proven to be extremely powerful for studying the genetic architectures of complex biological traits and diseases.

Nevertheless, the disadvantages of the traditional candidate gene approach are also obvious. The traditional approach lacks a definitive functional confirmation of the target candidate, and often encounters a high occurrence of spurious association and interstudy discrepancy in practice. In particular, the practicability of the traditional candidate gene approach is largely limited by its reliance on the existing knowledge about the known or presumed genetics of target traits, which is usually finite or sometimes not available at all and results in an information bottleneck. This makes it difficult to identify the most likely disease-related genes and genes controlling other traits using the traditional candidate gene approach. However, as it profited from the high flexibility in the actual application, large efforts have been focused on breaking the restriction of the information bottleneck. Consequently, a number of strategies have been developed. These strategies mainly include a position-dependent strategy, a function-dependent strategy, a comparative genomics strategy and a combined strategy (4). Using these strategies, many candidates including biomedically, economically, agriculturally, and evolutionarily important genes have been convincingly identified. However, the volume of the already identified genes responsible for the biological traits and genetic diseases of interest is still small and there is an urgent need to accelerate the rapidity of gene discovery by applying new strategies and methods.

2.2. Trends in Candidate Gene Approach Studies

The candidate gene approach is experiencing an increasing application in a wide spectrum of scientific fields due to its advantageous features, and the shortcomings faced by the traditional one are being overcome. Besides the above-discussed strategies for breaking the information bottleneck, some new trends in the current candidate gene approach studies have occurred. An ongoing revolution in this field is represented by the integration of enormous amounts of data being produced from various novel high-throughput techniques. Among them some national and international co-operations on mega initiatives such as the genome sequence project, the SNPs project, the epigenetic genome project, the phenome project, and the protein function and biochemical pathways (PFBP) project for race-based or personalized care have been launched from model organisms to human beings (Cancer Genome Atlas Research Network, 2008) (10–13). This has produced a magnitude of data on the Internet and has provided opportunities and possibilities to a massive collection of the biological and disease data for improving candidate gene analyses.

Under these circumstances, which are similar to the whole genome association study but working in a hypothesis-driven manner, the large-scale candidate gene study or comprehensive candidate gene study for simultaneously detecting many selected candidate genes has been launched to identify disease susceptibility genes such as dementia, cancer, diabetes, asthma, and hypertension-susceptible genes (14–16). Hereinto, the large-scale attempt has been achieved usually through association studies in the two-stage, three-stage or multi-stage designs (17–20). In recent association studies, however, the substitution of single locus SNPs by the previously-infrequent marker types has gradually become a common occurrence and involves the combined genotype, the haplotype, and even the haplotype block, as well as the non-DNA sequence variants such as the alternative splicing mRNA, the mRNA abundance, the circulating molecule concentration, and the protein profile (21–24). Another trend in this field is the methodological integration with other quantitative methods and biotechnologies, for examples, genome-wide scans, the genetic epidemiological method, expression microarray, SNP chips, and protein chips, which is also spurring the in-depth development of the candidate gene approach. Taken together, the new trends in recent developments of the candidate gene approach could be summarized as the ones with high-throughput, integrative, and multiple digital resources-dependent characteristics.

3. Digital Candidate Gene Approach

3.1. Background and Definition

As discussed above, various international genome projects from model animals to human beings have provided access to a vast amount of biological data sources, which has greatly accelerated the research advancements in life sciences. As more and more biological data in public databases have become available, various new utilizations of digital resources have been developed for different research purposes. Hereinto, the rapidly growing biological resources enable a large-scale and effective utilization to prioritize candidate genes. The reliable digital deposits in public databases that are dynamically updated by the practical experimental data submitted from the world's researchers or teams, either on a small scale or on a large scale, are allowing the dissection of the molecular architectures underlying complex biological traits and diseases. In theory, the integration analyses of larger data sets pooled from different sources could increase the identification capability of the as yet undiscovered genes with small effect sizes. At the forefront of the candidate gene approach research is to work with the multitude of available data resources from public databases. Many recent studies employing a variety of biological data sources from the Web, in which more and more computational methods emerge to identify the most likely candidate genes underlying biological traits and diseases, have primarily highlighted the web resources-related new feature of the candidate gene approach.

From the standpoint of scientific philosophy, the new development of a scientific field (subfield) often requires the development of a new concept. According to this, we have proposed the term DigiCGA to generalize the web sources-related development of the candidate gene approach (4). As a development of the candidate gene approach, DigiCGA was defined by us previously as a novel gene discovery approach for complex traits and diseases that is realized through extracting, filtering, (re)assembling, or (re)analyzing all possible available data sources derived from the public databases. This is done following objective principles, in which cross and species specific genome-wide structural and functional data, the biological ontologies (e.g., anatomy ontology, cell and tissue ontology, developmental ontology, gene ontology, and phenotype and trait ontology), and certain algorithms are usually utilized to make a computational prioritization of the potential candidates underlying the biological traits or diseases of particular interest. As an extension, all digital resources-based analyses for biological traits and diseases can be regarded as the generalized DigiCGA analyses. In our opinion, strengthened with the new concept, the emergence of DigiCGA would increase the efficiency of utilizing all available digital data sources and become one of the most remarkable progresses in the candidate gene approach.

3.2. Principles and Classifications for DigiCGA

Despite the explosion of a large amount of genomic data from many organisms, converting genomic data into biological knowledge to identify genes involved in a particular process or disease remains a major challenge (25). This urgent requirement to develop novel strategies and methods for identifying trait or disease genes accelerates the development of DigiCGA. Knowledge of the technologies and principles supporting DigiCGA is widely involved in the fundamentals and applications of biology, computer, and bioinformatics.

In our opinion, the reported approaches related with DigiCGAs could be primarily classified as the ontology-based identification approach, computation-based identification approach, and integrated identification approach (including literature-based meta-analysis) (4). The ontology-based identification approach mainly involves bioinformatic analyses for the in *silico* identification of candidate genes using varieties of biological ontology resources available through the Internet. Computation-based identification makes gene discoveries by using the biological functions of genes or proteins through mathematical models. Usually, the computation-based identification approach, by using certain algorithms and a variety of web-based data sets, includes those computational candidate gene identification methods that describe a computational framework or model to prioritize the most likely candidate genes underlying the biological traits or diseases. The integrated identification approach comprises most of the combined methods for prioritizing candidate genes, including converging actual experimental data, web database-based resources (including literature-based resources (26) and biological ontology resources) or the theoretical assembling of molecular features or molecular interaction principles, for example, gene structure variation, homologs, orthologs, SNPs data, protein–DNA interactions, protein–protein interactions (interactome), molecular module, and pathway and gene regulatory network (27–31).

There have been a series of studies falling into the different categories of DigiCGAs. An example of the ontology-based identification approach is the prioritization of positional candidate genes by using gene ontology (32). In computation-based identification, many statistical algorithms or computational methods have been reported, which include data-mining analysis (33), hidden Markov analysis (34), cluster analysis (35), kernel-based data fusion analysis (36), machine learning (37), KNN classification algorithm from the machine learning techniques (38), and others. Tiffin et al. (39) compared seven independent computational methods for disease gene identification (39). There were also many candidate genes prioritized by the integrative approach for gene discovery such as the combined pathway and gene ontology analysis (40), text and data mining (41), combined genetic maps and QTL analysis (42), combination analysis of functional annotations, protein–protein interactions, regulatory information, expression data, sequence-based data and literature mining data (43), and mutome network modeling integrative analysis (44).

Of course, there are other criteria for classifying DigiCGA that can be put into different categories. According to the data types or properties, DigiCGA could be mainly classified into the DNA information-based approach, mRNA information-based approach, protein information-based approach, and multiple information-based approach. Another suggestion was to classify the gene identification algorithms according to the theory basis that DigiCGA follows, in which four classifications were divided into an ab initio algorithm, a homological algorithm, a cross-species algorithm, and an other algorithm (45). As digital data resources increase, more effective methods for DigiCGA will be developed.

3.3. Software and Online Tools Related to DigiCGA

Currently, some application software or online tools for prioritizing candidate genes such as GFSST, Endeavour, POCUS, G2D, TOM, FunMap, eVOC, DGP, QTL Mixer, SUSPECTS, DEEP, and other tools have been developed and released to the public, many of which are used purely for disease-specific purposes, and a few for general purpose. In addition, other tools such as GeneMark, Glimmer, ORFGENE, AthaMap web tools, ESTminer, Rank Gene and Target Explorer mainly enable pure gene identification without using special phenotypes but their core thoughts may potentially contribute to the future developments of DigiCGA. Some software and tools for the prioritization of candidate genes are summarized in Table 1.

3.3.1. TOM

This tool uses the information stored in online databases and the filtering ability of known biological principles to output a list of candidate genes responsible for multigenic diseases (http://www-micrel.deis.unibo.it/~tom/). The database resources using this tool include NCBI Gene Expression Omnibus, a gene expression and hybridization array data repository; NCBI GEO, an expression profiles database; ArrayExpress, a public repository for microarray gene expression data at the EBI; the ArrayExpress gene expression database and Gene Ontology. The rationale behind TOM is based upon the combination of gene mapping, expression profiling and functional annotations, in which the following three steps are followed:

1. Gene mapping contrast;
2. Expression profiling analysis to extract; and
3. Functional annotations filtration.

3.3.2. BioMercator

BioMercator is a general rather than disease-specific tool for candidate gene discovery. BioMercator automatically performs the task of candidate gene discoveries through integrating genetic maps

Table 1
Software and online tools related to DigiCGA

Name	Literature source	Website
GeneSeeker	Nucleic Acids Res. 2005; 33, W758–W761	http://www.cmbi.ru.nl/GeneSeeker
GFSST	BMC Bioinformatics. 2006; 7, 135	http://www.gfsst.nci.nih.gov
Endeavour	Nat Biotechnol. 2006; 24, 537–544	http://www.esat.kuleuven.be/endeavour
POCUS	Genome Biol. 2003; 4, R 75	http://www.hgu.mrc.ac.uk/Users/Colin.Semple
G2D	Nucleic Acids Res. 2007; 35, W212–W216	http://www.ogic.ca/projects/g2d_2
SUSPECTS	Bioinformatics. 2006; 22, 773–774	www.genetics.med.ed.ac.uk/suspects
TOM	Nucleic Acids Res. 2006; 34, W285–W292	http://www-micrel.deis.unibo.it/~tom
BioMercator	Bioinformatics. 2004; 20, 2324–2326	www.moulon.inra.fr/~bioinfo/BioMercator
FunMap	Bioinformatics. 2004; 20, 1808–1811	Link disabled
GFINDer	Nucleic Acids Res. 2005; 33, W717–W723	http://www.bioinformatics.polimi.it/GFINDer
PROSPECTR	BMC Bioinformatics. 2005; 6, 55	http://www.genetics.med.ed.ac.uk/prospectr
eVOC	Nucleic Acids Res. 2005; 33, 1544–1552	Link disabled
QTL Mixer	Bioinformatics. 2005; 21, 1737–1738	http://www.qtl.pzr.uni-rostock.de/qtlmix.php
DGP	Nucleic Acids Res. 2004; 32, 3108–3114	Link disabled
CoGenT++	Bioinformatics. 2005; 21, 3806–3810	http://www.cgg.ebi.ac.uk/cogentpp.html
KNN classifier	Bioinformatics. 2006; 22, 2800–2805	Available on request: jianzxu@hotmail.com
SNPs3D	BMC Bioinformatics. 2006; 7, 166	http://www.SNPs3D.org
PhD-SNP	Bioinformatics. 2006; 22, 2729–2734	http://www.gpcr.biocomp.unibo.it/cgi/predictors/PhD-SNP/PhD-SNP.cgi

Ref. (4)

and quantitative trait loci (QTLs). This enables the visualization of co-location between genes and QTL through a graphical interface. BioMercator mainly involves:

1. A map projection algorithm for the prior QTL information; and
2. Meta-analysis.

When analyzing a task, the user is allowed to input QTL data in a dialog window. The common loci (sharing the same name) in each pair of homologous chromosomes are listed and the interval between two common loci is computed into a specific distance ratio, in which the inverted pairs can be automatically discarded from the list of common loci and are then computed by application of the appropriate distance ratio through a homothetic projection process. Meta-analysis is based on the automatically processed QTL data sets. Concomitant with the QTL imputed by the user, meta-analysis algorithm can help to determine if N-QTL detected from independent experiments in the same region of a chromosome are consistent with 1, 2, 3, 4-, or N-QTL models. The maximum likelihood method is employed to substantiate the most concord QTL distribution and determine the best model among the five.

3.3.3. eVOC

eVOC is a sharp tool to identify disease candidate genes (41, 46, 47). The principle of eVOC is largely based on the fundamental issue that the expression of disease genes is often dys-regulated in affected tissues. eVOC integrates text-mining of bio-medical literature and data-mining of available human gene expression data to identify the possible disease candidate genes. Here are some of the main running steps followed by eVOC:

1. Use text mining of PubMed abstracts to identify association between the disease name and anatomy terms;
2. Use the identified anatomy terms to independently identify genes that are expressed in the related tissues from the Ensemble genomic database. Here, the terms in the anatomical system ontology provide a human readable description of the terms commonly used in the annotation of samples taken for expression studies;
3. Annotation of the publicly available EST and mRNA data with terms from the ontology provide a means to connect expressed sequences with terms describing the location and timing of expression; and
4. Use the eVOC anatomical ontology to link expression phenotype and genomic sequence.

3.3.4. PROSPECTR

PROSPECTR (PRiOrization by Sequence and Phylogenetic Extent of CandidaTe Regions) uses an alternating decision tree, which has been trained to differentiate between genes likely to be involved in disease and genes unlikely to be involved in disease (http://www.genetics.med.ed.ac.uk/prospectr/). The resource databases that PROSPECTR uses are mainly found in Ensembl and Online Mendelian Inheritance in Man (OMIM), in which thousands of known genes involved in human disease are deposited. PROSPECTR relies on:

1. Disease genes sharing patterns of sequence-based features;
2. Significant differences between the sets of genes known to be involved in human hereditary disease and those not known to be involved in disease; and
3. WEka as a platform for machine-learning experiments.

PROSPECTR is an automatic classifier using the alternating decision tree algorithm, which ranks genes in the order of the likelihood that they are involved in disease. This algorithm uses an iterative fashion to create the trees by adding rules, and the rules are automatically derived from the differences between the disease and control gene sets, in which a new rule is added to the tree either as a new node or as a child of an existing node (37). From the enriched lists of genes at the suspected disease loci, a ranked list ordered by the likelihood of involvement in disease is returned.

3.3.5. Endeavour

As described by the authors, Endeavour is a multiple databases-based and multiple species-supported online tool, which is free and open to all users. This tool uses a training set of genes known to be involved in a biological process of interest and is based on the similarity of identified target genes to known genes underlying biological processes or disease (43). Endeavour proceeds by:

1. Inferring several models (based on various genomic data sources);
2. Applying each model to the candidate genes to rank those candidates against the profile of the known genes; and
3. Merging the several rankings into a global ranking of the candidate genes.

4. DigiCGA for Cancer Gene Identification

4.1. General Consideration

It has been proven that the biological essence of cancer is a genetic disease and that carcinogenesis occurs, at least in part, due to the accumulation of mutations in critical genes that control the mechanisms of cell proliferation, differentiation, and death (48).

As a consequence, the individual and family susceptibility to cancer is closely associated with the polymorphisms of cancer susceptibility genes, and even the cancer types also have a direct association with the polymorphisms of certain locus such as TERT-CLPTM1L (49). In theory, the prevention and treatment of cancer diseases heavily rely on understanding the molecular mechanisms of various phases of the cancerogenic process, for which the identification of cancer genes is the first step. Currently, the genetics of cancer is still not well understood and the identification of cancer genes is a major bottleneck. Usually, there are three main aspects of cancer gene identification, which are identifying cancer therapeutic targets, searching for cancer diagnostic biomarkers, and discovering genetic risk markers for individual and family cancer risk assessment.

The methods for cancer gene discovery include the identification of viral oncogenes, identification of genes associated with recurrent chromosomal aberrations and screening for genes capable of the transformation of cells in culture. In recent years, the completed genome sequence of human and model organisms has markedly enhanced the efficiency of cancer gene identification (50). The analysis of publicly available databases can help to identify potential candidates for genes or mutations specifically related to the cancer phenotype (51). As Hanauer et al. (52) stated, with the generation of massive amounts of global data and development of new computational algorithms, bioinformatics is renovating the approaches to studying the genetic basis of cancer (52). Gene discovery made by DigiCGA is essentially a bioinformatics-based discovery. Like other biological traits or genetic diseases, the formerly mentioned strategies and methods provided by DigiCGA are also suited for identifying potential genes driving carcinogenesis. For example, the determination of which genes are differentially expressed between normal and disease states can be used to identify diagnostic and therapeutic targets for cancer research. As an important component of bioinformatics approaches, the generalized DigiCGA has already shown some success in cancer gene identification (53, 54). Nevertheless, a systematical discussion for applying DigiCGA in cancer gene identification has not yet been addressed. In the subsequent subsections of this section, we will discuss relative issues under this subject.

4.2. Public Web Resources for Cancer Genes

Digital resources for cancer offer an attractive starting point for cancer gene discovery. Cancer gene resources have been widely deposited on the Web, including the general databases like GenBank, SWISS_PROT, and EMBL as well as the subject-specialized databases such as the GO consortium and KEGG database. Moreover, numerous studies on cancer have led to the generation of a large amount of cancer gene data, and the creation and maintenance of cancer-specific databases. For instance, SAGEmap, as a component of the Cancer Genome Anatomy Project, provides a central location for depositing, retrieving and analyzing human gene expression data, which uses serial analysis of gene expression to quantify transcript levels in both malignant and normal human tissues (55). In the daily updated KEGG database, there are many pathways responsible for various cancer diseases, including colorectal cancer, pancreatic cancer, glioma, thyroid cancer, acute myeloid leukemia, chronic myeloid leukemia, basal cell carcinoma, melanoma, renal cell carcinoma, bladder cancer, prostate cancer, endometrial cancer, small cell lung cancer and non-small cell lung cancer, etc. Accumulating work on cancer pathways would be very useful for the research on candidate gene discoveries. Up to now, a series of public web resources, special for cancer genes, have been created (see Table 2), which provide the available data resources for the applications of DigiCGA in cancer gene research. Hereinto, the Cancer Gene Anatomy Project (CGAP) database of the National Cancer Institute has prevailed in the majority of reported studies.

4.3. Status Quo of Applying DigiCGA for Cancer Gene Identification

4.3.1. A Glance of Research Progress

The bioinformatic computational techniques derived from DigiCGA have a high potential for discovering aberrantly expressed cancer-related genes or identifying causal genes involved in the various stages of carcinogenesis. In fact, recent studies have demonstrated the broadness of digital application in the identification of new potential targets for cancer prevention and therapy (53, 56). All digital resource-based analyses of cancer-related cases are cataloged as part of the generalized DigiCGA analysis, where not only cancer genes but also hallmarks such as the expression patterns may be involved. To date, a number of cancer-related genes and their hallmarks have been identified by DigiCGA digitally using expression databases (57). Some of them may have a major function in regulating the initiation, development, and progression of cancer and provide potential targets or markers for cancer prognostication, diagnosis, prevention and treatment.

In this field, many studies have used genome-wide and multitissue screening of cancer genes with in *silico* transcriptome analysis. This can identify genes differentially expressed in normal and tumor tissues by comparing cancer libraries deposited in publicly available databases (58). In research reported by Scheurle et al. (59), the data mining tool called Digital Differential Display (DDD) from the CGAP was chosen to analyze the differential expressions of ESTs from different solid tumor types. Genes from six classes of ribosomal proteins, enzymes, cell surface molecules, secretory proteins, adhesion molecules and immunoglobulins were found to be differentially expressed in tumor-derived libraries of breast, colon, lung, ovary, pancreas and prostate. Besides the application of DDD in cancer gene discovery, the research of

Table 2
Some web resources associated with cancer gene

Web resources (databases) name	Description	URL
CGAP (cancer genome anatomy project)	An interdisciplinary program established and administered by NCI to generate the gene expression information and technological tools needed to decipher the molecular anatomy of the cancer cell	http://www.cgap.nci.nih.gov
Cancer genome project	Use the human genome sequence and high throughput mutation detection techniques to identify somatically acquired sequence variants/mutations and hence identify genes critical in the development of human cancers	http://www.sanger.ac.uk/genetics/CGP
TCGA (the cancer genome atlas)	A comprehensive and coordinated effort to accelerate our understanding of the molecular basis of cancer through the application of genome analysis technologies	http://www.cancergenome.nih.gov
caBIG (cancer biomedical informatics grid)	Represents a colossal initiative involving virtually all aspects of cancer research	http://www.cabig.cancer.gov
ICGC (the international cancer genome consortium)	Aim at obtaining a comprehensive description of genomic, transcriptomic, and epigenomic changes in 50 different tumor types and/or subtypes	http://www.icgc.org
TGDBs (tumor gene family databases)	Contains information about genes which are targets for cancer-causing mutations, proto-oncogenes and tumor suppressor genes	http://www.tumor-gene.org/tgdf.html
SNP500Cancer	Re-sequenced SNPs from 102 reference samples	http://www.snp500cancer.nci.nih.gov
RTCGD (retrovirus tagged cancer gene database)	Aim at providing a potent cancer gene discovery tool	http://www.rtcgd.abcc.ncifcrf.gov
c-Myc cancer gene	Essential for the understanding of the genetic regulatory networks underlying the genesis of cancers	http://www.myccancergene.org

(continued)

Table 2
(continued)

Web resources (databases) name	Description	URL
CT (cancer/testis) gene database	Provides information about gene structure, chromosomal mapping, proteins, immunoreactivity in cancer patients and mRNA expression	http://www.cancerimmunity.org/CTdatabase
CGED (cancer gene expression database)	A database of gene expression profile and accompanying clinical information which includes data on breast, colorectal, hepatocellular, esophageal, thyroid, and gastric cancers	http://www.lifesciencedb.jp/cged
Breast cancer gene database	Information and data of breast cancer genes	http://www.bcm.edu/test-bcgd
Tumor associated gene database	Contains information for oncogenes and tumor suppressor genes involved in the tumorigenesis in at least one cancer type, as well as the unidentified cancer genes	http://www.binfo.ncku.edu.tw/TAG/GeneDoc.php
SV40 large T-antigen mutant database	Mutations in SV40 large T-antigen gene	http://www.supernova.bio.pitt.edu/pipaslab
PubMeth/methycancer	Links between DNA methylation levels and cancer	http://www.matrix.ugent.be/pubmeth/ or http://www.methycancer.genomics.org.cn
OncoDB.HCC	Oncogenomic database of hepatocellular carcinoma	http://www.oncodb.hcc.ibms.sinica.edu.tw
ITTACA	Contains both microarray gene expression and clinical data of tumors currently focusing on breast carcinoma, bladder carcinoma, and uveal melanoma	http://www.bioinfo.curie.fr/ittaca
IARC TP53 database	Compiles data on human somatic and germline TP53 genetic variations based on literatures	http://www.iarc.fr/p53
Human p53, human hprt, rodent lacI and rodent lacZ databases	DNA mutations at the human p53 gene, the human hprt gene and both the rodent transgenic lacI and lacZ locus have been created	http://www.ibiblio.org/dnam/mainpage.html
HPTAA	Human potential tumor-associated antigens	http://www.bioinfo.org.cn/hptaa/

(continued)

Table 2 (continued)

Web resources (databases) name	Description	URL
EHCO (the encyclopedia of hepatocellular carcinoma genes online)	An integrative platform for the pileup of unsorted HCC-related studies by using natural language processing and softbots	http://www.ehco.iis.sinica.edu.tw
COSMIC (catalogue of somatic mutations in cancer)	Sequence data, samples and publications	http://www.sanger.ac.uk/perl/CGP/cosmic
CanGEM	Gene copy number changes in cancer	http://www.cangem.org/
CancerGenes	Gene selection and prioritization in large collaborative projects	http://www.cbio.mskcc.org/cancergenes
Atlas of genetics and cytogenetics in oncology and haematology	Cards on cancer-related genes, chromosomal abnormalities, cancers, and cancer-prone diseases	http://www.atlasgeneticsoncology.org/
NCI60 cancer microarray project	Survey of gene expression in a panel of 60 NCI cancer cell lines exhibiting patterns related to their tissue of origin	http://www.genome-www.stanford.edu/nci60/index.shtml
Oncomine/GEO (gene expression omnibus)	A research platform global collection of cancer profiling data	http://www.oncomine.org

Note: some resources are interoverlapped, interincluded or interlinked

Scheurle et al. (59) also created a solid tumor DDD database which helps to facilitate target identification for cancer diagnostics and therapeutics (59). On the basis of this study, one colon tumor-specific EST was validated by Reverse Transcriptase Polymerase Chain Reaction (RT-PCR) analysis (60). Narayanan (61) provided another example of cancer gene discovery by using bioinformatics approaches, in which the CGAP database and data-mining tool were employed (61). On the basis of the functional candidate gene approach, the utilization of gene expression data resources not only facilitates gene discovery but also identifies the cancer-specific hallmarks such as molecular "modules" underlying malignancies. For example, the gene module map algorithm was used to perform an integrated analysis of 1,975 published microarrays spanning 22 tumor types. The results revealed that a growth-inhibitory module is specifically repressed in acute lymphoblastic leukemia. This suggests that cancer types can be classified in terms of the behavior of gene expression profiles (62). On the basis of the collected 1,551 gene expression sets (1,256 gene sets derived from Gene Ontology and 295 data sets of human primary breast cancers from the Netherlands Cancer Institute), Wong et al. (63) also utilized the module maps to find that the activation of a poor prognosis "wound signature" is strongly associated with the induction of both a mitochondria gene module and a proteasome gene module in human breast cancers (63).

Alternative splicing is an important phenomenon in cancer and the genome-wide computational screen has been used to detect the novel splice forms of cancer-specific transcript variants (64–66). In addition, SNP data in publicly accessible databases can also prioritize the cancer genes by the DigiCGA analysis. For example, Qiu et al. (48) successfully identified several SNP tumor associations through in *silico* association analysis (48). Aouacheria et al. (51) conducted a more recent study based on in *silico* whole genome screening to find that the UTR SNPs were significantly associated with the tumors (51). Moreover, Peeper and Berns (67) revealed that the integrative cross-species analysis is a powerful strategy to identify the responsible genes and assess their oncogenic capacity in the appropriate genetic context (67). Other informatic approaches such as text mining and semantic analysis were also used to analyze cancer-related genes, for example, Chen and Wen (68) have developed a biomedical literature-based integrated system for mining the information of cancer genetics (68).

4.3.2. Platforms, Algorithms/Tools for Cancer-Related Gene Analysis

Specialized platforms and algorithms/tools for cancer gene identification are relatively rare but some specialized ones still exist. There are many analytical strategies, algorithms and software/tools not specific to cancer but suited for the analysis of cancer genes, for example, PIANA software, the genome-scale in *silico* analysis of genes co-expressed with the target (69) and the computer-based differential display strategy (also referred to as in *silico* subtraction, DDD or DigiNorthern/electronic northern) (58). Besides the computational and bioinformatic approaches already discussed in DigiCGA, the core elements of many strategies and methods applied in the "wet" laboratory experiments can also be used to develop novel digital analysis approaches, some of which are indeed derived from the ones that were historically and are presently utilized in wet-laboratory experimental data.

Current approaches for digital analyses of cancer-related genes mainly include two classes: the pure bioinformatic methods and the combination of wet experiment-based methods with web resources. There are also some platform integrated tools for cancer-related gene analysis, for example, the tools in CGAP databases (70).

Several platforms, algorithms, and/or tools that have been reported to perform cancer-related gene analyses using web resources are briefly summarized below.

4.3.2.1. Module Maps

Under the frame of DigiCGA, the module maps algorithm could be taken as a meta-analysis of expression profiles from multiple cancer gene sources, in which a series of common microarray analysis tools such as GeneXPress are usually involved. The gene module maps can make a good delineation of common patterns of gene expression across heterogeneous tissue types and disease processes for cancer. In module maps, a module is a set of genes that act in concert to carry out a specific function. There are usually activated and deactivated modules. The gene expression profiles of certain cancer types could be considered as the consequence of combining activated and deactivated modules. The process of gene module maps is as follows (62):

1. Collecting web data sets of gene expression profiles from the available databases or platforms containing cancer gene resources.

2. Defining module or core module and allocating each module with an expression signature: classifying genes into different gene sets, including clusters of co-expressed genes, genes expressed in specific tissue types and genes belonging to the same functional category or pathway. A gene set reflects a module that participates in a specific biological process such as metabolism, transcription, translation, degradation, cellular and neural signaling, growth, cell cycle, apoptosis and extracellular matrix, and cytoskeleton components, the information of which usually comes from the well-annotated databases such as Gene Ontology and KEGG databases.

3. Mapping of modules: identifies the gene sets that are significantly associated with particular clinical annotations such as tissue and tumor type, diagnostic and prognostic information, and molecular markers according to the combination of modules that are activated and deactivated in them. The shared and unique characteristic between modules is denoted "specific" and "general."

4. Paired annotations: localize modules to the more strict category with crossed annotations.

4.3.2.2. Cancer Outlier Profile Analysis

Cancer Outlier Profile Analysis (COPA), an R package developed by MacDonald and Ghosh (71) as a part of the BioConductor project according to the method proposed by Tomlins et al. (72), is a tool using expression data sets to find candidate genes involved in recurrent translocations in carcinomas for a particular cancer type. There is also a web-based COPA procedure on the Oncomine database that provides a data mining platform specific to oncology-related microarray analysis.

The idea behind COPA is that genetic translocations occur in cancer cells, and that these translocations can result in the upregulation of oncogenes that may affect the progression of the cancer. This idea can be used to both pre-filter genes as well as find interesting genes that may be involved in translocations. In order to identify genes or outlier expression profiles that might be lowly and only expressed in a subset of tumor samples, the COPA procedure uses the median and median average difference (MAD) to detect those genes overexpressed only in a subset of the analytical samples, where, according to the number of outliers, the candidate genes are ranked based on the sum of outlier samples for each pair.

4.3.2.3. GeneHub-GEPIS

GeneHub-GEPIS is a bioinformatics tool for inferring gene expression patterns in a large panel of normal and cancer tissues based on human and mouse EST sequence abundance (http://www.cgl.ucsf.edu/Research/genentech/genehub-gepis/). Zhang et al. (73) reported the application of GeneHub-GEPIS to perform digital expression analysis in cancer tissues (73). For a given set of genes, they reported a change in expression in about 40 different types of normal and cancerous tissues. The GeneHub database integrates gene and protein information from several databases including GenBank, RefSeq, Ensembl, Fantom, Entrez Gene, UniGene, miRBase, protein databases (PDB, UniProt) and commercial microarray platforms (Affymetrix and Agilent). The GEPIS (gene expression profiling in *silico*) server utilizes EST abundance information to calculate gene expression levels in a panel of normal and cancerous human tissues for a given input DNA sequence. The application is composed of two parts: a front-end web interface for user input, text- and cDNA sequence-based data retrieval, display and download, and a backend engine to perform GeneHub-GEPIS analysis and data storage. The back-end expression analysis relies on an integrated gene database we constructed that stores gene definitions and cross-references.

4.3.2.4. Repair-FunMap

More as data repository rather than as tools related to cancer genes, Repair-FunMap is a functional platform of the DNA repair systems. It uses an iterative procedure that employs an automatic literature data mining algorithm and manual curation. The Repair-FunMap, as a protein compendium for cancer research, provides clues to understanding the inter-relationship between proteins in the network, and builds scientific models of the DNA repair processes (74). The data sources of Repair-FunMap come from the publicly available human DNA repair databases. The biological principle utilized by Repair-FunMap is that proteins involved in cell-cycle regulation are considered to be part of the mechanism that controls the cellular response to DNA damages. The Repair-FunMap database contains not only the proteins directly involved in DNA repair, but also the proteins that interact with the DNA repair proteins. The protein interaction network with graphics display associated with the human DNA repair processes was established to represent the current knowledge on the intrinsic signaling pathways related to DNA repair and provides direct links to the literature that describe experimental evidence supporting the interaction.

4.3.2.5. Tools in CGAP Database

The CGAP database (http://cgap.nci.nih.gov/) is a commonly used platform for cancer-related gene analyses. Tools in the CGAP database have been classified into five groups: tools to find genes, tools to find cDNA libraries, tools to examine gene expression, tools to examine chromosomes and tools to find SNPs.

1. Tools to find genes: There are five tools, Clone Finder, Gene Finder, Batch Gene Finder, GO Browser, and Nucleotide Blast. Clone Finder generates a list of the most reliable clones from a list of UniGene clusters. Gene Finder finds genes based on various search criteria and links to gene information in the NCBI and NCI databases. Batch Gene Finder finds genes from a list of UniGene cluster numbers, GenBank accessions, or LocusLink identifiers, and links to gene information in the NCBI and NCI databases. GO Browser classifies human and mouse genes by molecular function, biological process, and cellular component. Nucleotide Blast finds genes based on nucleotide sequence similarities.

2. Tools to find cDNA libraries: The CGAP Library Finder Tools can find any cDNA library from dbEST. Hereinto, the cDNA Library Finder can find a single cDNA library or a group of libraries depending on the search criteria selected. The SAGE Absolute Level Lister lists all SAGE Genie libraries and breaks down the total number of tags in a single library into various expression levels from lowest to highest and lists the distinct tags in each expression level.

3. Tools to examine gene expression: They include the cDNA Digital Gene Expression Displayer (DGED), cDNA xProfiler, Gene Library Summarizer (GLS), SAGE Absolute Level Lister, SAGE Anatomic Viewer and SAGE Digital Gene Expression Displayer. DGED is a tool that compares gene expression between two pools of libraries. cDNA xProfiler compares gene expression between two pools of cDNA libraries. In contrast to DGED, for xProfiler to identify a gene to be "present" in a library pool, there must be at least one EST sequence found in the UniGene cluster for that gene. GLS generates unique and non-unique gene lists for a single cDNA library or library group, and finds all the genes expressed in a single cDNA library or group of cDNA libraries. SAGE Absolute Level Lister shows the distribution of transcript

expression levels in any particular SAGE library. SAGE Anatomic Viewer displays gene expression in human normal and malignant tissues by shading each organ in one of ten colors, each representing a different level of gene expression. SAGE Digital Gene Expression Displayer distinguishes significant differences in gene expression profiles between two pools of SAGE libraries.

4. Tools to examine chromosomes: There are six tools included in this category: Expression-Based SNP Imagemaps, which finds SNPs based on cancer type and chromosome; FISH-mapped BACs, which finds BAC clones, available to the public, that integrate the cytogenetic and physical maps of the human genome; Genetic and Physical SNP Maps, which reveal genetic and physical locations of confirmed, validated, and predicted SNPs; the web-based Mitelman Database Tool, which searches the Mitelman Database (a genome-wide map of chromosomal breakpoints in human cancer); Recurrent Aberrations CGAP, a tool to search the Mitelman data of Recurrent Aberrations in cancer; and SNP500Cancer, which finds SNPs that are of immediate importance to molecular epidemiology studies in cancer.

5. Tools to find SNPs: There are five tools: CGAP SNP Index, which searches for candidate SNPs by gene name, gene symbol, or GenBank accession number; Expression-Based SNP Imagemaps, which find SNPs based on cancer type and chromosome; Genetic and Physical SNP Maps, which show genetic and physical locations of confirmed, validated, and predicted SNPs; SNP Gene Viewer, which views maps of SNPs on human reference sequences and MGC sequences and gives predictions of protein coding changes; and SNP500Cancer as reviewed above.

5. Challenges

There is no doubt regarding the feasibility of applying DigiCGA in cancer gene research but DigiCGA is still an expanding field in which many puzzles remain to be solved. For the application of DigiCGA in cancer gene identification, sufficient data resources are of high necessity and the first problem comes from the web data resources that DigiCGA uses. The efficiency of application of DigiCGA for identifying cancer genes relies heavily on the characteristics and qualities of web data resources. With further development of cancer biology, new high-throughput technologies, data repository and analytical techniques, there has been, and will be more, available data resources for cancer research but the large volume and multiple source characteristics of these data resources unavoidably produce strong interference to the veracity and accuracy of DigiCGAs results due to the high level of noise. How to deal with the high diversity and heterogeneity of data sets remains a large challenge for DigiCGA.

In our opinion, one very important aspect of the future applications of DigiCGA is to consider the generality and specialty of cancers. At present, the digital identification of cancer gene does not distinguish the types and properties of genes. Cancer genes are widely involved in xenobiotic metabolism, in replication and repair of the DNA, in the control of cell cycle and cellular proliferation, apoptosis, the inflammation process, etc. In already reported DigiCGA analyses, the difference between carcinogenic genes and antitumoral genes, development genes, progression genes, transformation genes and so on was not reflected in the current frame of strategies and methods. In addition, understanding which mechanisms are general and which are specific has important therapeutic implications to cancers. Furthermore, there have been no cancer type-specific applications of DigiCGA, and current research does not address the commonalities and variations between different types as well as the mechanism underlying the transformation to malignant tumor.

6. Prospects

One of the future directions for DigiCGA research is to integrate all available information resources, including all available web data sources derived from general, specialized, and cancer-specific database/literatures, "wet" data sets directly produced from laboratory experiments, and simulation data sets. As pointed out by Attur et al. (75), the post-genomic era of functionomics will facilitate to narrow the bridge between correlative data and causative data by quaint hypothesis-driven research using a system approach integrating "intercoms" of interacting and interdependent disciplines. Forming a unified whole will govern the coming era. Systems biology ultimately aims to delineate and comprehend the functioning of complex biological systems in such detail that the predictive models of human diseases could be developed (76). The development of digital strategies in the system biology era will also lie on the holistic strategy and integrated data. For the future development of DigiCGA, the multiple source and multiple level data resources need complex systemic modeling which would address cancer problems from a holistic viewpoint accordant with the thoughts of systems biology. Many new thoughts and methods would be brought into the process of systemic modeling. In our opinion, the most prominent change of DigiCGA would be the theorem transformation from the empirical hypothesis driven mode to the ab initio mode.

7. Conclusions

In this chapter, we have introduced the synoptic knowledge about traditional candidate gene approach and DigiCGA. The reported applications of DigiCGA in cancer-related gene analyses, as well as issues concerning web resources and tools for cancer have also been summarized. Cancer mechanistically results from the abnormal expressions of certain genes, to which the cancer gene identification is a prerequisite. Currently, the identification of genes involved in cancer remains a challenge. It is still largely dependent on molecular biology technologies for cancer gene identification. However, as we have demonstrated, digital strategies are having more impact and further accumulation of digital resources will facilitate the developments of digital strategies for cancer gene identification. It is anticipated that the combination of digital strategies with more computational, bioinformatic, and biological technologies would be heralded as the next major breakthrough for candidate gene identification, and this will play a more intensive and active role in the field of cancer research.

Acknowledgments

This work was supported by National Natural Science Foundation of China (U0631005, 30901021).

References

1. Magrath, I., and Litvak, J. (1993) Cancer in developing countries: opportunity and challenge. *J. Natl. Cancer Inst.* **85**, 862–874
2. Vogelstein, B., and Kinzler, K.W. (2004) Cancer genes and the pathways they control. *Nat. Med.* **10**, 789–799
3. Hanahan, D., and Weinberg, R.A. (2000) The hallmarks of cancer. *Cell* **100**, 57–70
4. Zhu, M.J., and Zhao, S.H. (2007) Candidate gene identification approach: progress and challenges. *Int. J. Biol. Sci.* **3**, 420–427
5. Tabor, H.K., Risch, N.J., and Myers, R.M. (2002) Candidate-gene approaches for studying complex genetic traits: practical considerations. *Nat. Rev. Genet.* **3**, 391–397
6. Kwon, J.M., and Goate, A.M. (2000) The candidate gene approach. *Alcohol Res. Health* **24**, 164–168
7. Daly, A.K. (2003) Candidate gene case-control studies. *Pharmacogenomics* **4**, 127–139
8. Yochum, G.S., Cleland, R., and Goodman, R.H. (2008) A genome-wide screen for beta-catenin binding sites identifies a downstream enhancer element that controls c-Myc gene expression. *Mol. Cell Biol.* **28**, 7368–7379
9. Flanagan, J.M., Funes, J.M., Henderson, S., Wild, L., Carey, N., and Boshoff, C. (2009) Genomics screen in transformed stem cells reveals RNASEH2A, PPAP2C, and ADARB1 as putative anticancer drug targets. *Mol. Cancer Ther.* **8**, 249–260
10. Heng, H.H. (2007) Cancer genome sequencing: the challenges ahead. *Bioessays* **29**, 783–794
11. Esteller, M. (2006) The necessity of a human epigenome project. *Carcinogenesis* **27**, 1121–1125
12. Varki, A., Wills, C., Perlmutter, D., Woodruff, D., Gage, F., Moore, J., et al. (1998) Great ape phenome project? *Science* **282**, 239–240

13. Freimer, N., and Sabatti, C. (2003) The human phenome project. *Nat. Genet.* **34**, 15–21
14. Yoshida, T., and Yoshimura, K. (2003) Outline of disease gene hunting approaches in the Millennium Genome Project of Japan. *Proc. Jpn. Acad.* **79**, 34–50
15. Schubert, K., von Bonnsdorf, H., Burke, M., Ahlert, I., Braun, S., Berner, R., et al. (2006) A comprehensive candidate gene study on bronchial asthma and juvenile idiopathic arthritis. *Dis. Markers* **22**, 127–132
16. Miyata, T. (2008) Large-scale candidate gene approach to identifying hypertension-susceptible genes. *Hypertens Res.* **31**, 173–174
17. Sato, Y., Suganami, H., Hamada, C., Yoshimura, I., Yoshida, T., and Yoshimura, K. (2004) Designing a multistage, SNP-based, genome screen for common diseases. *J. Hum. Genet.* **49**, 669–676
18. Thomas, D., Xie, R., and Gebregziabher, M. (2004) Two-stage sampling designs for gene association studies. *Genet. Epidemiol.* **27**, 401–414
19. Beckly, J.B., Hancock, L., Geremia, A., Cummings, J.R., Morris, A., Cooney, R., et al. (2008) Two-stage candidate gene study of chromosome 3p demonstrates an association between nonsynonymous variants in the MST1R gene and Crohn's disease. *Inflamm. Bowel Dis.* **14**, 500–507
20. Li, J. (2008) Prioritize and select SNPs for association studies with multi-stage designs. *J. Comput. Biol.* **15**, 241–257
21. Zhang, K., Calabrese, P., Nordborg, M., and Sun, F. (2002) Haplotype block structure and its applications to association studies: power and study designs. *Am. J. Hum. Genet.* **71**, 1386–1394
22. Sironen, A., Thomsen, B., Andersson, M., Ahola, V., and Vilkki, J. (2006) An intronic insertion in KPL2 results in aberrant splicing and causes the immotile short-tail sperm defect in the pig. *Proc. Natl. Acad. Sci. USA* **103**, 5006–5011
23. Schadt, E.E., Lamb, J., Yang, X., Zhu, J., Edwards, S., Guhathakurta, D., et al. (2005) An integrative genomics approach to infer causal associations between gene expression and disease. *Nat. Genet.* **37**, 710–717
24. Stylianou, I.M., Affourtit, J.P., Shockley, K.R., Wilpan, R.Y., Abdi, F.A., Bhardwaj, S., et al. (2008) Applying gene expression, proteomics and single-nucleotide polymorphism analysis for complex trait gene identification. *Genetics* **178**, 1795–1805
25. Tranchevent, L.C., Barriot, R., Yu, S., Van Vooren, S., Van Loo, P., Coessens, B., et al. (2008) Endeavour update: a web resource for gene prioritization in multiple species. *Nucleic Acids Res.* **36**, W377–W384
26. Hristovski, D., Peterlin, B., Mitchell, J.A., and Humphrey, S.M. (2005) Using literature-based discovery to identify disease candidate genes. *Int. J. Med. Inform.* **74**, 289–298
27. Sugaya, N., Ikeda, K., Tashiro, T., Takeda, S., Otomo, J., Ishida, Y., et al. (2007) An integrative in silico approach for discovering candidates for drug-targetable protein–protein interactions in interactome data. *BMC Pharmacol.* **7**, 10
28. Franke, L., van Bakel, H., Fokkens, L., de Jong, E.D., Egmont-Petersen, M., and Wijmenga, C. (2006) Reconstruction of a functional human gene network, with an application for prioritizing positional candidate genes. *Am. J. Hum. Genet.* **78**, 1011–1025
29. Rossi, S., Masotti, D., Nardini, C., Bonora, E., Romeo, G., Macii, E., et al. (2006) TOM: a web-based integrated approach for identification of candidate disease genes. *Nucleic Acids Res.* **34**, W285–W292
30. George, R.A., Liu, J.Y., Feng, L.L., Bryson-Richardson, R.J., Fatkin, D., and Wouters, M.A. (2006) Analysis of protein sequence and interaction data for candidate disease gene prediction. *Nucleic Acids Res.* **34**, e130
31. Yonan, A.L., Palmer, A.A., Smith, K.C., Feldman, I., Lee, H.K., Yonan, J.M., et al. (2003) Bioinformatic analysis of autism positional candidate genes using biological databases and computational gene network prediction. *Genes Brain Behav.* **2**, 303–320
32. Harhay, G.P., and Keele, J.W. (2003) Positional candidate gene selection from livestock EST databases using gene ontology. *Bioinformatics* **19**, 249–255
33. Perez-Iratxeta, C., Bork, P., and Andrade, M.A. (2002) Association of genes to genetically inherited diseases using data mining. *Nat. Genet.* **31**, 316–319
34. Pellegrini-Calace, M., and Tramontano, A. (2006) Identification of a novel putative mitogen-activated kinase cascade on human chromosome 21 by computational approaches. *Bioinformatics* **22**, 775–778
35. Freudenberg, J., and Propping, P. (2002) A similarity-based method for genome-wide prediction of disease-relevant human genes. *Bioinformatics* **18**, S110–S115
36. De Bie, T., Tranchevent, L.C., van Oeffelen, L.M., and Moreau, Y. (2007) Kernel-based data fusion for gene prioritization. *Bioinformatics* **23**, i125–i132
37. Adie, E.A., Adams, R.R., Evans, K.L., Porteous, D.J., and Pickard, B.S. (2005)

Speeding disease gene discovery by sequence based candidate prioritization. *BMC Bioinformatics* **6**, 55

38. Xu, J., and Li, Y. (2006) Discovering disease-genes by topological features in human protein–protein interaction network. *Bioinformatics* **22**, 2800–2805

39. Tiffin, N., Adie, E., Turner, F., Brunner, H.G., van Driel, M.A., Oti, M., et al. (2006) Computational disease gene identification: a concert of methods prioritizes type 2 diabetes and obesity candidate genes. *Nucleic Acids Res.* **34**, 3067–3081

40. Feng, Z., Davis, D.P., Sásik, R., Patel, H.H., Drummond, J.C., and Patel, P.M. (2007) Pathway and gene ontology based analysis of gene expression in a rat model of cerebral ischemic tolerance. *Brain Res.* **1177**, 103–123

41. Tiffin, N., Kelso, J.F., Powell, A.R., Pan, H., Bajic, V.B., and Hide, W.A. (2005) Integration of text- and data-mining using ontologies successfully selects disease gene candidates. *Nucleic Acids Res.* **33**, 1544–1552

42. Arcade, A., Labourdette, A., Falque, M., Mangin, B., Chardon, F., Charcosset, A., et al. (2004) BioMercator: integrating genetic maps and QTL towards discovery of candidate genes. *Bioinformatics* **20**, 2324–2326

43. Aerts, S., Lambrechts, D., Maity, S., Van Loo, P., Coessens, B., De Smet, F., et al. (2006) Gene prioritization through genomic data fusion. *Nat. Biotechnol.* **24**, 537–544

44. Hernández, P., Solé, X., Valls, J., Moreno, V., Capellá, G., Urruticoechea, A., et al. (2007) Integrative analysis of a cancer somatic mutome. *Mol. Cancer* **6**, 13

45. Chen, Y.P., and Chen, F. (2008) Using bioinformatics techniques for gene identification in drug discovery and development. *Curr. Drug Metab.* **9**, 567–573

46. Tang, S., Zhang, Z., Tan, S.L., Tang, M.H., Kumar, A.P., Ramadoss, S.K., et al. (2007) KBERG: knowledgebase for estrogen responsive genes. *Nucleic Acids Res.* **35**, D732–D736

47. Ceresa, M., Masseroli, M., and Campi, A. (2007) A web-enabled database of human gene expression controlled annotations for gene list functional evaluation. *Conf. Proc. IEEE Eng. Med. Biol. Soc.* **2007**, 394–397

48. Qiu, P., Wang, L., Kostich, M., Ding, W., Simon, J.S., and Greene, J.R. (2004) Genome wide in silico SNP-tumor association analysis. *BMC Cancer* **4**, 4

49. Rafnar, T., Sulem, P., Stacey, S.N., Geller, F., Gudmundsson, J., Sigurdsson, A., et al. (2009) Sequence variants at the TERT-CLPTM1L locus associate with many cancer types. *Nat. Genet.* **41**, 221–227

50. Collier, L.S., and Largaespada, D.A. (2006) Transforming science: cancer gene identification. *Curr. Opin. Genet. Dev.* **16**, 23–29

51. Aouacheria, A., Navratil, V., López-Pérez, R., Gutiérrez, N.C., Churkin, A., Barash, D., et al. (2007) In silico whole-genome screening for cancer-related single-nucleotide polymorphisms located in human mRNA untranslated regions. *BMC Genomics* **8**, 2

52. Hanauer, D.A., Rhodes, D.R., Sinha-Kumar, C., and Chinnaiyan, A.M. (2007) Bioinformatics approaches in the study of cancer. *Curr. Mol. Med.* **7**, 133–141

53. Kim, B., Lee, H.J., Choi, H. Y., Shin, Y., Nam, S., Seo, G., et al. (2007) Clinical validity of the lung cancer biomarkers identified by bioinformatics analysis of public expression data. *Cancer Res.* **67**, 7431–7438

54. Kirschbaum-Slager, N., Parmigiani, R.B., Camargo, A.A., and de Souza, S.J. (2005) Identification of human exons overexpressed in tumors through the use of genome and expressed sequence data. *Physiol. Genomics* **21**, 423–432

55. Lal, A., Lash, A.E., Altschul, S.F., Velculescu, V., Zhang, L., McLendon, R.E., et al. (1999) A public database for gene expression in human cancers. *Cancer Res.* **59**, 5403–5407

56. Mello, B.P., Abrantes, E.F., Torres, C.H., Machado-Lima, A., Fonseca, R.D., Carraro, D.M., et al. (2009) No-match ORESTES explored as tumor markers. *Nucleic Acids Res.* **37**, 2607–2617

57. Brentani, H., Caballero, O.L., Camargo, A.A., da Silva, A.M., da Silva, W.A. Jr., Dias Neto, E., et al. (2003) The generation and utilization of a cancer-oriented representation of the human transcriptome by using expressed sequence tags. *Proc. Natl. Acad. Sci. USA* **100**, 13418–13423

58. Aouacheria, A., Navratil, V., Barthelaix, A., Mouchiroud, D., and Gautier, C. (2006) Bioinformatic screening of human ESTs for differentially expressed genes in normal and tumor tissues. *BMC Genomics* **7**, 94

59. Scheurle, D., DeYoung, M.P., Binninger, D.M., Page, H., Jahanzeb, M., and Narayanan, R. (2000) Cancer gene discovery using digital differential display. *Cancer Res.* **60**, 4037–4043

60. DeYoung, M.P., Tress, M., and Narayanan, R. (2003) Identification of Down's syndrome critical locus gene SIM2-s as a drug therapy target for solid tumors. *Proc. Natl. Acad. Sci. USA* **100**, 4760–4765

61. Narayanan, R. (2007) Bioinformatics approaches to cancer gene discovery. *Methods Mol. Biol.* **360**, 13–31

62. Segal, E., Friedman, N., Koller, D., and Regev, A. (2004) A module map showing conditional

activity of expression modules in cancer. *Nat. Genet.* **36**, 1090–1098

63. Wong, D.J., Nuyten, D.S., Regev, A., Lin, M., Adler, A.S., Segal, E., et al. (2008) Revealing targeted therapy for human cancer by gene module maps. *Cancer Res.* **68**, 369–378

64. Roy, M., Xu, Q., and Lee, C. (2005) Evidence that public database records for many cancer-associated genes reflect a splice form found in tumors and lack normal splice forms. *Nucleic Acids Res.* **33**, 5026–5033

65. Wang, Z., Lo, H.S., Yang, H., Gere, S., Hu, Y., Buetow, K.H., et al. (2003) Computational analysis and experimental validation of tumor-associated alternative RNA splicing in human cancer. *Cancer Res.* **63**, 655–657

66. Xu, Q., and Lee, C. (2003) Discovery of novel splice forms and functional analysis of cancer-specific alternative splicing in human expressed sequences. *Nucleic Acids Res.* **31**, 5635–5643

67. Peeper, D., and Berns, A. (2006) Cross-species oncogenomics in cancer gene identification. *Cell* **125**, 1230–1233

68. Chen, S.N., and Wen, K.C. (2006) An integrated system for cancer-related genes mining from biomedical literatures. *Int. J. Comput. Sci. Appl.* **3**, 26–39

69. Benbow, L., Wang, L., Laverty, M., Liu, S., Qiu, P., Bond, R.W., et al. (2002) A reference database for tumor-related genes co-expressed with interleukin-8 using genome-scale in silico analysis. *BMC Genomics* **3**, 29

70. Riggins, G.J., and Strausberg, R.L. (2001) Genome and genetic resources from the Cancer Genome Anatomy Project. *Hum. Mol. Genet.* **10**, 663–667

71. MacDonald, J.W., and Ghosh, D. (2006) COPA: cancer outlier profile analysis. *Bioinformatics* **22**, 2950–2951

72. Tomlins, S.A., Rhodes, D.R., Perner, S., Dhanasekaran, S.M., Mehra, R., Sun, X.W., et al. (2005) Recurrent fusion of TMPRSS2 and ETS transcription factor genes in prostate cancer. *Science* **310**, 644–648

73. Zhang, Y., Luoh, S.M., Hon, L.S., Baertsch, R., Wood, W.I., and Zhang, Z. (2007) GeneHub-GEPIS: digital expression profiling for normal and cancer tissues based on an integrated gene database. *Nucleic Acids Res.* **35**, W152–W158

74. Wen, L., and Feng, J.A. (2004) Repair-FunMap: a functional database of proteins of the DNA repair systems. *Bioinformatics* **20**, 2135–2137

75. Attur, M.G., Dave, M.N., Tsunoyama, K., Akamatsu, M., Kobori, M., Miki, J., et al. (2002) "A system biology" approach to bioinformatics and functional genomics in complex human diseases: arthritis. *Curr. Issues Mol. Biol.* **4**, 129–146

76. Mohammad, F., Singh, P., and Sharma, A. (2009) A Drosophila systems model of pentylenetetrazole induced locomotor plasticity responsive to antiepileptic drugs. *BMC Syst. Biol.* **3**, 11

Part II

Screening Cancer Susceptibility Genes

Chapter 8

The Use of Denaturing High Performance Liquid Chromatography (DHPLC) for Mutation Scanning of Hereditary Cancer Genes

Deborah J. Marsh and Viive M. Howell

Abstract

Denaturing high performance liquid chromatography (DHPLC) facilitates automated mutation scanning of PCR products with the ability to detect nearly 100% of sequence variants including single nucleotide substitutions and small insertions or deletions. It has particular application for genetic screening in inherited conditions; both for the initial identification of a mutation in disease carriers followed by sequence analysis, and for screening "at-risk" individuals prior to the development of disease in families with a known mutation. Specifically, in familial cancer syndromes, DHPLC has been reported as a genetic screening tool for the risk of developing breast and ovarian cancer (*BRCA1*), von Hippel Lindau disease (*VHL*), Cowden syndrome (*PTEN*), and Multiple Endocrine Neoplasia types 1 and 2 (*MEN1* and *RET*). This chapter focuses on the methodologies specific to the WAVE® System for Mutation Detection 2100 (Transgenomic Inc., Omaha, NE, USA) and highlights the use of Navigator™ software (Transgenomic Inc.), including data analysis with scatter graphs.

Key words: Denaturing high performance liquid chromatography, Mutation scanning, Heteroduplex, Homoduplex, Familial cancer genes, Hereditary cancer genes, GC-clamp, Partial denaturation, Scatter graphs, Navigator™ software

1. Introduction

Denaturing high performance liquid chromatography (DHPLC) facilitates high throughput scanning for sequence variants. It is commonly used to identify single nucleotide substitutions, as well as small insertions and deletions for mutation detection and genotyping (1). It is not suitable for analysing large gene deletions, homozygous mutations, or multiple copy number aberrations. DHPLC can be applied to methylation analyses (2). DNA fragments between ~150 and 600 bp (and in some cases up to 1.5 kb (3)) are amplified from genomic DNA by PCR followed by a heteroduplex enhancement cycle consisting of denaturation followed by temperature slow reannealing, to assist in the formation of mismatched strands of DNA in samples heterozygous for a variant allele (4, 5). Reannealed PCR amplicons are injected into the flow path of a reversed-phase high performance liquid chromatography column in the presence of the ion-pairing reagent triethylammonium acetate (TEAA) that binds to hydrophobic beads on a stationary phase column. The negatively charged phosphate backbones of partially denatured DNA fragments are attracted to the positively charged ammonium groups on the TEAA and so are captured on the column.

Under partial denaturation temperature conditions predicted by melt profile software, homo- and heteroduplex samples are differentially retained on the column. The less stable, more denatured, heteroduplexes are eluted from the column earlier than the more stable homoduplexes. At increasing concentrations of acetonitrile, the TEAA-DNA attraction is diminished, fragments begin to elute from the column, and are identified by UV detection. Elution profiles are presented as chromatograms. When no sequence variants are present, the DHPLC profile will show a single peak. A heterozygous sample will show up to four peaks, representing the two heteroduplex and the two homoduplex populations present after denaturation and reannealing. Profiles that deviate from a single peak should be sequenced to determine the exact sequence variant.

DHPLC has been compared to other mutation scanning techniques, including single-strand conformation polymorphism (SSCP), conformation sensitive gel electrophoresis (CSGE), protein truncation test (PTT) and two dimensional gene scanning (TDGS), and found to have the highest sensitivity, with the detection of almost 100% of sequence variants (6, 7). Numerous familial cancer genes have now been interrogated by DHPLC using constitutive DNA from known mutation carriers and at-risk members of families with inherited cancer syndromes. These include *BRCA1* (6, 7), *PTEN* (8), *RET* (8), *HRPT2* (5), *MEN1* (5, 9), *VHL* (8, 10), *SDHB* (10), *SDHD* (10), and *NF1* (11).

When designing a germline genetic screening programme for a familial cancer syndrome that incorporates DHPLC, it is important to acknowledge the spectrum of reported mutations, including gross germline deletion and polymorphisms, in order to accurately interpret DHPLC elution profiles. DHPLC is suitable for genetic scanning of familial syndromes where mutations are either clustered in residues, for example, *RET* proto-oncogene mutations in Multiple Endocrine Neoplasia Type 2 (MEN 2; OMIM#171400) that are located in mutation "hot-spots," or spread throughout the entirety of a gene such as *PTEN* in Cowden Syndrome (CS; OMIM#158350). For syndromes where gross germline deletion is reported in a percentage of families, for example, complete loss of *VHL* in some patients with von Hippel Lindau Disease (VHL; OMIM#193300), DHPLC can still be used as the first mutation scanning strategy to identify substitutions or small insertions or deletions if present, before progressing to alternative mutation strategies to identify large gene deletions (see Note 1).

An inherent problem of many mutation scanning techniques, including DHPLC, is interference from common polymorphisms although the influence of these can be minimised (see Subheading 3.1, step 3). A further problem can be the presence of multiple melt domains in single amplicons that can often be addressed by the incorporation of GC-clamped primers (see Subheading 3.1, step 5) (8, 12, 13). Technological platforms that enable DHPLC are essentially offered by three companies – the Helix™ System (Varian Inc., Palo Alto, CA, USA), Hewlett-Packard HP 1100 Series HPLC System (Agilent Technologies Inc., Santa Clara, CA, USA), and the WAVE® System for Mutation Detection (Transgenomic Inc., Omaha, NE, USA). This chapter focuses on the WAVE® System and linked software. A schematic of this system is shown in Fig. 1.

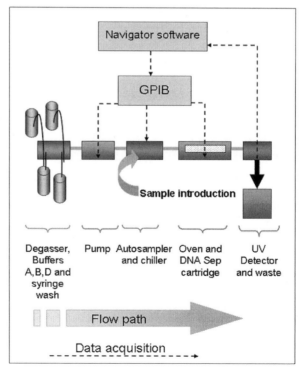

Fig. 1. Schematic of the WAVE system, showing the relative placement of hardware components, the direction of the flow of the mobile phase, point of introduction of the sample and the transfer or acquisition of data. GPIB, General Purpose Interface Board.

2. Materials

2.1. Generation and Assessment of PCR Products

1. Genomic DNA samples known to be either wild-type or variant for the gene of interest, in addition to unknown test samples that may be unscreened affected family members or individuals at-risk of developing disease, should be selected for PCR.
2. Standard PCR stock reagents, including PCR-quality deionised H_2O, 10× reaction buffer (e.g. Geneamp® PCR Buffer II, Applied Biosystems, Foster City, CA, USA), 25 mM or 50 mM $MgCl_2$ (e.g. from Applied Biosystems), 2.5 mM of each deoxynucleotide (dATP, dTTP, dGTP, dCTP) (e.g. from Roche Applied Science, Indianapolis, IN, USA), 200 µM stocks of forward and reverse primers (e.g. from Sigma-Genosys, Sydney, Australia), and polymerase (e.g. AmpliTaq GOLD DNA polymerase, Applied Biosystems) (see Note 2).
3. Standard PCR Thermal Cycler (e.g. MJ Research Tetrad, Bio-Rad Laboratories, Hercules, CA, USA).
4. Standard ultrapure agarose (e.g. from Progen Industries, QLD, Australia) or polyacrylamide gels (e.g. pre-cast gels from Bio-Rad Laboratories).

2.2. DHPLC Using the WAVE® System for Mutation Detection 2100

1. DHPLC Instrumentation – WAVE® System for Mutation Detection 2100 (Transgenomic Inc.).
2. DHPLC Analysis Column – DNASep® cartridge (Transgenomic Inc.).
3. WAVE Optimised™ Buffer A (Transgenomic Inc.), a solution of 0.1 M TEAA (pH 7).
4. WAVE Optimised™ Buffer B (Transgenomic Inc.), a solution of 0.1 M TEAA (pH 7), 25% acetonitrile.
5. WAVE Optimised™ Buffer D (Transgenomic Inc.), a solution of 75% acetonitrile.
6. Transgenomic Wave Size Standard: a HaeIII digest of pUC18 plasmid DNA in a 10 mM Tris-HCl, 1.0 mM EDTA solution, pH 7.4.
7. WAVE® High Range Mutation standard, 70°C; WAVE® Mid Range Mutation standard, 64°C; WAVE® Low Range Mutation standard, 56°C (Transgenomic Inc.). Standards are the hybridisation of wild-type and mutant alleles differing by a single base pair in a 10 mM Tris-HCl (pH 8.8), 75 mM potassium chloride solution.

3. Methods

3.1. Primer Design and Melt Profiles

1. Published primers available from other mutation scanning technologies such as SSCP or denaturing gradient gel electrophoresis (DGGE) may be suitable for DHPLC. It is suggested that melt profiles are generated using these primers in the first instance (8).

2. If primers need to be designed specifically for DHPLC, it is recommended that they amplify fragments between 150 and 600 bp. In our hands, amplicons in the range of ~200–400 bp have been successfully used for DHPLC (5) (see Note 3). Standard primer design software (e.g. Primer Express®, Applied Biosystems; or freeware Primer3, http://primer3.sourceforge.net/) can be used for initial primer design prior to analysis of the melt profile of the fragment.

3. Primers, where possible, should be designed to exclude common polymorphisms from the PCR amplicon. If this is not possible, primers may be designed and temperatures selected to locate common polymorphisms in a fully denatured region of the melt profile, thus excluding them from detection in the elution profile (8).

4. The melt profile of a fragment is generated using Navigator™ Software. This software constructs melt profiles for each amplicon to predict the temperature (T_m) of 75% helicity, where 75% of the amplicon is doublestranded (i.e. partially denatured conditions). Alternatively, the optimal temperature for DHPLC of a fragment can be predicted by the freeware DHPLC Melt Programme (http://insertion.stanford.edu/melt.html). Figure 2a illustrates a Navigator™ Software predicted melt profile for a PCR amplicon. Melt profiles of 1°C and 2°C above and below the optimum T_m are also mapped. The most optimal fragments will have a single melt domain enabling accurate detection of variants at a single T_m; however, this is not always possible and if more than one melt domain is present in the fragment, multiple temperatures may need to be analysed for each amplicon to ensure the detection of all variants (see Note 4).

5. The use of guanine-cytosine (GC)-clamped primers for DHPLC should be considered if there are multiple melt domains in a fragment and/or if it is anticipated that variants will be scattered along the entirety of the amplicon (see Note 5).

3.2. PCR and Heteroduplex Enhancement

1. Primers should be diluted to a working concentration of 20 μM and 1 μM of each primer used in a 50 μL PCR reaction. A 50 μL reaction volume is preferred in order to allow

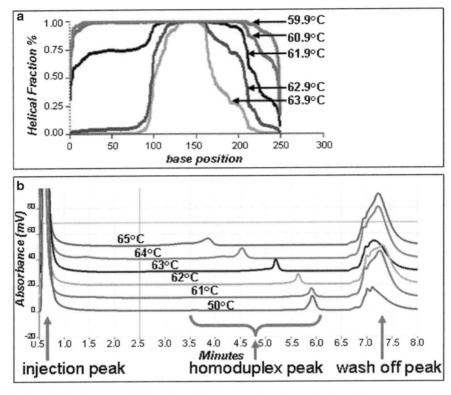

Fig. 2. (**a**) Navigator™ Software predicted melt profile for an amplicon. The optimal predicted temperature for mutation detection is 61.9°C. Melt profiles for temperatures 1°C and 2°C above and below this temperature are also mapped. (**b**) Chromatograms of optimisation of this amplicon with pooled normal DNA graphed as Absorbance at 260 nm as millivolts vs. Time in minutes. The injection peak at the start, the homoduplex peak of interest and wash off peak at the end of each injection are shown. As partially denaturing conditions are reached, the homoduplex peak shifts to the left towards the injection peak. As the temperature increases above the predicted optimal temperature, the peak starts to broaden and collapse indicating temperatures approaching denaturing conditions.

for some evaporation, thus ensuring sufficient volume for multiple injections if required.

2. Template concentrations of 10–100 ng of genomic DNA extracted from blood lymphocytes are recommended in order to minimise the risk of impurities that may remain after DNA extraction with some commercial systems that can inhibit PCR (see Note 6). At least one known wild-type (preferably multiple), as well as known variant, should be included along with samples to be tested. In cases where blood is not available from affected family members (e.g. deceased individuals), analyses can be performed on DNA from tumour or non-tumour tissue if stored. Special considerations must be taken into account if using tumour DNA to scan for variants in a tumour suppressor gene (see Note 7).

3. Some commercial polymerase buffers may contain additives that have an adverse, and likely cumulative effect on the DNASep® cartridge, so careful selection of a polymerase is recommended (see Note 2). PCR reactions must not contain oil.

4. PCR is carried out in a standard thermal cycler followed by the assessment of PCR products on standard agarose or polyacrylamide gels for the presence of a single band.

5. PCR products should undergo heteroduplex enhancement to facilitate the formation of homo- and heteroduplexes in heterozygous samples for a sequence variant following PCR by the performance of a denaturation step of 94°C for 5 min followed by ramping to 25°C over 45 min in a thermal cycler. This step can occur immediately following the reaction PCR and products stored, or alternatively performed prior to DHPLC analysis.

6. PCR products should be stored at 4°C until injection onto the HPLC column.

3.3. Optimisation of Partially Denaturing Conditions

1. Initially, run PCR products on the WAVE® System for mutation detection under non-denaturing conditions (50°C) to assess the quality of the peak, with a single, narrow peak being the optimal.

2. Wild-type PCR products should be analysed between 1 and 5 temperatures, 0.5°C–2°C above and below the predicted optimal T_m to confirm partially denaturing conditions. Partially denaturing conditions are indicated by a left shift of the peak (towards the injection peak) of ~1 min (Fig. 2b). Wild-type DNA is expected to present with a single homoduplex peak under partially denaturing conditions.

3. Once partially denaturing conditions are established for the wild-type DNA, prepared PCR products heterozygous for previously identified sequence variants should be run under these conditions. Before scanning for unknown variants, known variants should be analysed at all temperatures within the predicted range for partial denaturation for their ability to resolve homo- and heteroduplexes. A single temperature should be chosen where all variants can be resolved; however, this is not always possible and on occasion certain PCR amplicons may need to be injected and analysed at more than one temperature to ensure that no variants are missed (see Note 4).

4. Results are analysed using Navigator™ Software.

3.4. DHPLC Using the WAVE

The WAVE® System for Mutation Detection 2100 (Transgenomic Inc.) consists of a L7300+ high precision peltier oven, single plate autosampler with peltier controlled chiller module, programmable UV detector, quaternary gradient solvent delivery system, four line degasser, General Purpose Interface Board (GPIB) control module, computer system with remote system control, and Navigator™ Software. The arrangement and interaction of these modules, including sample introduction, mobile phase flow path and data acquisition is presented in Fig. 1.

The stationary phase in the WAVE is a DNASep® cartridge (Transgenomic Inc.) consisting of polystyrene-divinylenzene copolymer beads. The beads are alkylated with C-18 chains that form C–C bonds. The mobile phase consists of a combination of two buffers in varying concentrations; WAVE Optimised™ Buffer A (Transgenomic) is a solution of 0.1 M TEAA (pH 7) and WAVE Optimised™ Buffer B (Transgenomic) is a solution of 0.1 M TEAA (pH 7) and 25% acetonitrile. WAVE Optimised™ Buffer D (Transgenomic) is a solution of 75% acetonitrile used to clean the column following each injection.

For sizing purposes, the Transgenomic Wave Size Standard should be run through the instrument. For the purpose of controlling for DNA variant detection, two to three controls (WAVE low-range mutation standard, WAVE mid-range mutation standard, and WAVE High-Range Mutation Standard, Transgenomic Inc.) are injected onto the column and analysed prior to scanning samples in order to determine the quality of the column with regard to high resolution outputs.

1. Apart from the heteroduplex enhancement step noted above (see Subheading 3.2, step 5), no additional steps or purification of PCR amplicons is required. A volume of heteroduplex enhanced PCR product suitable for the number of injections to be performed, including dead volume, is placed in the instrument's chiller. A 2–5 µL aliquot is aspirated with a feed volume of 25 µL by the autosampler and injected into the mobile phase in the direction of the flow path of the DNASep® cartridge (Fig. 1).

2. The mobile phase has a constant flow rate of 0.9 mL/min with a linear acetonitrile gradient determined by Navigator™ software according to the size and GC content of the amplicon. This gradient is achieved by combining 0.1 M TEAA buffer (pH 7) (Buffer A, Transgenomic Inc.) and 0.1 M TEAA with 25% acetonitrile (Buffer B) where the percentage of Buffer A equals 100% minus the percentage of Buffer B. The time for processing consists of 0.5 min for injection with a 5% decrease in Buffer B (identified by the injection peak), followed by a linear gradient (which includes a 2.2 min lag time for detection) with a slope of 2% increase in Buffer B per minute, a 0.5 min cleaning stage starting at 6.7 min using 100% buffer D (identified by a wash off peak), and a 0.9 min equilibration before the next injection. The elution and detection of homo- and heteroduplex peak occurs during the linear gradient.

3. Eluted DNA fragments are detected by the system's UV detector and analysed as chromatograms. Homo- and heteroduplex peaks are detected between the initial injection peak, produced by residual nucleotides and primers in the reaction, and the wash peak, produced by the acetonitrile flush at the end of each analysis. Given that heteroduplexes are less stable, they denature earlier than the homoduplexes and so are seen first in the elution profile.

3.5. Data Analysis Using Navigator™ Software

1. Chromatograms are normalised against a wild-type PCR product, and the resulting peaks assessed both visually and by Navigator™ Software using the scatter graph function. The scatter graph function allows automated discriminant analysis of DHPLC chromatograms. Using this function, chromatograms with similar features are grouped into a cluster and each cluster is assigned a colour identifier. These clusters are represented in three-dimensional space so that the further apart the two clusters are, the further apart their points appear on the scatter graph. The axes represent the three-dimensions and may be manually rotated for different views of the data. The percentage of variance (variability) in the data is indicated on the three axes. For the scatter graph function to be most useful in the discrimination of variant samples, multiple wild-type samples should be injected and analysed to form a tight wild-type cluster. An example scatter graph is shown in Fig. 3.

2. All variants should be confirmed by the purification of PCR products, using a method such as the Wizard PCR Preps DNA Purification System (Promega Corporation, Madison, WI, USA) and sequencing.

4. Notes

1. Gross germline deletion of some tumour suppressor genes has been reported in patients with certain familial cancer syndromes, e.g. *VHL* in affected members of families with von Hippel Lindau disease. DHPLC is an unsuitable mutation scanning technique for these cases as the presence of only one wild-type allele precludes the formation of heteroduplexes and thus a definitive elution profile. In syndromes such as these, DHPLC may be suitable as an initial screen for germline intragenic mutations (substitutions, small insertions, and deletions). If mutations are not identified in this initial DHPLC screen, DNA from the probands of these families could undergo alternative screening to detect putative large gene deletions such as Southern blotting, fluorescence

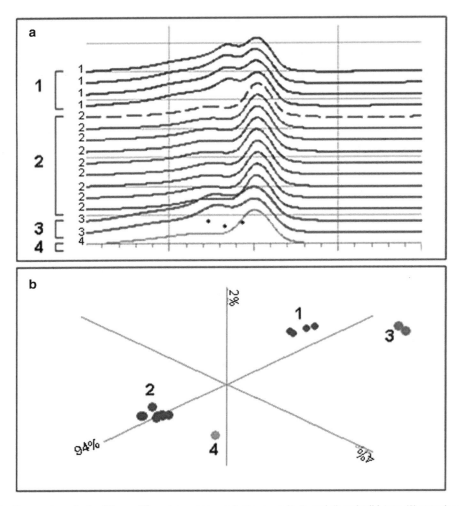

Fig. 3. Scatter graph analysis of three different sequence variant groups (1, 3, and 4) and wild-type (2) samples. Profiles have been numbered to indicate colour groupings by Navigator™ software. (**a**) The chromatograms are grouped into four different clusters. Profiles have been normalised to a wild-type sample in cluster 2 (indicated by the *dotted line*). (**b**) Scatter graph in three-dimensional space with clear separation of the four different clusters representing wild-type and three variant groups.

in situ hybridisation or multiplex ligation-dependent probe amplification. DHPLC is also not suitable for the detection of homozygous mutations given the presence of only a single allele type; however, this rarely occurs in constitutive DNA of patients with a familial cancer syndrome. Germline mosaicism such as that seen on occasion in *TSC2* in patients with Tuberous Sclerosis (OMIM:#191100) and *APC* in Familial Adenomatous Polyposis Coli (OMIM:#175100) can be detected by DHPLC, reportedly at mutant allele frequencies as low as 5%; however, care should be taken in interpretation of such data and more than one mutation scanning methodology is recommended (14).

2. A list of suitable polymerases for DHPLC can be obtained from Transgenomics. We have found that AmpliTaq GOLD DNA polymerase (Applied Biosystems) is suitable and does not compromise the life of the DNASep® cartridge (5, 8). Transgenomics also recommend Optimase® Polymerase (Transgenomic, Inc.). Furthermore, the PCR enhancing agents betaine or dimethyl sulfoxide (DMSO) may be used to minimise the formation of secondary structure in GC-rich regions but not in amounts exceeding up to 0.8–1.6 M or 10%, respectively. However, additional cleaning of the cartridge may still be required if these additives are used.

3. DNA fragment lengths up to 1.5 kb have been successfully used for mutation scanning by DHPLC; however, detection sensitivity decreases as the amplicon size increases above 700 bp (1). Additionally, detection sensitivity is also decreased in small amplicons, likely due to the inability of DHPLC to detect variants in the highest T_m domain of an amplicon (13). We have shown accurate detection of variants using amplicons in the range of 200–400 bp (5, 8).

4. Multiple melt domains are a common feature of PCR amplicons, especially as size increases. In the case of genes where scanning is for specific known variants or there are "hot-spot" areas of mutation, PCR amplicons can be tailored for the detection of variants in targeted regions. However, for the majority of cancer-associated genes, mutations are spread throughout the gene making efficient detection at a single temperature for each specific amplicon almost impossible due to variation of the fragment's melt profile. For reliable mutation detection under these circumstances, analyses should be performed at multiple temperatures to ensure the detection of all variants. Another option may be the use of GC-clamped primers (see Note 5).

5. GC-clamps artificially increase the T_m of the fragment close to the clamp, thus locating the sequence of interest in a lower T_m domain of the amplicon. Therefore, higher temperatures can be used to resolve variants prior to temperature-induced collapse of a peak due to full denaturation. This can be especially helpful when there are multiple melt domains in a fragment. It is more likely that a single denaturation temperature will be sufficient to detect all variants in a fragment. This can be of particular benefit when mutations are expected to be scattered along the entire length of exons rather than clustered in specific residues or "hot-spots" (i.e. more likely to be located in different melt domains of the fragment). Clamps may be located at the 5′, 3′ or both ends of the PCR amplicon. Clamps may be between 2 and 50 bps in length. Clamps previously designed for DGGE may be suitable for DHPLC. Examples of clamps used for DHPLC scanning of *PTEN*

include: 5'-CG-3', 5'-GCGCG-3', 5'-CGTCCCGC-3', 5'-CGCCCGCCGCGCCCCGCGCCCGGCCCGCCGCCCCGCCCG-3', and 5'-CGCCCGCCGCGCCCCGCGCCCGGCCCGCCGCCCCCGCCCGAAATAATAAA-3' (8).

6. On occasion, artefact peaks may occur before the appearance of homo- and heteroduplex peaks in the elution profile that are likely due to the method of sample preparation. These artefact peaks can be decreased relative to true peaks of interest by dilution of the template DNA prior to PCR amplification. This does, however, highlight the importance of including wild-type DNA controls in each experiment.

7. DHPLC can be used to scan tumour tissue from patients with familial syndromes in order to identify a mutation that may then be assessed in the germline of other family members, e.g. tumour tissue from a deceased relative. However, as there is often only one tumour suppressor gene allele in somatic DNA from a tumour due to loss of the wild-type allele, heteroduplex peaks are unable to form. Amplicons which include common polymorphisms can be utilised to assess for the presence of a wild-type allele in DNA extracted from tumour tissue if the polymorphism is heterozygous in the germline. If this is not found to be the case, one solution to this issue is to mix a wild-type PCR product in approximately equal amounts with the tumour DNA PCR product, in order to mimic the presence of a wild-type allele, then denature, perform heteroduplex enhancement and screen for the presence of both homo- and heteroduplex peaks by DHPLC.

Acknowledgements

DJM and VMH are Cancer Institute NSW Fellows (Australia). The Humpty Dumpty Foundation, Australia, is acknowledged for the donation of DHPLC equipment.

References

1. Xiao, W., and Oefner, P.J. (2001) Denaturing high-performance liquid chromatography: a review. *Hum. Mutat.* 17, 439–474
2. Perry, A.S., Liyanage, H., Lawler, M., and Woodson, K. (2007) Discovery of DNA hypermethylation using a DHPLC screening strategy. *Epigenetics* 2, 43–49
3. Oefner, P.J., and Underhill, P.A. (1998) DNA mutation detection using denaturing high performance liquid chromatography, in *Current Protocols in Human Genetics*, Wiley, New York, pp. 7.10.1–7.10.12
4. Kuklin, A., Munson, K., Gjerde, D., Haefele, R., and Taylor, P. (1997) Detection of single-nucleotide polymorphisms with the WAVE DNA fragment analysis system. *Genet. Test.* 1, 201–206
5. Howell, V.M., Cardinal, J.W., Richardson, A.L., Gimm, O., Robinson, B.G., and Marsh, D.J. (2006) Rapid mutation screening for

HRPT2 and MEN1 mutations associated with familial and sporadic primary hyperparathyroidism. *J. Mol. Diagn.* **8**, 559–566

6. Eng, C., Brody, L.C., Wagner, T.M., Devilee, P., Vijg, J., Szabo, C., Tavtigian, S.V., Nathanson, K.L., Ostrander, E., Frank, T.S., and Steering Committee of the Breast Cancer Information Core (BIC) Consortium. (2001) Interpreting epidemiological research: blinded comparison of methods used to estimate the prevalence of inherited mutations in BRCA1. *J. Med. Genet.* **38**, 824–833

7. Gerhardus, A., Schleberger, H., Schlegelberger, B., and Gadzicki, D. (2007) Diagnostic accuracy of methods for the detection of BRCA1 and BRCA2 mutations: a systematic review. *Eur. J. Hum. Genet.* **15**, 619–627

8. Marsh, D.J., Theodosopoulos, G., Howell, V.M, Richardson, A.L., Benn, D.E., Proos, A.L., et al. (2001) Rapid mutation scanning of genes associated with familial cancer syndromes using denaturing high-performance liquid chromatography. *Neoplasia* **3**, 236–244

9. Crepin, M., Pigny, P., Escande, F., Bauter, C.C., Calendar, A., Lefevre, S., et al. (2006) Evaluation of denaturing high performance liquid chromatography for the mutational analysis of the MEN1 gene. *J. Mol. Endocrinol.* **36**, 369–376

10. Meyer-Rochow, G.Y., Smith, J.M., Richardson, A.L., Marsh, D.J., Sidhu, S., Robinson, B.G., and Benn, D.E. (2009) Denaturing high performance liquid chromatography detection of SDHB, SDHD, and VHL germline mutations in pheochromocytoma. *J. Surg. Res.* **157**(1), 55–62

11. Han, S.S., Cooper, D.N., and Upadhyaya, M.N. (2001) Evaluation of denaturing high performance liquid chromatography (DHPLC) for the mutational analysis of the neurofibromatosis type 1 (NF1) gene. *Hum. Genet.* **109**, 487–497

12. Greiner, T.C. (2007) Enhanced detection of TP53 mutations using a GC-clamp in denaturing high performance liquid chromatography. *Diagn. Mol. Pathol.* **16**, 32–37

13. Wurzburger, R.J., Gupta, R., Parnassa, A.P., Sargam, J., Wexler, J.A., Chu, J.L., et al. (2003) Use of GC clamps in DHPLC mutation scanning. *Clin. Med. Res.* **1**, 111–118

14. Rohlin, A., Wernersson, J., Engwall, Y., Wiklund, L., Bjork, J., and Nordling, M. (2009) Parallel sequencing used in detection of mosaic mutations: Comparison with four diagnostic DNA screening techniques. *Hum. Mutat.* **30**, 1–9

Chapter 9

Enhanced Mismatch Mutation Analysis: Simultaneous Detection of Point Mutations and Large Scale Rearrangements by Capillary Electrophoresis, Application to *BRCA1* and *BRCA2*

Claude Houdayer, Virginie Moncoutier, Jérôme Champ, Jérémie Weber, Jean-Louis Viovy, and Dominique Stoppa-Lyonnet

Abstract

We present the routine diagnostic application of EMMA (Enhanced Mismatch Mutation Analysis®, Fluigent), a new, fast, reliable, and cost-effective method for mutation screening. This method is based on heteroduplex analysis by capillary electrophoresis and relies on the use of innovative matrices increasing the electrophoretic mobility differences between homoduplex and heteroduplex DNA, which is further enhanced by the addition of nucleosides in the separation matrix. Nucleosides interact with heteroduplex mismatched bases, hence increasing mobility difference with homoduplex. As separations are performed by multi-capillary electrophoresis, it allows for high automation, low cost, and high throughput. Moreover, EMMA, in combination with limiting PCR conditions, can be used to achieve the simultaneous detection of point mutation and large scale rearrangement in a single run.

We now report on the routine diagnostic use of this method for *BRCA1* and *BRCA2* screening. The coding sequence and exon–intron junctions of *BRCA1* and *BRCA2* were amplified in 24 multiplex PCRs using a single condition. PCRs were electrophoresed with a single analytical condition on an ABI3100, and data were analyzed using dedicated software (Emmalys).

The strength of this new method relies on the following assets: (1) a single condition of analysis: modeling related to melting domain is not required (2) simultaneous detection of point mutations and large scale rearrangements, (3) optimized and ready-to-use polymer that can be used on various ABI sequencers, (4) easy to use, (5) low reagent costs, and (6) throughput.

Key words: EMMA, Mutation, Screening, Capillary electrophoresis, Heteroduplex

1. Introduction

It is now well established that our understanding of genetic diseases and cancers implies the analysis of DNA. Unfortunately, despite the benefits for patient's health, a large number of genes are not screened on a routine, diagnostic basis for reasons of cost, technical difficulty, and equipment availability. Moreover, most of these genetic diseases are very polyallelic, and the nature of the mutation on the gene for a given patient is generally unknown. Thus, mutation search has to be conducted on the whole coding sequence and intron/exon junctions. Developing fast, reliable, and inexpensive methods for searching such mutations is thus an important issue for medicine.

Two main strategies are used to search for unknown mutations: direct sequencing and screening. The first one is presently considered as the most reliable, although not totally flawless. More specifically, reliable chemistry and software are prominent points to consider.

The second strategy involves screening for sequence variations and then only the fragment(s) in which a variation is detected is sequenced to characterize the variation. This reduces dramatically the number of fragments to be sequenced. These screening strategies are mainly based on heteroduplex analysis (HDA) by using a dedicated liquid chromatographic system (Denaturing High Performance Liquid Chromatography, DHPLC (1)) or a real-time PCR machine (High Resolution Melting curve analysis, HRM (2)). During a slow cool-down performed at the end of the PCR cycling, two homoduplex fragments (corresponding to the normal and mutated allele, respectively) and two heteroduplexes (with mismatched strands due to the hybridization of a wild-type strand with a mutant strand) are obtained. The aim of HDA is to separate the homoduplexes from the heteroduplexes. DHPLC, for instance, offers good sensitivity, is rather low cost, and is widely used in diagnostic laboratories. It remains, however, rather labor intensive. In particular, analysis conditions depend on the melting domains of the sequence under study and distinct analysis parameters may be necessary for the same fragment (3). Consequently, its implementation may prove cumbersome. HRM is a very fast and elegant method; however, analysis conditions also depend on melting domains, and therefore optimization is required for each PCR fragment.

HDA can also be performed by electrophoresis (EHDA): homoduplexes are separated from heteroduplexes, thanks to a difference in electrophoretic mobility. Separations are nowadays performed mostly by multicapillary electrophoresis, allowing for high automation, low cost, and high throughput. A novel method based on HDA, with improved resolution for the detection of unknown point mutation detection has been recently developed. This method, termed Enhanced Mismatch Mutation Analysis (EMMA), relies on the use of innovative matrices that increase the electrophoretic mobility differences between homoduplex and heteroduplex DNA. More interesting, sensitivity is improved further by using nucleosides as additives to enhance single base substitution detection (4). Nucleosides are supposed to interact with the heteroduplexes mismatched bases hence increasing mobility difference with homoduplexes. As a result, EMMA combines high throughput, low cost and sensitivity at least equal to that of DHPLC. Moreover, this method, in combination with adapted semiquantitative PCR conditions for the preparation of the sample, can be used to achieve the simultaneous detection of point mutations and large scale rearrangements in a single run (5, 6). This new feature, combined with the use of a single set of separation conditions for all fragments and with the multiplexing capability of the method, leads to a considerable simplification and cost reduction with regards to previous methods.

The use of EMMA for high-throughput screening of *BRCA1* and *BRCA2* point mutations and large rearrangements is described below. Using this protocol, two technicians were able to screen 400 patients on both *BRCA1* and *BRCA2*, in 6 months and with one ABI3100. Constitutional mutations of the *BRCA1* [MIM 113705] and *BRCA2* [MIM 600185] genes are associated with a predisposition to breast and ovarian cancer. It is essential to identify *BRCA* mutations to provide appropriate genetic counseling in patients and relatives, but this represents an extremely challenging task, as the vast majority of mutations are unique and spread over the entire coding sequence (see http://www.umd.be/BRCA1/ and http://www.umd.be/BRCA2). Gross rearrangement screening is mandatory in *BRCA1* analysis, as an average, 10% of the mutational spectrum consists of large deletions (6). Individual written consent for molecular analysis was obtained from each subject sampled.

2. Materials

2.1. DNA (See Note 1)

1. DNA calibrated to 50 ng/µL by UV spectrophotometric assay (Nanodrop, Thermo Scientific, Wilmington, DE, USA). Absorbance ratios (260/280) and (230/260) should be in the 1.8–2.0 and 2.0–2.2 ranges, respectively.

2.2. PCR

1. QIAGEN Multiplex PCR Master Mix (Qiagen, Courtaboeuf, France, ref. 206145).
2. Primers (6FAM-labeled), all sequences are displayed Tables 1–3 (see Note 2).
3. Microtubes (200 µL).
4. Pipette tips. Pipette tips are fitted with a cotton filter, and the pipettes are used specifically for the preparation of mixes and for the manipulation of DNA.
5. Thermocycler.

Table 1
Primer sequences for BRCA1 analysis

Multiplex	Primer name	Amplicon	Forward/reverse	Amplicon size (bp)	Primers	Nb of bases	Primer labeling
1	BC1_6F*	6	F	332	AGAGGTTTTCTACTGTTGCTG	21	6FAM
1	BC1_11.5F*	11.5	F	517	ATACTTTCCCAGAGCTGAAGT	21	6FAM
1	BC1_19F*	19	F	266	AAGGACCTCTCCTCTGTCAT	20	6FAM
1	BC1_22F*	22	F	431	GTGGCAAATTGACTTAAAATCC	22	6FAM
1	BC1_6R	6	R	332	CAGAACTAAAATTAACCTAGACT	23	None
1	BC1_11.5R	11.5	R	517	TGGCGCTTTGAAACCTTGAAT	21	None
1	BC1_19R	19	R	266	TGTGCATTGTTAAGGAAAGTG	21	None
1	BC1_22R	22	R	431	CAGTTCTCAAATCCTTACCCA	21	None
2	BC1_11.1F*	11.1	F	552	GTTTATGAGGTTAGTTTCTCTAA	23	6FAM
2	BC1_11.9F*	11.9	F	457	TGGTGAAATAAAGGAAGATACTA	23	6FAM
2	BC1_12F*	12	F	317	TGTGTGACATGAAAGTAAATCC	22	6FAM
2	BC1_13F*	13	F	405	TTGTAGTTCCATACTAGGTGAT	22	6FAM
2	BC1_11.1R	11.1	R	552	TCTCTAGGATTCTCTGAGCAT	21	None
2	BC1_11.9R	11.9	R	457	TGCAGTCAAGTCTTCCAATTC	21	None
2	BC1_12R	12	R	317	CCATTAATTCAAAGAGATGATGT	23	None
2	BC1_13R	13	R	405	CTGAGCAAGGATCATAAAATGT	22	None
3	BC1_2F*	2	F	314	CCTTCCAAATCTTAAATTTACTTT	24	6FAM
3	BC1_8F*	8	F	368	TGTGTAAATTCCTGGGCATT	20	6FAM

Enhanced Mismatch Mutation Analysis: Simultaneous Detection of Point Mutations 151

3	BCL_11.10F*	11.10	F	424	CATTGAAGAATAGCTTAAATG	21	6FAM
3	BCL_11.2F*	11.2	F	522	AAGGAGCCAACATAACAGATG	21	6FAM
3	BCL_2R	2	R	314	AATCTTACTAGACATGTCTTTC	23	None
3	BCL_8R	8	R	368	CAAAGCTGCTACCACAAATA	21	None
3	BCL_11.10R	11.10	R	424	CAGTTCCTTAACTATACTTGG	22	None
3	BCL_11.2R	11.2	R	522	GTAACAAATGCTCCTATAATTAG	23	None
4	BCL_11.4F*	11.4	F	521	CCTAACCCAATAGAATCACTC	21	6FAM
4	BCL_14R*	14	R	373	AATGCCTGTATGCAAAAACTG	22	6FAM
4	BCL_20F*	20	F	449	ATGAGGTTTCACCATGTTGGT	21	6FAM
4	BCL_11.4R	11.4	R	521	GACACTTAACTGTTTCTAGTTT	23	None
4	BCL_14F	14	F	373	TCTGCCTGATATACTTGTTAAA	23	None
4	BCL_20R	20	R	449	GAAGAGTGAAAAAGAACCTGT	22	None
5	BCL_5F*	5	F	316	GCCATTACTTTTAAATGGCTC	22	6FAM
5	BCL_15F*	15	F	447	TGCCAGTCATTCTGATCTCT	21	6FAM
5	BCL_16F*	16	F	549	ATTCATGTACCCATTTTTCTCTT	23	6FAM
5 et 9	BCL_7F*	7sT et 7T	F	275 et 379	GGTAACCTTAATGCATTGTCTT	22	6FAM
5	BCL_5R	5	R	316	TTATAAATTTTTCTGATGAATGGTT	25	None
5	BCL_15R	15	R	447	GTGGGCTTAATTAAGTATAACA	22	None
5	BCL_16R	16	R	549	GTGATTGTTTTCTAGATTTCTTC	23	None
5	BCL_7sTR	7sT	R	275	ATGGTTTTACCAAGGAAGGATT	22	None

(continued)

Table 1 (continued)

Multiplex	Primer name	Amplicon	Forward/reverse	Amplicon size (bp)	Primers	Nb of bases	Primer labeling
6	BC1_10F*	10	F	307	CTAAATAAGATTGGTCAGCTTTCT	24	6FAM
6	BC1_11.3F*	11.3	F	526	TAAAAGTGAAAGAGTTCACTCC	22	6FAM
6	BC1_23F*	23	F	488	AGGGGTGGTGTACGTGTCT	20	6FAM
6	BC1_10R	10	R	307	TTTTGTGGGTTGTAAAGGTCC	21	None
6	BC1_11.3R	11.3	R	526	GTAGAAGACTTCCTCCTCAG	20	None
6	BC1_23R	23	R	488	CCATGGAAACAGTTCATGTATT	22	None
7	BC1_3F*	3	F	419	TTCCTGACACAGCAGACATTT	21	6FAM
7	BC1_9F*	9	F	299	CCACAGTAGATGCTCAGTAAA	21	6FAM
7	BC1_11.8F*	11.8	F	553	TTAGCCGTAATAACATTAGAGAA	23	6FAM
7	BC1_24F*	24	F	353	TTAGCTTCTACCTCATTAATCC	22	6FAM
7	BC1_3R	3	R	419	ATGTCAAAACTTTACCAGGAAC	22	None
7	BC1_9R	9	R	299	AACAAACTGCACATACATCCC	21	None
7	BC1_11.8R	11.8	R	553	TCTAATTTCTTGGCCCCTCTT	21	None
7	BC1_24R	24	R	353	AGGACAGTAGAAGGACTGA	19	None
8	BC1_11.7F*	11.7	F	440	TCAGAAAGATAAGCCAGTTGAT	22	6FAM
8	BC1_17F*	17	F	352	ATAGTTCCAGGACACGTGTA	20	6FAM
8	BC1_21F*	21	F	284	AAGAAAAGCTCTTCCTTTTTGAA	23	6FAM
8	BC1_11.7R	11.7	R	440	ATTTTGGCCCTCGTTTCTAC	21	None
8	BC1_17R	17	R	352	CGATCTCCTAATCTCGTG	18	None

8	BCl_21R	21	R	284	TCTAGAACATTTCAGCAATCTG	22	None
9	BCl_11.6F*	11.6	F	520	CTAATTCATGGTTGTTCCAAAG	22	6FAM
9	BCl_18F*	18	F	300	ATAAATCCAGATTGATCTTGG	21	6FAM
9	BCl_11.6R	11.6	R	520	TGATGGGAAAAGTGGTGGTA	21	None
9	BCl_18R	18	R	300	GTAACTCAGACTCAGCATCA	20	None
9	BCl_7TR	7T	R	379	AAGGCAGGAGGACTGCTTCT	20	None

Table 2
Primer sequences for BRCA2 analysis

Multiplex	Primer name	Amplicon	Forward/ reverse	Amplicon size (bp)	Primers	Nb of bases	Primer labeling
1	BC2_11.12F*	11.12	F	538	CGCAAGACAAGTGTTTCTGA	21	6FAM
1	BC2_12F*	12	F	377	TAGGTCACTATTTGTTGTAAGTA	23	6FAM
1	BC2_14.2F*	14.2	F	320	CAGGACATCCATTTTATCAAGT	22	6FAM
1	BC2_25F*	25	F	485	GATTTGCTTTTATTATTAGCATATAC	26	6FAM
1	BC2_11.12R	11.12	R	538	ACTTTGGTTCCTAATACCAACT	22	None
1	BC2_12R	12	R	377	TAAAGAGGTCCTTGATTAGGC	21	None
1	BC2_14.2R	14.2	R	320	AATTGTCATACAATACCTAAAGG	23	None
1	BC2_25R	25	R	485	AAACTTTACCTCACATACTACC	22	None
2	BC2_4F*	4	F	350	AACTCCCTATACATTCTCATTC	22	6FAM
2	BC2_8F*	8	F	288	TGTTTCAAATGTGTCATGTAATC	23	6FAM
2	BC2_10.2F*	10.2	F	462	TTTCCATGAAGCAAACGCTGA	21	6FAM
2	BC2_11.9F*	11.9	F	543	CCACCTAAGCTCTTAAGTGAT	21	6FAM
2	BC2_4R	4	R	350	AGATCTTCTACCAGGCTCTTA	21	None
2	BC2_8R	8	R	288	GACTTTCTCAAAGGCTTAGATA	22	None
2	BC2_10.2R	10.2	R	462	TGCTTTACTGCAAGAATGCAG	21	None
2	BC2_11.9R	11.9	R	543	GGATATTACTTTGGAAAAACTAG	23	None
3	BC2_11.4F*	11.4	F	528	CGGACATCTCCTTGAATATAG	21	6FAM
3	BC2_14.1F*	14.1	F	320	ACAAAACAGTTACCAGAATAGTA	23	6FAM

3	BC2_27.1F*	27.1	F	476	GAGGGAGACTGTGTGTAATAT	21	6FAM
3	BC2_11.4R	11.4	R	528	TCTGGTTTCAGGCACTTCAA	21	None
3	BC2_14.1R	14.1	R	320	TTGGTCTGCCTGTAGTAATCA	21	None
3	BC2_27.1R	27.1	R	476	CTTTCCAAAAGAGAAATTTCATTG	24	None
4	BC2_2F*	2	F	342	AGGAGATGGGACTGAATTAGA	21	6FAM
4	BC2_6F*	6	F	279	ACATGTAACACCACAAAGAGAT	22	6FAM
4	BC2_11.8F*	11.8	F	527	GGAAACAGACATAGTTAAACAC	22	6FAM
4	BC2_22F*	22	F	442	ACACCCTTAAGATGAGCTCTA	21	6FAM
4	BC2_2R	2	R	342	CACATAAGGAACAGTTTATGG	21	None
4	BC2_6R	6	R	279	ATTGCCTGTATGAGGCAGAAT	21	None
4	BC2_11.8R	11.8	R	527	TTGTGTAACAAGTTGCAGGAC	21	None
4	BC2_22R	22	R	442	GTGGATTTGCTTCTCTGATAT	22	None
5	BC2_7F*	7	F	356	ATTCTGCCTCATACAGGCAAT	21	6FAM
5	BC2_10.1F*	10.1	F	457	TACTGATATGTAATATTTAGCACA	24	6FAM
5	BC2_11.3F*	11.3	F	530	TCAACCAAAACACAAATCTAAGA	23	6FAM
5	BC2_19.1F*	19.1	F	263	CTTCCTAAGACTTTTTAAAGTGA	23	6FAM
5	BC2_7R	7	R	356	CACACTTATCAAAGACATTATCT	23	None
5	BC2_10.1R	10.1	R	457	CAAAGGGCTTCTGATTTGCT	20	None
5	BC2_11.3R	11.3	R	530	GCTCTTCTTAATGTTATGTTCAG	23	None
5	BC2_19.1R	19.1	R	263	GAATAATTACATCAACACAACCA	23	None
6	BC2_11.13F*	11.13	F	484	TGTGTAAACTCAGAAATGGAAAA	23	6FAM

(continued)

Table 2
(continued)

Multiplex	Primer name	Amplicon	Forward/ reverse	Amplicon size (bp)	Primers	Nb of bases	Primer labeling
6	BC2_11.2F*	11.2	F	530	TAAAAGAAGAGGTCTTGGCTG	21	6FAM
6	BC2_13F*	13	F	310	CCGTTACATTCACTGAAAATTG	22	6FAM
6	BC2_18.1F*	18.1	F	396	GAAACAATATATTCCTAGCTACA	23	6FAM
6	BC2_11.13R	11.13	R	484	TAAGGGCTCTCCTCTTCTT	20	None
6	BC2_11.2R	11.2	R	530	ATTTCCTAAAGCAAGATTATTCC	23	None
6	BC2_13R	13	R	310	TAAAACGGGAAGTGTTAACTTC	22	None
6	BC2_18.1R	18.1	R	396	TTTAAGACAGCTAAGAGGGGA	21	None
7	BC2_3F*	3	F	490	CAAAAGTAATCCATAGTCAAGAT	23	6FAM
7	BC2_17F*	17	F	410	GAACTCATAAAAACTTAATGATCT	24	6FAM
7	BC2_24.1F*	24.1	F	275	AAAACTCAGTATCAACAACTACC	23	6FAM
7	BC2_11.10F*	11.10	F	534	GATACTTATTTAAGTAACAGTAGC	24	6FAM
7	BC2_3R	3	R	490	AGAGGCCAGAGAGACTGATT	20	None
7	BC2_17R	17	R	410	GATGGCAACTGTCACTGACAA	21	None
7	BC2_24.1R	24.1	R	275	ACTATATTGTGCATTACCTGTTT	23	None
7	BC2_11.10R	11.10	R	534	ACATTCATCATTATCTAGAGAG	22	None
8	BC2_11.5F*	11.5	F	509	TTTAACACCTAGCCAAAAGGC	21	6FAM
8	BC2_15F*	15	F	441	TGAACTCCCGACCTCAGAT	19	6FAM
8	BC2_24.2F*	24.2	F	287	TCTGTAGGTTTCAGATGAAATTTT	24	6FAM
8	BC2_11.5R	11.5	R	509	TTGAAACGACAGAATCATGACA	22	None

8	BC2_15R	15	R	441	ATTCATCCATTCCTGCACTA	20	None
8	BC2_24.2R	24.2	R	287	GAGGTTCAAAGAGGCTTACTT	21	None
9	BC2_11.6F*	11.6	F	529	GCACAAAACTGAATGTTTCTAC	22	6FAM
9	BC2_18.2F*	18.2	F	476	TCTGACATAATTCATTGAGCG	22	6FAM
9	BC2_19.2F*	19.2	F	303	CAATATATTTATTAATTTGTCCAG	24	6FAM
9	BC2_11.6R	11.6	R	529	TGACATGCTTCTTGAGCTTTC	21	None
9	BC2_18.2R	18.2	R	476	TGGAAATGCATTATTTAAGCTCA	23	None
9	BC2_19.2R	19.2	R	303	CTGCAGTGAACCAAGATCAC	20	None
10	BC2_10.3F*	10.3	F	430	TACTTCAGAGAATTCTTTGCCA	22	6FAM
10	BC2_11.14F*	11.14	F	310	TTGAAACAGAAGCAGTAGAAATT	23	6FAM
10	BC2_11.7F*	11.7	F	524	CGGACTTGCTATTTACTGATC	21	6FAM
10	BC2_26F*	26	F	394	AGGGTTTTTCATTCTTTTTTGGT	23	6FAM
10	BC2_10.3R	10.3	R	430	CAAAGTGGATATTAAACCTGCA	22	None
10	BC2_11.14R	11.14	R	310	TCCCCCAAACTGACTACACA	20	None
10	BC2_11.7R	11.7	R	524	GCTAGCTGTATGAAAACCCAA	21	None
10	BC2_26R	26	R	394	CCACATAACAACCACATTTTCT	22	None
11	BC2_14.3F*	14.3	F	277	ATGGACATGGCTCTGATGATA	21	6FAM
11	BC2_23F*	23	F	413	AAATCCACTACTAATGCCCAC	21	6FAM
11	BC2_27.2F*	27.2	F	490	GCTGCACAGAAGGCATTTCA	20	6FAM
11	BC2_14.3R	14.3	R	277	TTAAACCTAATCTTTGGATTTAGA	24	None
11	BC2_23R	23	R	413	GGCTGGTAAATCTGAAATAAAAT	23	None
11	BC2_27.2R	27.2	R	490	CTTTGCTCATTGTGCAACATAA	22	None

(continued)

Table 2
(continued)

Multiplex	Primer name	Amplicon	Forward/ reverse	Amplicon size (bp)	Primers	Nb of bases	Primer labeling
12	BC2_5F*	5	F	288	AATATCTAAAAGTAGTATTCCAAC	24	6FAM
12	BC2_11.11F*	11.11	F	532	ACAGACAGTTTCAGTAAAGTAA	22	6FAM
12	BC2_16F*	16	F	470	TGTTTTTGTAGTGAAGATTCTAG	23	6FAM
12	BC2_20F*	20	F	386	TAATCTCAGCCTCCCAAAGTT	21	6FAM
12	BC2_21F*	21	F	363	GCAGTTATATAGTTTCTTATCTTTA	25	6FAM
12	BC2_5R	5	R	288	TGTATGAAACAAACTCCCAC	20	None
12	BC2_11.11R	11.11	R	532	TTTGGGATATTAAATGTTCTGG	22	None
12	BC2_16R	16	R	470	TGCTTAACCATAATGCACTTAAAA	24	None
12	BC2_20R	20	R	386	TAAAGTCAATTTACTACTCAA	21	None
12	BC2_21R	21	R	363	ATCCCTTTTGAGAAATGCAGC	21	None
13	BC2_10.4F*	10.4	F	426	AAAGTGGACTGGAAATACATAC	22	6FAM
13	BC2_11.1iF*	11.1i	F	430	TCCCAAAAGTGCTGAGATTACAGG	24	6FAM
13	BC2_10.4R	10.4	R	426	GTATACAGATGATGCCTAAGAT	22	None
13	BC2_11.1iR	11.1i	R	430	CAGCCAAGACCTCTTCTTTTA	21	None
14	BC2_11.1F*	11.1	F	294	AGTAATCTCTCAGGATCTTGAT	22	6FAM
14	BC2_11.1R	11.1	R	294	ACATCCTTGGAAGTAGGAGTT	21	None
15	BC2_9F*	9	F	347	GACCTAGGTTGATTGCAGATA	21	6FAM
15	BC2_9R	9	R	347	AGAGGTTGCGGTAAACCGAG	20	None

Table 3
Primer sequences for internal control

Multiplex	Primer name	Amplicon	Forward/reverse	Amplicon size (bp)	Primers	Nb of bases	Primer labeling
M2BC1 – M1_M6_M7_M10_M11_M12BC2	ATM_15F*	ATM_15	F	349	AAGGCAAAGCATTAGGTACTTG	22	6FAM
M2BC1 – M1_M6_M7_M10_M11_M12BC2	ATM_15R	ATM_15	R	349	TTCTCCTTCCTAACAGTTTACC	22	None
M9BC1 – M4BC2	ATM_28F*	ATM_28	F	413	TATGATACTTTAATGCTGATGG	22	6FAM
M9BC1 – M4BC2	ATM_28R	ATM_28	R	413	GGTTATATCTCATATCATTCAG	22	None
M1_M3_M6_M7_M8BC1 – M5_M8_M9_M14_M15BC2	ATM_36F*	ATM_36	F	394	TCGGCCTTAAGGTTAATTCTTG	22	6FAM
M1_M6_M7_M8BC1 – M5_M8_M9_M14BC2	ATM_36R	ATM_36	R	394	GGACAAAGCTTTAGTTACTGAG	22	None
M3BC1 – M15BC2	ATM_36_2R	ATM_36_2	R	474	TCTGGCACAAGTAGGGTAAA	20	None
M4BC1	ATM_37F*	ATM_37	F	293	GGAGGTTAACATTCATCAAG	20	6FAM
M4BC1	ATM_37R	ATM_37	R	293	GCAATTTAACAGTCATGACC	20	None
M13BC2	ATM_48F*	ATM_48	F	330	CATTTCTCTTGCTTACATGAAC	22	6FAM
M13BC2	ATM_48R	ATM_48	R	330	TAATAAAGGAAAGTCAAGAGG	22	None
M5BC1 – M2_M3BC2	ATM_52F*	ATM_52	F	406	TTCCCTGGGATAAAAACCCAAC	22	6FAM
M5BC1 – M2_M3BC3	ATM_52R	ATM_52	R	406	GGTATACACGATTCCTGACATC	22	None

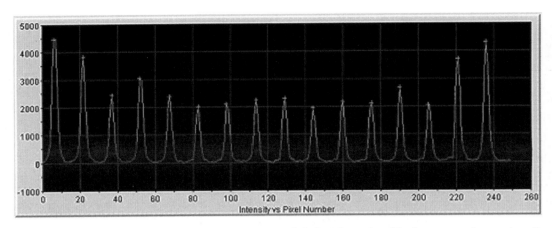

Fig. 1. Spatial calibration. The spatial map defines the number of pixels at the center of the fluorescence from each capillary in the spatial dimension of the Charged Coupled Device camera. Each peak corresponds to a capillary number. The smiley aspect is expected with EMMA and do not interfere with the quality of results.

2.3. EMMA

1. EMMA polymer (see Note 3) (Fluigent, Paris, France P/N: 15331103).
2. EMMA electrophoresis running buffer (see Note 4) (Fluigent, P/N: 5331101).
3. Fifty Centimeter length-to-detector array (Applied Biosystems, Courtaboeuf, France).
4. The ABI PRISM® 3100 Genetic Analyzer (Applied Biosystems). To calibrate the launch of the spatial calibration in *Spatial Run Schedules*, choose accept if the calibration is correct. The signal height of capillaries at the extremities of the array may be higher than those in the middle (see Fig. 1). This is a normal situation with EMMA 3100.
5. Emmalys software (Fluigent, P/N: 5331254102).

3. Methods

Data are collected using the Data Collection Software of the instrument and analyzed using Emmalys software.

3.1. Preparation of Primer Mixes and PCR

1. Prepare primer mixes as indicated in Tables 4 and 5. Mixes are prepared in a fume hood, and the DNA is added on a dedicated laboratory bench top.
2. Prepare 24 multiplex PCRs according to the conditions indicated in Table 6 and use the amplification protocols shown in Table 7.
3. On completion of the PCR, store at −20°C until elution.

Table 4
Primer mix preparation for BRCA1 multiplex PCRs

	Stock (μM)	Final concentration (μM)	Volume (μL)
Multiplex 1 (M1BC1)			
ATM_36F*	100	1.7	1.7
ATM_36R	100	1.7	1.7
BC1_19F*	100	1	1
BC1_19R	100	1	1
BC1_6F*	100	0.8	0.8
BC1_6R	100	0.8	0.8
BC1_22F*	100	2.5	2.5
BC1_22R	100	2.5	2.5
BC1_11.5F*	100	3.3	3.3
BC1_11.5R	100	3.3	3.3
TE buffer	10:1		81.4
Total volume			100
Multiplex 2 (M2BC1)			
ATM15F*	100	0.7	0.7
ATM15R	100	0.7	0.7
BC1_12F*	100	2	2
BC1_12R	100	2	2
BC1_13F*	100	1.8	1.8
BC1_13R	100	1.8	1.8
BC1_11.9F*	100	2	2
BC1_11.9R	100	2	2
BC1_11.1F*	100	2	2
BC1_11.1R	100	2	2
TE buffer	10:1		83
Total volume			100
Multiplex 3 (M3BC1)			
ATM36F*	100	1	1
ATM36_2R	100	1	1
BC1_8F*	100	1	1

(continued)

Table 4
(continued)

	Stock (μM)	Final concentration (μM)	Volume (μL)
BC1_8R	100	1	1
BC1_2F*	100	2	2
BC1_2R	100	2	2
BC1_11.10F*	100	1	1
BC1_11.10R	100	1	1
BC1_11.2F*	100	1	1
BC1_11.2R	100	1	1
TE buffer	10:1		88
Total volume			100
Multiplex 4 (M4BC1)			
ATM37F*	50	0.6	1.2
ATM37R	50	0.6	1.2
BC1_14F	100	2	2
BC1_14R*	100	2	2
BC1_20F*	100	3	3
BC1_20R	100	3	3
BC1_11.4F*	100	2	2
BC1_11.4R	100	2	2
TE buffer	10:1		83.6
Total volume			100
Multiplex 5 (M5BC1)			
BC1_7F*	100	1	1
BC1_7sTR	100	1	1
BC1_5F*	100	0.8	0.8
BC1_5R	100	0.8	0.8
ATM52F*	100	2	2
ATM52R	100	2	2
BC1_15F*	100	2	2
BC1_15R	100	2	2
BC1_16F*	100	2	2
BC1_16R	100	2	2

(continued)

Table 4
(continued)

	Stock (µM)	Final concentration (µM)	Volume (µL)
TE buffer	10:1		84.4
Total volume			100
Multiplex 6 (M6BC1)			
ATM_36F*	75	1.5	2
ATM_36R	75	1.5	2
BC1_10F*	100	2	2
BC1_10R	100	2	2
BC1_23F*	100	2	2
BC1_23R	100	2	2
BC1_11.3F*	100	2	2
BC1_11.3R	100	2	2
TE buffer	10:1		84
Total volume			100
Multiplex 7 (M7BC1)			
ATM_36F*	75	1	1.3
ATM_36R	75	1	1.3
BC1_9F*	100	0.8	0.8
BC1_9R	100	0.8	0.8
BC1_3F*	100	3	3.0
BC1_3R	100	3	3.0
BC1_24F*	100	1.5	1.5
BC1_24R	100	1,5	1.5
BC1_11.8F*	100	2	2.0
BC1_11.8R	100	2	2.0
TE buffer	10:1		82.7
Total volume			100
Multiplex 8 (M8BC1)			
ATM_36F*	75	1	1.3
ATM_36R	75	1	1.3
BC1_21F*	100	1.5	1.5

(continued)

Table 4 (continued)

	Stock (µM)	Final concentration (µM)	Volume (µL)
BC1_21R	100	1.5	1.5
BC1_17F*	100	2	2.0
BC1_17R	100	2	2.0
BC1_11.7F*	100	2	2.0
BC1_11.7R	100	2	2.0
TE buffer	10:1		86.3
Total volume			100
Multiplex 9 (M9BC1)			
ATM28F*	75	2	2.7
ATM28R	75	2	2.7
BC1_18F*	100	2	2.0
BC1_18R	100	2	2.0
BC1_7F*	100	3	3.0
BC1_7TR	100	3	3.0
BC1_11.6F*	100	2	2.0
BC1_11.6R	100	2	2.0
TE buffer	10:1		80.7
Total volume			100

For each primer a 100 µM stock solution is used. In the rightmost column is indicated the volume of stock solution for a 100 µL-primer mix final solution

3.2. Create Protocols and Plate Records for EMMA Analysis

EMMA analysis has to be performed using an EMMA module and EMMA protocol. The EMMA module is located on the provided CD. To create the EMMA protocol, follow the instructions below:

1. In the panel of the Data Collection software click GA Instruments>ga3100> Protocol Manager to open Protocol Manager window.
2. Click New.
3. Complete the Protocol Editor dialog box.
   Select REGULAR for type.

Table 5
Primer mix preparation for BRCA2 multiplex PCRs

	Stock (μM)	Final concentration (μM)	Volume (μL)
Multiplex 1 (M1BC2)			
ATM15F*	50	1	2
ATM15R	50	1	2
BC2_14.2F*	100	2	2
BC2_14.2R	100	2	2
BC2_12F*	100	1	1
BC2_12R	100	1	1
BC2_25F*	100	2	2
BC2_25R	100	2	2
BC2_11.12F*	100	2	2
BC2_11.12R	100	2	2
TE buffer	10:1		82
Total volume			100
Multiplex 2 (M2BC2)			
BC2_4F*	100	1	1
BC2_4R	100	1	1
ATM52F*	50	1	2
ATM52R	50	1	2
BC2_8F*	100	2	2
BC2_8R*	100	2	2
BC2_11.9F*	100	2	2
BC2_11.9R	100	2	2
BC2_10.2F*	100	2.5	2.5
BC2_10.2R	100	2.5	2.5
TE buffer	10:1		81
Total volume			100
Multiplex 3 (M3BC2)			
ATM52F*	75	2	2.7
ATM52R	75	2	2.7
BC2_14.1F*	100	2	2.0
BC2_14.1R	100	2	2.0

(continued)

Table 5
(continued)

	Stock (µM)	Final concentration (µM)	Volume (µL)
BC2_27.1F*	100	2	2.0
BC2_27.1R	100	2	2.0
BC2_11.4F*	100	2	2.0
BC2_11.4R	100	2	2.0
TE buffer	10:1		82.7
Total volume			100
Multiplex 4 (M4BC2)			
ATM28F*	50	1	2
ATM28R	50	1	2
BC2_6F*	100	2	2
BC2_6R	100	2	2
BC2_2F*	100	1.5	1.5
BC2_2R	100	1.5	1.5
BC2_22F*	100	3.5	3.5
BC2_22R	100	3.5	3.5
BC2_11.8F*	100	2	2
BC2_11.8R	100	2	2
TE buffer	10:1		78
Total volume			100
Multiplex 5 (M5BC2)			
BC2_19.1F*	100	2.5	2.5
BC2_19.1R	100	2.5	2.5
ATM36F*	50	1	2
ATM36R	50	1	2
BC2_7F*	100	3	3
BC2_7R	100	3	3
BC2_10.1F*	100	2.5	2.5
BC2_10.1R	100	2.5	2.5
BC2_11.3F*	100	2.5	2.5
BC2_11.3R	100	2.5	2.5

(continued)

Table 5
(continued)

	Stock (μM)	Final concentration (μM)	Volume (μL)
TE buffer	10:1		75
Total volume			100
Multiplex 6 (M6BC2)			
ATM15F*	50	1	2
ATM15R	50	1	2
BC2_13F*	100	2.5	2.5
BC2_13R	100	2.5	2.5
BC2_18.1F*	100	2.5	2.5
BC2_18.1R	100	2.5	2.5
BC2_11.13F*	100	3	3
BC2_11.13R	100	3	3
BC2_11.2F*	100	3	3
BC2_11.2R	100	3	3
TE buffer	10:1		74
Total volume			100
Multiplex 7 (M7BC2)			
ATM15F*	50	0.6	1.2
ATM15R	50	0.6	1.2
BC2_24.1F*	100	2	2
BC2_24.1R	100	2	2
BC2_17F*	100	3	3
BC2_17R	100	3	3
BC2_3F*	100	3	3
BC2_3R	100	3	3
BC2_11.10F*	100	3	3
BC2_11.10R	100	3	3
TE buffer	10:1		75.6
Total volume			100
Multiplex 8 (M8BC2)			
ATM_36F*	50	0.5	1

(continued)

Table 5
(continued)

	Stock (μM)	Final concentration (μM)	Volume (μL)
ATM_36R	50	0.5	1
BC2_24.2F*	100	1	1
BC2_24.2R	100	1	1
BC2_15F*	100	3.5	3.5
BC2_15R	100	3.5	3.5
BC2_11.5F*	100	3.5	3.5
BC2_11.5R	100	3.5	3.5
TE buffer	10:1		82
Total volume			100
Multiplex 9 (M9BC2)			
ATM_36F*	50	0.4	0.8
ATM_36R	50	0.4	0.8
BC2_19.2F*	100	3	3
BC2_19.2R	100	3	3
BC2_18.2F*	100	2	2
BC2_18.2R	100	2	2
BC2_11.6F*	100	2.5	2.5
BC2_11.6R	100	2.5	2.5
TE buffer	10:1		83.4
Total volume			100
Multiplex 10 (M10BC2)			
ATM15F*	50	0.75	1.5
ATM15R	50	0.75	1.5
BC2_11.14F*	100	2.5	2.5
BC2_11.14R	100	2.5	2.5
BC2_26F*	100	1.5	1.5
BC2_26R	100	1.5	1.5
BC2_10.3F*	100	2.5	2.5
BC2_10.3R	100	2.5	2.5
BC2_11.7F*	100	2	2

(continued)

Table 5
(continued)

	Stock (µM)	Final concentration (µM)	Volume (µL)
BC2_11.7R	100	2	2
TE buffer	10:1		80
Total volume			100
Multiplex 11 (M11BC2)			
ATM15F*	50	0.5	1
ATM15R	50	0.5	1
BC2_14.3F*	100	2	2
BC2_14.3R	100	2	2
BC2_23F*	100	1	1
BC2_23R	100	1	1
BC2_27.2F*	100	2.5	2.5
BC2_27.2R	100	2.5	2.5
TE buffer	10:1		87
Total volume			100
Multiplex 12 (M12BC2)			
ATM15F*	50	0.5	1
ATM15R	50	0.5	1
BC2_5F*	100	1.5	1.5
BC2_5R	100	1.5	1.5
BC2_21F*	100	2	2
BC2_21R	100	2	2
BC2_20F*	100	3.5	3.5
BC2_20R	100	3.5	3.5
BC2_16F*	100	2	2
BC2_16R	100	2	2
BC2_11.11F*	100	2	2
BC2_11.11R	100	2	2
TE buffer	10:1		76
Total volume			100
Multiplex 13 (M13BC2)			

(continued)

Table 5
(continued)

	Stock (µM)	Final concentration (µM)	Volume (µL)
ATM48F*	50	1	2
ATM48R	50	1	2
BC2_10.4F*	100	3	3
BC2_10.4R	100	3	3
BC2_11.1iF*	100	3	3
BC2_11.1iR	100	3	3
TE buffer	10:1		84
Total volume			100
Multiplex 14 (M14BC2)			
ATM_36F*	50	0.5	1
ATM_36R	50	0.5	1
BC2_11.1F*	100	1	1
BC2_11.1R	100	1	1
TE buffer	10:1		96
Total volume			100
Multiplex 15 (M15BC2)			
ATM36F*	100	2	2
ATM36_2R	100	2	2
BC2_9F*	100	2	2
BC2_9R	100	2	2
TE buffer	10:1		92
Total volume			100

For each primer a 100 µM stock solution is used. In the rightmost column is indicated the volume of stock solution for a 100 µL-primer mix final solution

Table 6
Composition of Multiplex PCR

Reagents	Concentration	Volume (µL)
Master mix	2×	5
Primer mix	10×	1
Water		2
ADN	50 ng/µL	2

Enhanced Mismatch Mutation Analysis: Simultaneous Detection of Point Mutations

Table 7
Amplification conditions for the 24 multiplex PCRs

Step	Temperature	Duration	Number of cycles
Enzyme activation/ denaturation	95°C	15 min	1
Denaturation	94°C	30 s	
Annealing	58°C	90 s	23
Elongation	72°C	90 s	
Final elongation	72°C	10 min	1
Heteroduplex formation	96°C	5 min	1
	Then −1°C/min to reach 25°C		
Hold	25°C		

Select EMMA for Run module.

Select Any4Dye or Any5Dye (depending on the Spectral Calibration) for Dye set.

4. Create a plate for EMMA analysis by following the instructions in the user guide of the instrument to open a new plate. Choose EMMA as the Instrument protocol.

3.3. Separation of Amplified Products on the ABI3100

1. Make the PCR reactions up to 20 µL with pure water (the minimum volume per tube is 20 µL). Wells in columns A and H have to be completed with 1 µL EMMA buffer 10×, in order to compensate for the higher intensity of the capillaries at the extremities of the array (see Fig. 1, spatial calibration).

2. Ensure that no air bubbles are present in the sample wells. Proceed as described in the instrument user guide for plate loading.

3. Launch the analyses. Proceed as described in the instrument user guide. Be careful to select "GenMapper Generic" as the "Application" and "EMMA High," or "EMMA low" for "Instrument Protocol" (see Note 5).

3.4. Interpretation of Data in Emmalys Software

3.4.1. Point Mutations (See Note 6)

For the analysis of point mutations using the Emmalys software follow the instructions below:

1. Index "sample selection" (see Fig. 2).
2. Select the run files (.fsa) to be analyzed (96 max).
3. Select a profile without variation.
4. Proceed to the next step.

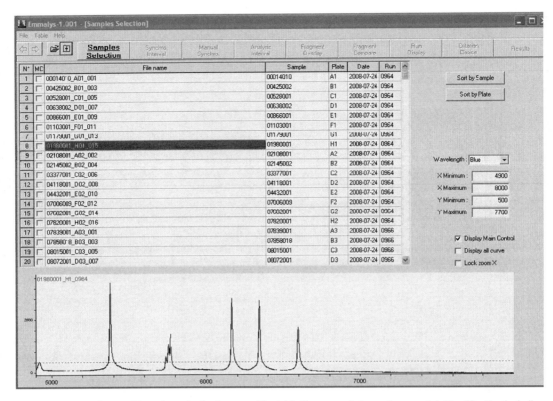

Fig. 2. Emmalys software: "Samples selection" screen. The table (*top screen*) shows the sample's identification including file name, sample number, position on the plate, and date of run. The bottom screen shows the profile of the selected sample. The user has to select a main control (i.e., a profile without variation) by ticking the box. This control is used as a reference for profile analyses.

5. Index "synchro interval" (see Fig. 3).
6. Select an interval with one well-separated peak.
7. Proceed to the next step.
8. Index "analysis interval" (see Fig. 4).
9. Select one interval for each peak.
10. Proceed to the next step.
11. Three screens are then available for result analysis/interpretation:
    (a) "Fragment overlay": superposition of all selected samples, for one peak: this screen allows a rapid detection of the variant samples (*see* Fig. 5).
    (b) "Fragment compare": superposition up to seven samples: this screen allows a more detailed view of each peak (*see* Fig. 6).
    (c) "Run display": samples are viewed by series of 16, for each peak (*see* Fig. 7).

Enhanced Mismatch Mutation Analysis: Simultaneous Detection of Point Mutations 173

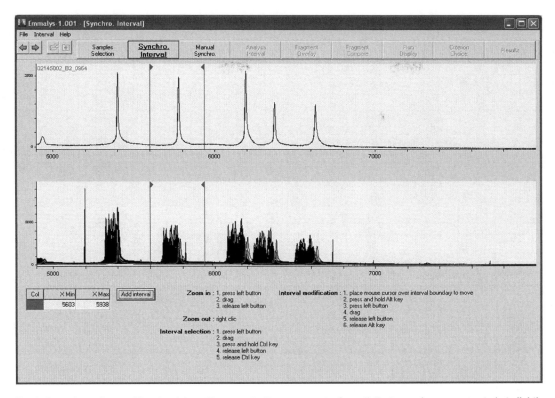

Fig. 3. Emmalys software: "Synchro interval" screen. As the same peaks from distinct samples are separated at slightly different scan numbers (a well-known phenomenon in capillary electrophoresis), the user should define an interval for one well-separated peak to ensure proper alignment. This procedure is described in the *bottom part* of the screen.

Note that all alignment parameters may be visualized and modified (for advanced users) in the "criterion choice" screen (Fig. 8). At last, the "results" screen shows the results by samples and following analysis parameters defined in the preceding steps (Fig. 9).

3.4.2. Large Scale Rearrangements (See Note 7)

The principle of the method involves quantitative evaluation of the relative proportion of a given fragment in the unknown sample with a normal control. In order to compare two fragments amplified in two different tubes, peak intensities are normalized to a nonmutated DNA fragment used as an internal control (ATM, see Table 3). Fluorescence intensities were then normalized by adjusting the peaks obtained for the control amplicons to the same level. The yield of each amplicon in the various samples was evaluated and deletions of one or more amplicons were revealed by a twofold decrease of the corresponding peak(s). High throughput data analysis is possible by automated profile analysis and ratio calculation. Hence, in order to determine the presence or absence of a large scale rearrangement, we use several

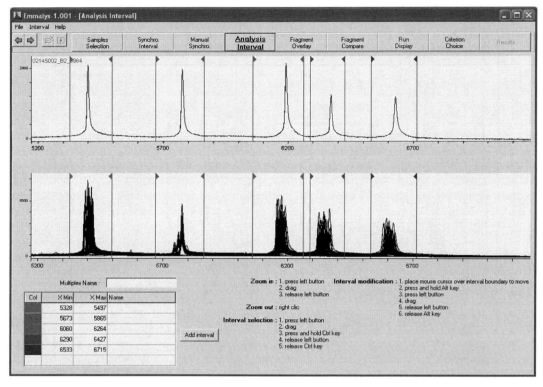

Fig. 4. Emmalys software: "Analysis interval" screen. The user should select one interval for each peak, following instructions in the *bottom part* of the screen.

ratios defined as follows: R1 is the ratio between peak intensity of fragment of interest over peak intensity of internal control. R2 is the ratio of R1 of sample of interest on R1 of control sample for a defined fragment (R1 of control sample may be a mean value over several control samples). If a region of the gene is duplicated, it will involve three initial copies of this region in the genome, hence leading to $R2 = 1.5$. In contrast, if a region of a gene is deleted, it will lead to one initial copy only and thus to $R2 = 0.5$. Always use normal and mutant controls to ensure the reliability of data interpretation.

For the analysis of large scale rearrangements using the Emmalys software follow the instructions below:

1. Index "large scale rearrangement."
2. Choose peak control (ATM).
3. Choose calculation mode: peak height or peak area.
4. Choose R2 calculation mode (one reference sample used as a control or all samples without variant profile are used to calculate a mean control which is used for R2).

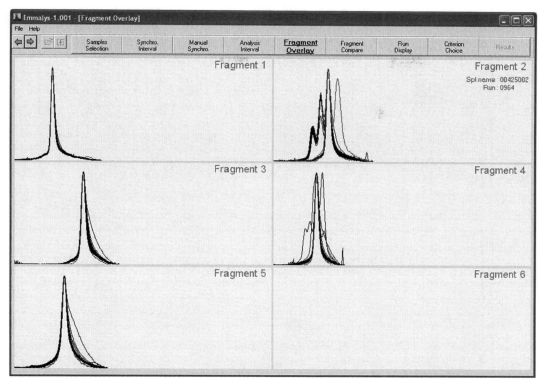

Fig. 5. Emmalys software: "Fragment overlay" screen. Following the alignment procedure (performed in previous steps), this screen displays superposition of all selected samples for one fragment (i.e., peak), thereby allowing a rapid detection of the variant samples.

4. Notes

1. DNA quality and quantity slightly impact on EMMA results for point mutation screening. On the other hand, as observed for all semiquantitative multiplex PCR techniques, results from large scale rearrangement screening are highly dependent on the quality of the DNA studied. Degraded DNA can be responsible for the loss of proportionality between signal intensity and copy number, particularly for large fragments, making the analysis uninterpretable. Contamination of DNA by phenol will have an even greater effect because it generates a random fluctuation of signal intensity. Phenol-free extraction techniques should therefore be preferred (perchlorate/chloroform or column-based commercial kits) or a system ensuring the absence of contamination by phenol such as the gel lock extraction system, which uses a gel-barrier system (Eppendorf). It is also essential to adjust all DNA samples studied to a suitable working concentration, classically

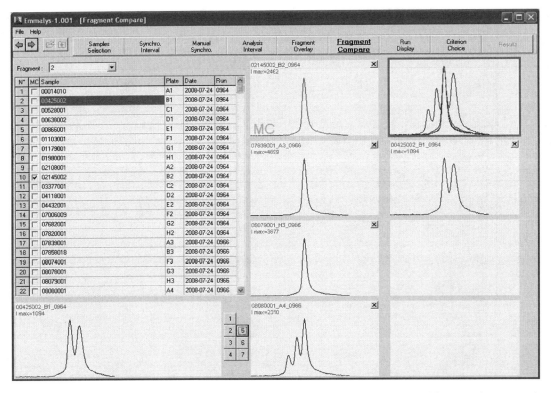

Fig. 6. Emmalys software: "Fragment compare" screen. Another analysis option is available on this screen, by superposition of up to seven samples. MC indicates the main control.

50 ng/μL. If the DNA concentration is too high, for example, the proportionality between signal intensity and copy number will be lost, particularly for small fragments. DNA calibration can be performed with: (1) a tube spectrophotometer (unsuitable for large series); (2) the NanoDrop from Thermo Scientific (which has the advantage of tracing the spectrum of the sample); or (3) a plate reader (rapid, but reading at only one wavelength at a time). In our experience, the use of fluorescent dyes for the assay, such as PicoGreen (Molecular Probes), is unnecessary for these applications. Finally, buccal swabs are poorly adapted to these analyses as DNA is often present in a low concentration and difficult to calibrate.

2. EMMA is sensitive to the position of the mutation along the fragment and mutations in the 0–70 bp region close to each extremity may go undetected. This must be taken into account when designing the primers. This sensitivity to mutation position is, however, compensated by the possibility of covering

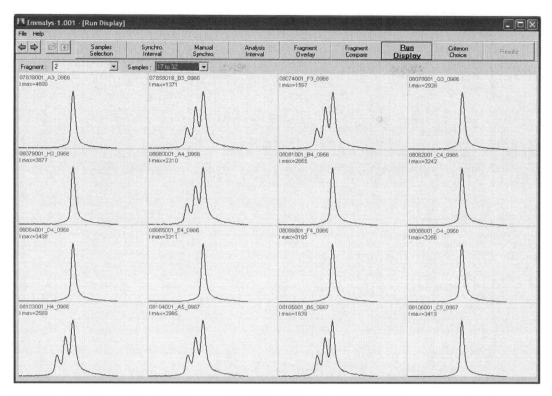

Fig. 7. Emmalys software: "Run display" screen. The third analysis option displays samples by series of 16. Two menus (*top screen*) allow the selection of fragments (i.e., peaks) and series of samples.

the gene of interest with larger and overlapping amplicons, since this technique can typically accommodate fragments up to 550 bp.

3. The bottle of EMMA polymer contains 7 mL of separation matrix, which is sufficient for about 50 runs on an Applied Biosystems 3100 instrument. The polymer is stable until expiration date (written on bottle) when stored at 2°C–8°C. DO NOT FREEZE. EMMA polymer is delivered ready to use. Remove polymer from the 2°C–8°C storage prior to utilization. Proceed as described in the 3,100 user manual for polymer replacement.

Viscosity of EMMA polymer is higher than other polymers usually used in the ABI instruments. EMMA protocols may thus vary from regular protocols, e.g., lead to longer array filling time. EMMA polymer must not stay more than 1 week in the instrument. An excessive temperature in the room may reduce EMMA polymer lifetime.

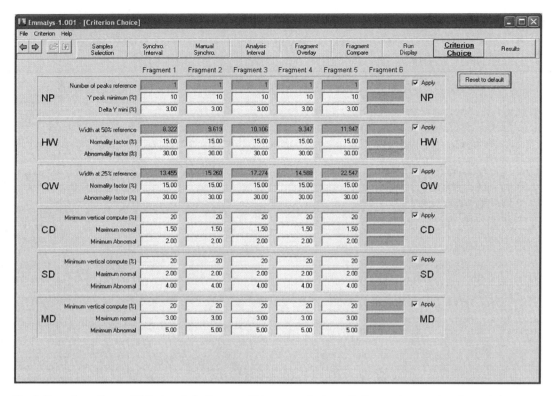

Fig. 8. Emmalys software: "Criterion choice" screen. This screen displays all alignment parameters for each fragment. Default parameters are recommended; however, each parameter may be modified by advanced users in capillary electrophoresis.

Read the EMMA polymer Material Safety Data Sheet (MSDS) and follow the handling instructions. Wear appropriate protective eyewear, clothing, and gloves.

Prior to use, the polymer should be gently mixed O/N (or at least 2 h) at room temperature, then put on the bench for 1 h to eliminate bubbles.

4. The EMMA buffer is delivered as a 10× buffer. It has to be use at 1× concentration in the instrument. Once prepared the 1× EMMA buffer can be stored for 1 week at room temperature and for 1 month at 2–8°C. 1× EMMA buffer has to be replaced daily in both the anode and cathode buffer reservoirs. Proceed as described in the instrument user guide for buffer replacement.

Not replacing EMMA buffer 1× daily may lead to loss in resolution or not interpretable data.

EMMA buffer 10× may cause eye, skin, and respiratory tract irritation. Please read the MSDS and follow the handling

Enhanced Mismatch Mutation Analysis: Simultaneous Detection of Point Mutations

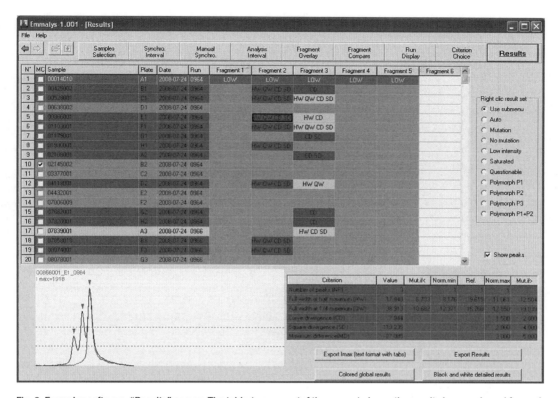

Fig. 9. Emmalys software: "Results" screen. The table (*upper part* of the screen) shows the results by sample and for each fragment using color and two-letter codes. Normal, variant, and questionable samples appear in *grey*, *dark grey*, and *light grey*, respectively. The two-letter code refers to the criterions as defined in the previous screen (Fig. 8.). Selected sample profile for each fragment are superposed to the corresponding one of the main control (*bottom left*).

   instructions. Wear appropriate protective eyewear, clothing, and gloves.

5. Distinct injections protocols are available to ensure optimum results (EMMA high-low). Samples can be injected for 10–20 s at 1–4 kV then electrophoresed at 15 kV for 45 min.
   It means that following a low-intensity run, the user may run the samples a second time using a "higher injection" protocol.

6. EMMA profiles are specific and reproducible, thereby allowing polymorphism interpretation without sequencing. We recommend working on series of 32 samples or more to achieve proper and easy interpretation of polymorphisms. Below this range, it may prove difficult to correctly interpret polymorphism profiles because of a too low number. Furthermore, there is no need to incorporate mutated

7. A classical trap in the interpretation of large scale rearrangement concerns the false-positive results generated by a PCR primer mismatch. Each deletion of a single exon must therefore be systematically checked by another technique (long range PCR, RNA studies, real-time PCR, for example) and/or by shifting the primers. Finally, duplication of an isolated exon is the most difficult case to characterize. The ideal situation is therefore to have a duplicated control of the sequence of interest, for example, DNA from a case of trisomy 13 in *BRCA2* analyses.

control samples when working on a large series of 30 samples or more because we are looking for rare events and the majority of samples will not display mutations.

Acknowledgments

Authors thank Medicen, la Région Ile de France and la Ville de Paris for grant support.

References

1. Xiao, W., and Oefner, P.J. (2001) Denaturing high-performance liquid chromatography: A review. *Hum. Mutat.* **17**, 439–474
2. Vandersteen, J.G., Bayrak-Toydemir, P., Palais, R.A., and Wittwer, C.T. (2007) Identifying common genetic variants by high-resolution melting. *Clin. Chem.* **53**, 1191–1198
3. Houdayer, C., Gauthier-Villars, M., Lauge, A., Pages-Berhouet, S., Dehainault, C., Caux-Moncoutier, V., et al. (2004) Comprehensive screening for constitutional RB1 mutations by DHPLC and QMPSF. *Hum. Mutat.*, **23**, 193–202
4. Weber, J., Looten, R., Houdayer, C., Stoppa-Lyonnet, D., and Viovy, J.L. (2006) Improving sensitivity of electrophoretic heteroduplex analysis using nucleosides as additives: Application to the breast cancer predisposition gene BRCA2. *Electrophoresis* **27**, 1444–1452
5. Weber, J., Miserere, S., Champ, J., Looten, R., Stoppa-Lyonnet, D., Viovy, J.L., and Houdayer, C. (2007) High-throughput simultaneous detection of point mutations and large-scale rearrangements by CE. *Electrophoresis* **28**, 4282–4288
6. Mazoyer, S. (2005) Genomic rearrangements in the BRCA1 and BRCA2 genes. *Hum. Mutat.* **25**, 415–422

Chapter 10

Economical Protocol for Combined Single-Strand Conformation Polymorphism and Heteroduplex Analysis on a Standard Capillary Electrophoresis Apparatus

Piotr Kozlowski and Wlodzimierz J. Krzyzosiak

Abstract

Combined single-strand conformational polymorphism (SSCP) and heteroduplex (HD) analysis (SSCP–HD) take advantage of parallel mutation detection in single-strand and duplex fraction during the single capillary electrophoresis (CE) run. The high mutation detection rate of individual SSCP and HD in CE guarantees almost a 100% success rate of combined SSCP–HD. Described here, the protocol for SSCP–HD–CE does not require dedicated instrumentation but can be applied for any commonly available CE DNA analyzer. We focused mostly on the sample preparation step that is critical for the stability of generated fractions and reproducibility of a generated result. The application of universal primer for fluorescent labeling and omitting the PCR purification step also greatly reduce the cost of mutation detection by SSCP–HD–CE.

Key words: SSCP, HD, Capillary electrophoresis, Heteroduplex analysis, Mutation detection

1. Introduction

Hundreds of genes and thousands of mutations implicated in inherited human diseases have been identified thus far in research and clinical laboratories. Cancer-related genes such as *BRCA1*, *BRCA2*, *ATM*, *TP53*, *MSH2*, and *MLH1* belong to the most extensively studied. Additionally, the identification of causative alleles modifying the risk and associating with common diseases will require detailed information about the polymorphism of numerous genomic areas where an association signal will be identified. This process is in its infancy. The facts presented above clearly indicate the need for an efficient, cost-effective and high throughput platform for the identification of new genetic alterations.

Among the various techniques developed for mutation detection, single-strand conformation polymorphism (SSCP) and heteroduplex analysis (HD) are widely used. SSCP detects base changes in single-stranded DNA, whereas HD does the same in double-stranded DNA subjected to electrophoresis in nondenaturing conditions. In the SSCP analysis initially described by Orita et al. (1, 2), the PCR product is denatured, and separated strands adopt folded structures determined by their nucleotide sequences. A single base alteration is detected by SSCP when the folding of the single-strand changes sufficiently to alter its electrophoretic mobility (see Fig. 1). In the HD analysis initially described by Keen et al. and Nagamine et al. (3, 4), the PCR-amplified DNA fragments are denatured and reannealed to give a mixture of four duplexes: two homoduplexes and two heteroduplexes in the heterozygote samples. Heteroduplexes have an aberrant, distorted structure with bubbles or bulges at the sites of mismatched bases, and generally move more slowly in gel than homoduplexes (see Fig. 1).

Many modifications and alternative protocols for SSCP and HD have been proposed; one of the most important is the adaptation of these methods to the capillary electrophoresis (CE) platform (5–9). CE is a modern analytical platform that significantly reduces sample-handling steps (almost full automation), shortens and facilitates analysis and allows for more precise control of electrophoresis conditions. The multicolor detection and multicapillary systems guarantee high throughput analysis where it is necessary, and efficient heat dissipation allows for rapid DNA fragment separations at a high voltage.

Another important improvement is the combination of SSCP and HD (5, 10, 11). This modification allows for simultaneous mutation detection in single-strand and duplex fractions. The combination of these two methods was possible because the electrophoretic conditions (separation in nondenaturing medium) used in both methods are very similar in which duplexes migrate much faster than single-strand conformers of the same length. Assuming that the chance of mutation detection by SSCP and HD is independent (i.e., they follow different principles of mutation detection; SSCP detects better substitutions and HD detects better insertions and deletions (indels)) and that the mutation detection rate of each method is about 80%, one can calculate that the mutation detection rate of combined SSCP–HD should be close to 100%. This high mutation detection rate was confirmed in several reports by independent researchers (5, 10, 12).

We propose here the protocol for combined SSCP–HD in CE. Our protocol is focused mostly on the pre-CE steps such as study design and sample preparation. CE steps can be performed on any CE apparatus equipped with a fluorescence detection system.

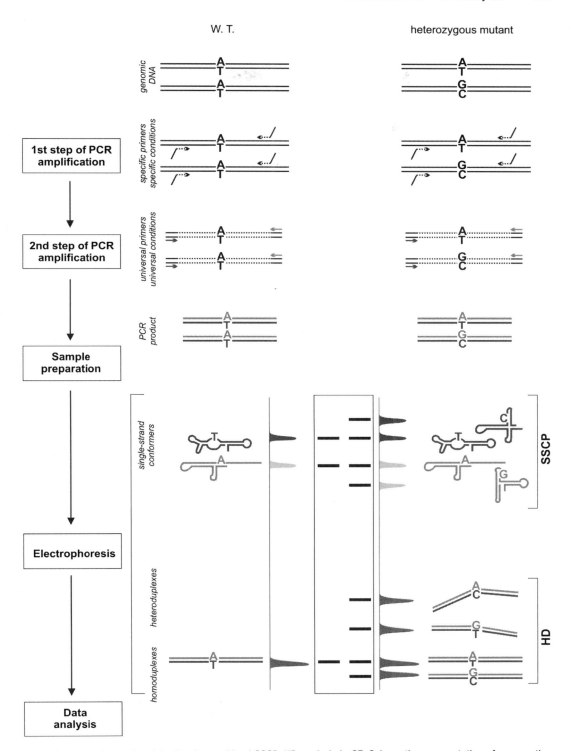

Fig. 1. Strategy of mutation detection by combined SSCP–HD analysis in CE. Schematic representation of consecutive analysis steps (PCR amplification, sample preparation, electrophoresis, and data analysis) of the wild-type (WT) and heterozygous mutant sample is shown on the left- and the right-hand side, respectively.

Although, in our protocol, we recommend using unpurified PCR products, the use of purified PCR products is also described. Omitting the purification procedure greatly simplifies analysis and reduces its cost. After minor modifications, our protocol can also be applied for individual SSCP or HD analysis. The proposed protocol is mostly dedicated for detecting new mutations in large multiexon genes and searching for the new polymorphisms (including SNPs) in different genomic regions – candidate for association study. Alternatively, SSCP–HD–CE can be also applied for the genotyping of known polymorphisms. Although there are several well-established platforms for the genotyping of known polymorphisms on an individual, medium-throughput or high-throughput scale, these platforms are usually dedicated for bi-allelic SNPs and are less suitable, or not applicable at all, for the genotyping of indels or more complex polymorphisms. Thus, the combined SSCP–HD in CE can be highly sensitive, high-throughput mutations/polymorphisms detection platform, comparable with denaturing HPLC (13) or the high-resolution melting method (14). The important advantage of the SSCP–HD–CE method is that it does not require dedicated instrumentation. Array CE apparatus are commonly used for sequencing or STR genotyping and are available in many research and service laboratories.

2. Materials

2.1. PCR Amplification

1. 10× PCR buffer, dNTP set (100 mM solutions of dATP, dCTP, dGTP, dTTP), Taq polymerase (5 U/μL) (Promega, Madison, WI, USA).
2. HPLC-purified PCR universal primers 5'-labeled with FAM or JOE; unlabeled PCR primers (MWG-Biotech Ebensburg, Germany; http://www.mwg-biotech.com).
3. Deionized water (resistivity <18 MΩ cm).

2.2. PCR Product Purification

1. Microcon centrifugal filter device YM-100 (Millipore, Bedford, MA, USA).
2. Deionized water (resistivity <18 MΩ cm).

2.3. CE Analysis

1. GeneScan polymer (Applied Biosystems).
2. Glycerol, 87% (w/v) (Merck).
3. GeneScan ROX-500 size standard (Applied Biosystems).
4. 10× TAE buffer (Applied Biosystems).
5. Deionized water (resistivity <18 MΩ cm).

3. Methods

3.1. Amplicons Design

1. Design the PCR primers for the sequence of interest; any primer picking program can be used; e.g., primer3 http://frodo.wi.mit.edu(15). The amplicons should not be longer than 300 bp (12). In most cases, one amplicon covers one exon. In the case of exons longer than ~250 bp, an array of overlapping amplicons, covering the total exon length should be designed. The polymorphisms databases should be investigated to avoid fragments containing more than two common polymorphisms (see Note 1). As the mutation detection rate is lower in the flanking region, the analyzed DNA fragment should be at least 50 bp from the amplicon ends (including total primer sequences).

2. To reduce the cost of analysis, add universal sequences to the 5′ ends of the forward and reverse primers. In our laboratory for forward and reverse universal sequences, we use: GTC CTG CCA ATG AGA AGA AA and GAG ACC ATT TTC CCA GCA TC, respectively (12). In subsequent steps, these sequences will be used for the reamplification of all designed amplicons in identical conditions with a universal pair of fluorescently labeled primers.

3.2. PCR Amplification

As only a minute amount of PCR product is sufficient even for many capillary runs, the PCR is carried out in the lowest possible volume. Here we propose the protocol for the 5 µL PCR, carried out in the 96-well standard thermocycler GeneAmp PCR System 9700 (Applied Biosystems, Foster City, CA, USA).

3.2.1. First Step of Amplification: PCR with Specific Primers

1. Prepare an adequate volume of PCR premixture containing all reagents except template DNA. For 20 reactions (total volume 100 µL), add and mix up well the following components: 10 µL 10× PCR buffer (100 mM Tris-HCl, pH 8.3, 500 mM KCl, 15 mM MgCl$_2$), 2 µL each of dNTP (10 mM), 2.5 µL Taq polymerase (5 U/µL) (Promega, Madison, WI, USA), and 57.5 µL deionized H$_2$O (see Note 2).

2. Add 8 µL of PCR premixture to empty tubes in 96-well plate, 8-strip or individual tube format.

3. To each tube with the PCR premixture, add 1 µL of genomic DNA (~5 ng/µL); close tubes tightly and spin down to collect all aliquots at the bottom and remove all bubbles or foam.

4. Place tubes carefully in the thermocycler and start the cycling program: 35 cycles of the following steps; denaturation 1 s at 94°C, annealing 1 s at 55°C and extension 1 s at 72°C (see Note 3).

3.2.2. Second Step of Amplification: PCR with Universal Pair of Primers

The second step of amplification is the same as the first one (steps 1–4, Subheading 3.2.1) with two exceptions:

- (step 1) Instead of template specific primers use fluorescently labeled universal primers. In our experiment, we use 5′-FAM – GTC CTG CCA ATG AGA AGA AA and 5′-JOE – GAG ACC ATT TTC CCA GCA TC as forward and reverse universal primers, respectively.
- (step 3) Instead of 1 μL of genomic DNA, use 1 μL of 1,000× water dilution of the first PCR product.

3.3. Sample Preparation

After the amplification reaction, the PCR product is accompanied by unreacted nucleotides, primers, and salts present in the PCR buffer. Most of these components are low molecular weight ions that are preferentially electroinjected to the capillary, decreasing the signal from PCR products. To reduce this effect, the PCR product may be purified from primers and desalted before CE analysis. Below we present the sample preparation protocol for SSCP–HD analysis using both purified and unpurified PCR products (see Fig. 2).

1. Although most PCR products are present in the duplex fraction, we recommend starting sample preparation with reduplexing procedure. It improves the quality of duplex fraction (peaks sharpness) during CE. Reduplex the PCR product by incubating the post-PCR mixture for 10 min at 94°C

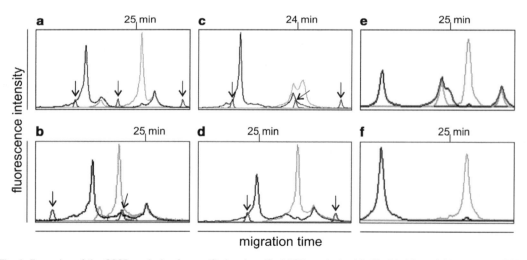

Fig. 2. Examples of the SSCP analysis of unpurified and purified PCR products. (**a**), (**b**), (**c**), (**d**), and (**e**) represent SSCP analysis of amplicons 263, 263, 251, 273, and 276 bp in length, respectively. (**e**) and (**f**) show the direct comparison of SSCP analysis of unpurified (**e**) and purified (**f**) PCR product 276 bp in length. The SSCP pattern of purified PCR product is composed only of single-color-labeled peaks while the SSCP pattern of an unpurified PCR product includes also double-color-labeled peaks. It was shown that double-color-labeled peaks are single-strand conformers with hybridized excessive primers (16). *Dark-gray*, *light-gray*, and *arrow head*-indicated peaks represent the FAM-labeled strand, JOE-labeled strand, and DNA size standard (ROX-labeled), respectively.

followed by 60 min at 64°C. To reduce the sample-handling steps, the reduplexing procedure can be performed in the thermocycler immediately after PCR (see Note 4).

2. [optional] Purify the PCR product using the Microcon centrifugal filter device YM-100 (Millipore, Bedford, MA, USA), according to the manufacturer's recommendations. After purification, dilute the sample again in deionized water to the original volume (5 µL) (see Note 5).

3. Dilute unpurified (step 1, Subheading 3.3) or purified (step 2, Subheading 3.3) PCR samples in deionized water. We found that the optimal dilution factor for a typical PCR product (yield ~100 ng/µL; length ~300 bp) is 40× and 120× for an unpurified and purified PCR product, respectively (16). However, if the signal from the PCR product is too low or exceeds the upper detection limit an additional optimization step is necessary to find the optimum dilution factor for the analyzed amplicon. In this case, prepare and test the serial dilutions of selected PCR samples (test the dilution range 10× to 120× for unpurified and 30× to 480× for purified products). Select the dilution where the signal strength from the SSCP and duplex fractions is high but within the dynamic detection range.

4. Divide the diluted PCR product into two portions. One of them is the duplex portion and the other serves for the generation of single-strand conformers. To prepare single-strand conformers, denature one portion at 95°C for 30 s. After denaturation, leave the sample at RT for 2 min (see Note 6).

5a. Prepare the sample for HD analysis in CE – add 1 µL of a duplex portion and 1 µL 40× diluted ROX-500 size standard to 10 µL of deionized water (see Note 7).

5b. Prepare sample for SSCP analysis in CE –add 1 µL SSCP portion and 1 µL 40× diluted ROX-500 size standard to 10 µL of deionized water (see Note 7).

5c. Prepare sample for combined SSCP–HD analysis in CE –add 1 µL of a duplex portion, 1 µL SSCP portion, and 1 µL 40× diluted ROX-500 size standard to 10 µL of deionized water (see Fig. 3) (see Note 7).

6. Mix samples well, spin them down and place into the CE analyzer.

3.4. Capillary Electrophoresis

Analysis can be performed on any standard single- or multicapillary DNA analyzer (e.g., ABI-Prism 310, 3100, 1700 (Applied Biosystems), CEQ-2000, 8000, 8800 (Beckman)). The general strategy for CE analysis and signal detection is similar in most commonly available apparatus but the detailed procedure differs

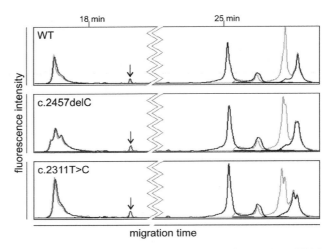

Fig. 3. Examples of the combined SSCP–HD–CE analysis of 290 bp long DNA fragment. Duplex and SSCP fraction are presented on the left- and right-hand side, respectively. Electrophoregrams represent the wild-type (WT) sequence and two sequence alterations located in the exon 11 of *BRCA1* gene. Color labels are the same as described in the legend to Fig. 2.

from apparatus to apparatus and is described in detail in appropriate manufacturers' manuals.

1. Analyze the SSCP, HD, or combined SSCP–HD samples in nondenaturing CE following the manufacturer's protocol for nondenaturing CE analysis.

2. Typical CE analysis of HD, SSCP, or combined SSCP–HD samples is performed in the following conditions: capillary length ~42 cm; electroinjection voltage 15 kV; electroinjection time 5 s; nondenaturing polymer (5.5% GeneScan (Applied Biosystems) with 1× Tris-borate-EDTA (TBE) buffer and 10% glycerol); run temperature 30°C; run voltage 13 kV; and electrophoresis time ~22 min for HD or 27 min for SSCP and combined SSCP–HD analysis (see Note 8).

3. Align the electrophoregrams according to the migration of the DNA size standard to minimize run-to-run and capillary-to-capillary differences in migration (see Fig. 4).

4. Identify sample/fragments showing a changed pattern (e.g., additional peaks) of SSCP or HD fraction.

5. To identify the exact nucleotide change responsible for altered duplex or single-strand conformer migration, reamplify and sequence the PCR product. Resequencing is a separate procedure routinely used in many laboratories and described in detail in many protocols.

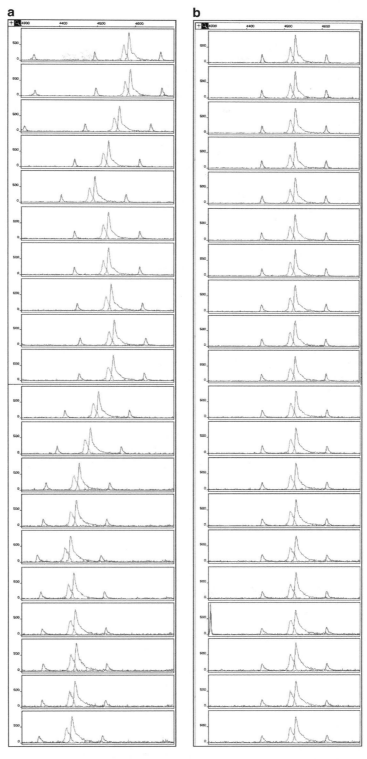

Fig. 4. Examples of the HD analysis of two multiplexed PCR fragments before (**a**) and after (**b**) calibration against DNA size standard ROX-500. Calibration was made using the Local Southern interpolation method. Grey peaks represent the homoduplexes of two PCR products of the same length (211 bp).

4. Notes

1. Each polymorphism occurring in an analyzed fragment can interfere with mutation detection and lower detection rate. The information about common SNPs can be found in databases such us: dbSNP (http://www.ncbi.nlm.nih.gov/snp) and HapMap (http://www.hapmap.org).

2. All reagents listed here can be replaced by adequate reagents from other companies. In some cases, the change of reagent may require a minor adjustment of the procedure to optimize the results.

3. The annealing temperature may differ depending on the melting properties of primers and sometimes has to be determined experimentally. In most of our experiments, the annealing temperature was 55°C. Extension time depends on fragment length but our experiments show that fragments up to 300 bp can be effectively amplified in PCR with a 1 s extension step (17).

4. Always perform the reduplexing procedure before sample purification (step 2, Subheading 3.3) or dilution (step 3, Subheading 3.3). Too low salt concentration in a diluted or purified sample can completely prevent duplex formation. On the other hand, low salt concentration stabilizes single-strand conformers formed after heat denaturation.

5. Other filtration or precipitation procedures can also be used for sample purification. We found the Microcon YM-100 filter device, a relatively easy and effective way for both the purification and desalting of the PCR products up to 600 bp.

6. Both fractions can be safely stored for at least 1 day at RT or for several days at 4°C. It enables the sequential analysis of many samples in automatic analyzers and minimizes sample-to-sample variation (16).

7. Most DNA size standards are mixtures of DNA duplexes of different length. For analysis in nondenaturing CE conditions, DNA size standards can be used both nondenatured (duplexes) and denatured (mixture of single-strands and duplexes). Although the spectrum of DNA size standard signals is much wider after denaturation (ranging from fast migrating duplexes to slow migrating single-strand conformers), their strength is very uneven and migration is less reproducible than the spectrum of signals of a nondenatured size standard. Thus, we recommend using nondenatured DNA size standard both for SSCP and HD analysis. As the migration of single-strand conformers is much slower than duplexes of corresponding length, the longest fragment of the DNA

size standard used for SSCP analysis has to be adequately longer than an analyzed PCR fragment. The ROX-500 size standard with fragments up to 500 bp is sufficient for the SSCP analysis of DNA fragments length up to ~250 bp.

8. The rate at which DNA fragments migrate in CE strongly depends on temperature, and even subtle temperature variation can influence this rate and thus can reduce the reproducibility of the analysis. To minimize the room temperature variation in the area in which the analyzer is located, the apparatus should be turned on about ~60 min ahead of the start of the analysis to allow temperature equilibration.

Acknowledgments

This work was supported by funding under the Sixth Research Framework Programme of the European Union, Project RIGHT (LSHB-CT-2004-005276) and by the Ministry of Science and Higher Education, grants: PBZ-KBN-124/P05/2004 and PBZMNii-2/1/2005.

References

1. Orita, M., Iwahana, H., Kanazawa, H., Hayashi, K., and Sekiya, T. (1989) Detection of polymorphisms of human DNA by gel electrophoresis as single-strand conformation polymorphisms. *Proc. Natl. Acad. Sci. U S A.* **86**, 2766–2770.
2. Orita, M., Suzuki, Y., Sekiya, T., and Hayashi, K. (1989) Rapid and sensitive detection of point mutations and DNA polymorphisms using the polymerase chain reaction. *Genomics* **5**, 874–879.
3. Keen, J., Lester, D., Inglehearn, C., Curtis, A., and Bhattacharya, S. (1991) Rapid detection of single base mismatches as heteroduplexes on Hydrolink gels. *Trends Genet.* **7**, 5.
4. Nagamine, C.M., Chan, K., and Lau, Y.F. (1989) A PCR artifact: generation of heteroduplexes. *Am. J. Hum. Genet.* **45**, 337–339.
5. Kozlowski, P., and Krzyzosiak, W.J. (2001) Combined SSCP/duplex analysis by capillary electrophoresis for more efficient mutation detection. *Nucleic Acids Res.* **29**, E71.
6. Inazuka, M., Wenz, H.M., Sakabe, M., Tahira, T., and Hayashi, K. (1997) A streamlined mutation detection system: multicolor post-PCR fluorescence labeling and single-strand conformational polymorphism analysis by capillary electrophoresis. *Genome Res.* **7**, 1094–1103.
7. Larsen, L.A., Christiansen, M., Vuust, J., and Andersen, P.S. (1999) High-throughput single-strand conformation polymorphism analysis by automated capillary electrophoresis: robust multiplex analysis and pattern-based identification of allelic variants. *Hum. Mutat.* **13**, 318–327.
8. Ren, J., and Ueland, P.M. (1999) Temperature and pH effects on single-strand conformation polymorphism analysis by capillary electrophoresis. *Hum. Mutat.* **13**, 458–463.
9. Tian, H., Brody, L.C., and Landers, J.P. (2000) Rapid detection of deletion, insertion, and substitution mutations via heteroduplex analysis using capillary- and microchip-based electrophoresis. *Genome Res.* **10**, 1403–1413.
10. Kourkine, I.V., Hestekin, C.N., Buchholz, B.A., and Barron, A.E. (2002) High-throughput, high-sensitivity genetic mutation detection by tandem single-strand conformation polymorphism/heteroduplex analysis capillary array electrophoresis. *Anal. Chem.* **74**, 2565–2572.
11. Hestekin, C.N., Jakupciak, J.P., Chiesl, T.N., Kan, C.W., O'Connell, C.D., and Barron, A.E. (2006) An optimized microchip electrophoresis

system for mutation detection by tandem SSCP and heteroduplex analysis for p53 gene exons 5–9. *Electrophoresis* **27**, 3823–3835.

12. Kozlowski, P., and Krzyzosiak, W.J. (2005) Structural factors determining DNA length limitations in conformation-sensitive mutation detection methods. *Electrophoresis* **26**, 71–81.

13. Underhill, P.A., Jin, L., Lin, A.A., Mehdi, S.Q., Jenkins, T., Vollrath, D., et al. (1997) Detection of numerous Y chromosome biallelic polymorphisms by denaturing high-performance liquid chromatography. *Genome Res.* **7**, 996–1005.

14. Reed, G.H., and Wittwer, C.T. (2004) Sensitivity and specificity of single-nucleotide polymorphism scanning by high-resolution melting analysis. *Clin. Chem.* **50**, 1748–1754.

15. Rozen, S., and Skaletsky, H. (2000) Primer3 on the WWW for general users and for biologist programmers. *Methods Mol. Biol.* **132**, 365–386.

16. Kozlowski, P., and Krzyzosiak, W.J. (2004) Optimum sample medium for single-nucleotide polymorphism and mutation detection by capillary electrophoresis. *Electrophoresis* **25**, 990–998.

17. Sobczak, K., Kozlowski, P., and Krzyzosiak, W.J. (1995) Faster and cheaper PCR on a standard thermocycler. *Acta. Biochim. Pol.* **42**, 363–366.

Chapter 11

Mutational Screening of *hMLH1* and *hMSH2* that Confer Inherited Colorectal Cancer Susceptibility Using Denature Gradient Gel Electrophoresis (DGGE)

Tao Liu

Abstract

Hereditary nonpolyposis colorectal cancer syndrome (HNPCC) is primarily due to heterozygous germline mutations in one of the mismatch repair (MMR) genes. Mutation screening for MMR genes with various techniques revealed that the majority of mutations identified are small DNA variations (83.8% in hMLH1 and 73% in hMSH2). Denaturing gradient gel electrophoresis (DGGE) is a sensitive, robust and powerful technique to detect small nucleotide variations and has been used for mutation screening for many years. The separation principle of DGGE is based on the melting behaviour of DNA molecules. In a denaturing gradient acrylamide gel, double-stranded DNA is subjected to a denaturant environment and will melt in discrete segments called melting domains. The melting temperature (T_m) of these domains is sequence-specific. Therefore, DNA containing a mutation will have a different mobility compared to the wild type. DGGE is the perfect method for mutation screening of large samples for unknown mutations. This is because it is user friendly, non-radioactive, cost-effective, less labour intensive and, more importantly, it is reliable and has a very high mutation detection rate. We have used DGGE to screen hMLH1 and hMSH2 mutations and have shown high detection rate.

Key words: HNPCC, MMR, DGGE, Gradient, Melting temperature, GC-clamp, Heteroduplex strand

1. Introduction

Hereditary nonpolyposis colorectal cancer syndrome (HNPCC) occurs primarily due to heterozygous germline mutations in one of the mismatch repair (MMR) genes; hMLH1, hMSH2, hMSH6 and hPMS2. HNPCC accounts for 5–8% of all colorectal cancer (CRC) cases in western countries (1). Applied mutation screening for MMR genes with various techniques revealed that the majority of mutations identified are small DNA variations (73% in hMSH2; 83.8% in hMLH1, 94.5% in hMSH6 and 94.1% in hPMS2) (2–9).

A number of techniques such as single stranded conformation polymorphism (SSCP), heteroduplex analysis (HA), protein truncation test (PTT), direct sequencing and denaturing gradient gel electrophoresis (DGGE) are available to identify these small nucleotide variations (2–4, 6, 7). However, in our experience, DGGE is the best choice to identify small mutations in MMR genes, as other techniques show either lower mutation detection rate or are too expensive (10). DGGE is a sensitive, robust technique that allows the separation of DNA molecules differing by as little as a single base change and has been used for mutation screening for many years (10). DGGE is a polymerase chain reaction (PCR)-based method and it can detect nearly 100% of small DNA alterations such as point mutations, small deletion/insertions as well splice site variants (11). The principle of this method is based on the melting properties of DNA in solution. DNA molecules melt in discrete segments, called melting domains, when the temperature or denaturant concentration is raised. In the DGGE system, DNA fragments are electrophoresed through a polyacrylamide gel that contains a liner gradient, from top to bottom, of increasing DNA denaturant concentration. When a DNA fragment enters the gel and reaches the concentration of denaturant equivalent to the T_m of its weakest melting domain, the domain melts and the DNA molecule forms a branched structure that has a retarded mobility in the gel matrix. DNA fragments differing by a single base change begin branching at different concentrations of denaturant and their migration will be retarded at different positions in the gel, resulting in the separation of the DNA fragment. DGGE can be used to detect single base changes in all melting domains of a DNA fragment except the highest T_m domain due to the loss of sequence-dependent migration of the DNA fragment upon complete strand dissociation. In order to overcome this problem and increase the sensitivity, a 40 base GC-rich sequence (GC-clamp) is added to one of the primers used to generate the template. The optimal position of the GC-clamp, either the 5'- or 3'-end of the template, can be determined using a computer program such as MELT95.

DGGE has been widely used for mutation screening in many different genes (12–14). In the practical sense, DGGE methodology comprises straightforward procedures such as fragment melting temperature prediction, primers design, run denaturant gel, and analysis of samples with aberrant band by DNA sequencing.

2. Materials

2.1. DNA Isolation from Lymphocytes

1. Lysis buffer (1 L): 8.29 g NH_4Cl (155 mM), 1 g $KHCO_3$ (10 mM), 0.034 g Na_2EDTA or 200 µL EDTA 0.5 M (0.1 mM). Fill to 1,000 mL with distilled water, adjust to pH 7.4 with 1 M HCl or NaOH for each use.

2. Chloroform/isoamyl alcohol 24:1.
3. SE-buffer: 4.39 g NaCl (75 mM), 8.41 g Na$_2$EDTA or 50 mL EDTA 0.5 M (25 mM). Fill to 1 L with distilled water and adjust to pH 8.0 with 1 M NaOH.
4. 3 M Sodium acetate: 246 g/L. Adjust to pH 5.2 with CH$_3$COOH.
5. 100× Tris–EDTA buffer: pH 8.0, 1.0 M Tris–HCl, containing 0.1 M EDTA.
6. Proteinase K (10 mg/mL): Dissolve 100 mg proteinase K in 10 mL TE for 30 min at room temperature. Aliquot and store at –20°C.

2.2. PCR

1. Sterilized distilled H$_2$O.
2. Genomic DNA sample 200 ng/µL. Store at –20°C.
3. AmpliTaq DNA polymerase (Perkin Elmer), 5 U/µL. Store at –20°C.
4. 10× Taq PCR buffer (Sphero-Q): 100 mM Tris–HCl. pH 9.0, 500 mM KCl, 15 mM MgCl$_2$, 0.1% gelatin and Triton X-100. Store at –20°C.
5. dNTP mix (Perkin Elmer): 10 mM of each dNTP. Store at –20°C.
6. 25 mM MgCl$_2$ solution (Perkin Elmer). Store at –20°C.
7. Oligonucleotide primers (Tables 1 and 2, see Note 1); 20 µM.

2.3. Polyacrylamide Gel Electrophoresis

1. 100% Denaturant polyacrylamide solution stock: 6.5% acrylamide/bisacrylamide (37.5:1), 7 M urea and 40% formamide. For 1 L, dissolve the following: 38.5% acrylamide/bisacrylamide (37.5:1) 168.8 mL, 400.42 g urea, 400 mL deionized formamide (see Note 2), 50× TAE-buffer 20 mL and distilled water up to 1,000 mL. Store at 4°C for 3 months.
2. 0% Denaturant polyacrylamide solution stock: 6.5% acrylamide/bisacrylamide (37.5:1), For 1 L, dissolve the following: 38.5% acrylamide/bisacrylamide (37.5:1) 168.8 mL, 50× TAE-buffer 20 mL, and distilled water up to 1,000 mL. Store at 4°C for 3 months.
3. 50× Tris–acetate (TAE) buffer, pH 8.0: 2.0 M Tris base, 50 mM EDTA and 1 M sodium acetate. For 1 L, mix 242 g Tris base, 100 mL of 0.5 M EDTA (pH 8.0), 57.1 mL glacial acetic acid. Adjust pH to 8.0 and make up to 1 L with dH$_2$O. Store at room temperature.
4. Ammonium persulfate 10% (APS): Dissolve 1 g in 10 mL distilled water. Aliquot to single use and store at –20°C until required.

Table 1
PCR primers for *hMLH1*

Exon	Name	Primer sequence
1	hMLH1X1-F[a]	5'-[b]CAC TGA GGT GAT TGG CTG AAG
	hMLH1X1-R	5'-GGG GAA AGA GGC GTG TC
2	hMLH1X2-F	5'-[b]CTG TTT GAT TTG CCA GTT TAG
	hMLH1X2-R	5'-GCA CAA ACA TCC TGC TAC
3	hMLH1X3-F	5'-[b]GAT TTG GAA ATG AGT AAC ATG A
	hMLH1X3-R	5'-CAA TGT CAT CAC AGG AGG ATA T
4	hMLH1X4-F	5'-[b]TGT TGA GAC AGG ATT ACT CTG AGA C
	hMLH1X4-R	5'-AAC CTT TCC CTT TGG TGA GG
5	hMLH1X5-F	5'-[b]GAT TTT CTC TTT TCC CCT TGG
	hMLH1X5-R	5'-CTT CAA CAA TTT ACT CTC CAT GTA
6	hMLH1X6-F	5'-[b]CCA TCT TGG GTT TTA TTT TCA A
	hMLH1X6-R	5'-CAA CTG TTC AAT GTA TGA GCA CTA
7	hMLH1X7-F	5'-[b]ATA ACC TTA TCT CCA CCA GCA AAC
	hMLH1X7-R	5'-CTA GTG TGT GTT TTT GGC AAC TCT
8	hMLH1X8-F	5'-[b]TTT TTT TAT ATA GGT TAT CGA CAT AC
	hMLH1X8-R	5'-CTC AGC CAT GAG ACA ATA AAT C
9	hMLH1X9-F	5'-[b]AGC TTC AGA ATC TCT TTT CTA ATA G
	hMLH1X9-R	5'-TGT TTC CTG TGA GTG GAT TTC
10	hMLH1X10-F	5'-[b]AGG AGA GCC TGA TAG AAC ATC TG
	hMLH1X10-R	5'-CAT GAC TTT GTG TGA ATG TAC ACC
11	hMLH1X11-F	5'-[b]TGT TCT CTC TTA TTT TCC TGA CAG
	hMLH1X11-R	5'-CAG AGA AGT AGC TGG ATG AGA AG
12	hMLH1X12-F	5'-[b]TTT TTT TAA TAC AGA CTT TGC TAG C
	hMLH1X12-R	5'-CAG AAT AAA GGA GGT AGG CTG TA
13:A	hMLH1X13A-F	5'-[b]CCT CCA AAA TGC AAC CCA C
	hMLH1X13A-R	5'-GTC ATT TCC TTT CGG GAA TC
13:B	hMLH1X13B-F	5'-[b]GAT TCC CGA AAG GAA ATG AC
	hMLH1X13B-R	5'-GCT TTC TCC ATT TCC AAA AC
14	hMLH1X14-F	5'-[b]CTA TTA CTT ACC TGT TTT TTT GGT
	hMLH1X14-R	5'-ATT GTT GTA GTA GCT CTG CTT GT
15	hMLH1X15-F	5'-[b]AAA TGT CAG AAG TGA AAA GGA TCT
	hMLH1X15-R	5'-GTC TCC CAT TTG TCC AAC CT

(continued)

Table 1 (continued)

Exon	Name	Primer sequence
16	hMLH1X16-F	5'-[b]ACA ACA GAA GTA TAA GAA TGG CTG TC
	hMLH1X16-R	5'-CAT TTG GAT GCT CCG TTA AAG
17	hMLH1X17-F	5'-[b]GGG AAA GGC ACT GGA GAA AT
	hMLH1X17-R	5'-GCA TGT ACC GAA ATG CTT AGT ATC
18	hMLH1X18-F	5'-[b]TGA TGT CCG TTT AGA ATG AGA AT
	hMLH1X18-R	5'-AGA TGT ATG AGG TCC TGT CCT AGT
19	hMLH1X19-F	5'-[b]ACA CAT CCC ACA GTG CAT AAA
	hMLH1X19-R	5'-CTA GCC CAC AAG ATC CAC TTC

[a]F forward primer, R reverse primer
[b]GC-clamp (5'-GCG GCC GCC CGT CCC GCC GCC CCC GCC CCG CCG COG CCG C-3')

5. 6× DGGE gel loading buffer: 0.25% bromophenol blue (Sigma), 0.25% xylene cyanol (Sigma), 15% ficoll. Dissolve 250 mg bromophenol blue, 250 mg xylene cyanol, and 20 g ficoll in 100 mL distilled water. Store at 4°C.

6. Ethidium bromide (10 mg/mL): Dissolve 1 g ethidium bromide in 100 mL distilled water. Note ethidium bromide is a highly hazardous substance. Always wear a lab coat, safety glasses and protective gloves when working with ethidium bromide. Store at room temperature in a dark bottle.

7. N,N,N',N'-Tetramethylethylenediamine (TEMED) is extremely destructive to tissues of the mucous membranes and upper respiratory tract, eyes and skin. Wear appropriate gloves, safety glasses and other protective clothing. Store in the dark at room temperature.

2.4. DNA Sequencing Reactions

1. ABI PRISM™ BigDye™ terminator cycle sequencing ready reaction kit with AmpliTaq DNA polymerase (Perkin Elmer). The DNA double strand sequencing reactions are performed for ABI PRISM model 377, according to manufacturers' instructions. Amplified products can be stored at −20°C. Safety warnings are provided on the reagents' bottles and in the manufacturers' Material Safety Data Sheets (MSDS). Dispose of waste in accordance with all local, state and federal health and environmental regulations and laws.

Table 2
PCR primers for *hMSH2*

Exon	Name	Primer sequence
1	hMSH2X1-F[a]	5'-[b]CTT CAA CCA GGA GGT GAG GAG G
	hMSH2X1-R	5'-TCC CCA GCA CGC GCC GTC
2	hMSH2X2-F	5'-TTTAAG GAG CAAAGAATC TGC
	hMSH2X2-R	5'-[b]CCT TATATG CCAAAT ACC AAT C
3	hMSH2X3-F	5'-[b]GCT TCT CCT GGC AAT CTC TC
	hMSH2X3-R	5'-GAA TCT CCT CTATCA CTA GAC TC
4	hMSH2X4-F	5'-[b]GTA GTT TAAACTATT TCT TTC AAAAT
	hMSH2X4-R	5'-TAATTC ACA TTTATAATC CAT GTA C
5	hMSH2X5-F	5'-CCA GTG GTATAG AAATCT TCG
	hMSH2X5-R	5'-[b]CCAATC AAC ATT TTT AAC CC
6	hMSH2X6-F	5'-AGG GTT CTG TTG AAG ATA CCA C
	hMSH2X6-R	5'-[b]CTC TCC TCTATT CTG TTC TTATC
7	hMSH2X7-F	5'-CAA GTTAAT TTATTT CAG
	hMSH2X7-R	5'-[b]AAAACAAAAAAA CAAAAT CA
8	hMSH2X8-F	5'-[b]GTT TTA CTA CTT TCT TTTA
	hMSH2X8-R	5'-ATTAAAAAG TATATT GCA
9	hMSH2X9-F	5'-[b]TCT TTA CCC ATTATT TATAGG ATT T
	hMSH2X9-R	5'-AAT TAT TCC AAC CTC CAA TGA
10	hMSH2X10-F	5'-CTT TTT CTT TTC TTC TTG
	hMSH2X10-R	5'-[b]AATAAA GGG TTAAAAATA
11	hMSH2X11-F	5'-[b]ACT GTTATT TCG ATT TGC A
	hMSH2X11-R	5'-GCC AGG TGA CAT TCA GAA
12	hMSH2X12-F	5'-[b]TCC TGT GTA CAG TTT CTG TTT T
	hMSH2X12-R	5'-CAC AAA GCC CAAAAA CC
13	hMSH2X13-F	5'-CTT GCT TTC TGA TATAAT TTG T
	hMSH2X13-R	5'-[b]GGA CAG AGA CAT ACA TTT CTATC
14	hMSH2X14-F	5'-[b]CAC ATT TTATGT GAT GGG AAA
	hMSH2X14-R	5'-CAT TAC CAA GAT ACT GAATTT AGA
15	hMSH2X15-F	5'-TGC TGT CTC TTC TCA TGC TG
	hMSH2X15-R	5'-[b]TTAAAC TAT GAAAAC AAA CTG ACAA
16	hMSH2X16-F	5'-GGG ACA TTC ACA TGT GTT TC
	hMSH2X16-R	5'-[b]TTAAGT TGA TAG CCC ATG G

[a]*F* forward primer, *R* reverse primer
[b]GC-clamp 5 (5'-GCG GCC GCC CGT CCC GCC GCC CCC GCC CCG CCG CGG CCG C-3')

3. Methods

3.1. DNA Isolation from Whole Blood/ Lymphocytes

1. To 10 mL whole blood (EDTA, heparin, citrate), add 30 mL lysis buffer and shake gently.
2. Incubate for 30 min on ice, and centrifuge at 300×g for 10 min at 4°C.
3. Discard the supernatant, add 10 mL lysis buffer, resuspend the pellet and centrifuge at 300×g for 10 min at 4°C.
4. Discard the supernatant, add 5 mL SE-buffer, resuspend the pellet and centrifuge at 300×g for 10 min at 4°C.
5. Discard the supernatant, add 5 mL SE-buffer and resuspend the pellet.
6. Add 40 µL proteinase K (10 mg/mL) and 250 µL 20% SDS, shake gently.
7. Incubate overnight at 37°C in a water bath.
8. Add 5 mL SE-buffer and 10 mL phenol, shake by hand for 10 min and centrifuge at 2,000×g for 5 min at 10°C.
9. Transfer the supernatant into a new tube, add 10 mL phenol/chloroform/isoamyl alcohol (25:24:1), shake by hand for 10 min and centrifuge at 2,000×g for 5 min at 10°C.
10. Again transfer the supernatant into a new tube, add 10 mL chloroform/isoamylalcohol (24:1), shake by hand for 10 min and centrifuge at 2,000×g for 5 min at 10°C.
11. Transfer the supernatant into a new tube, add 300 µL 3 M sodium acetate (pH 5.2) and 10 mL isopropanol; shake gently until the DNA precipitates.
12. Wash the DNA in 70% ethanol.
13. Dissolve the DNA in 500–1,000 µL 1× TE-buffer overnight at 4°C.
14. Measure the DNA concentration in a spectrophotometer (Pharmacia, GeneQuant) and analyse 200 ng in a 1% agarose gel.

3.2. PCR

1. Prepare the following reaction (50 µL) by adding the reagents into a reaction tube: 10× *Taq* PCR buffer, 10 µM of each oligonucleotide primer (Tables 1 and 2, see Note 1), 200 ng of a genomic DNA from patient, 20 mM dNTPs, H$_2$O, 200 ng of genomic DNA, 1.5 mM MgCl$_2$ (see Note 3) and 1 U Ampli*Taq* DNA polymerase (5 U/µL).
2. PCR is performed in a thermal cycler (DNA Engine Tetrad, MJ Research) using the following program (see Note 4):

Initial denaturation	94°C, 4 min
Amplification (35 cycles)	94°C, 30 s denaturation
	55°C, 30 s annealing
	72°C, 1 min extension
Extension	72°C, 10 min
	4°C, soak

3. Store samples at 4°C.

3.3. Polyacrylamide Gel Electrophoresis (see Note 5)

1. Clean the spacers and glass plates with detergent, rinse thoroughly with distilled H_2O, then clean with 100% ethanol and air-dry.
2. Assemble the gel cassette and place the cassette in the gel casting device according to the manufacturers' instructions, so that the inner smaller plate faces inwards (to create an upper buffer chamber).
3. Mix 5.0 mL 6.5% acrylamide solution with 50 µL 10% APS and 5 µL TEMED, and using a Pasteur pipette pour into the gel cassette. Allow to polymerize for at least 15 min (see Note 6).
4. Cast the gradient-gel in the HOEFER SE 620 system plates that hold volumes of 55 mL (1.5 mm spacer). Therefore, freshly prepare 30 mL of both low and high denaturing solutions (see Tables 3–5).
5. Add 150 µL 10% APS and 15 µL TEMED to each solution and mix gently.
6. Place the gradient gel maker on a magnetic stirrer positioned 25–30 cm above the top edge of the glass plate sandwich. Pour both low and high denaturing solution in the appropriate chamber of the gradient gel maker.
7. Activate the magnetic bar to create a vortex, and fill the gel sandwich to the top of the glass plate. Insert a comb into each gel at the top, taking care not to trap any air bubbles below the teeth of the comb.
8. Allow the gel to polymerize for between 2 and 3 h.
9. In the meantime, fill the electrophoresis tank with electrophoresis buffer (10 L), heat the TAE buffer in the buffer tank to 60°C (see Note 7). TAE buffer can be used three times before being replaced.
10. Carefully remove the gel comb and rinse the slots with distilled H_2O.
11. Put the gel(s) in the gel holder and place the holder in the electrophoresis tank and fill the upper buffer compartment with 1× TAE running buffer.

Table 3
DGGE conditions for exons of *hMLH1*

Exon	Conditions[a] (°C)	PCR (bp)	Fragment length gradient (%)
1	57	272	20–80
2	55	142	10–60
3	55	202	10–50
4	50	237	10–60
5	55	180	10–60
6	55	237	10–50
7	55	128	10–50
8	55	165	10–60
9	55	182	10–60
10	55	238	45–85
11	55	210	20–80
12	55	428	20–80
13:1	55	144	10–60
13:2	55	177	40–70
14	55	196	10–60
15	55	175	45–85
16	55	247	10–60
17	55	214	10–60
18	55	238	45–80
19	55	335	10–50

[a]Annealing temperature °C

12. Mix 20 µL amplified PCR-product with 4 µL 6× DGGE gel loading buffer.
13. Rinse the slots again with 1× TAE running buffer and carefully load the samples (see Note 8).
14. Place the lid back on the electrophoresis tank and switch on the system; perform the run at 85 V constant voltage (20–40 mA for one gel), 60°C temperature for 16 h.
15. Disassemble the gel cassette and carefully remove one glass plate and stain gel with 200 mL EB-staining solution (20 µL EB in 200 µL distilled H_2O) on a tumbling-plateau for 15 min.
16. Destain the gel 3×2 min in distilled H_2O.
17. Analyse the gel on a UV-transilluminator (see Notes 9 and 10).

Table 4
DGGE conditions for exons of *hMSH2*

Exon	Conditions[a] (°C)	PCR (bp)	Fragment length gradient (%)
1	60	310	45–80
2	55	202	0–60
3	60	353	20–80
4	55	240	0–60
5	55	284	28 (CDGE)
6	55	176	0–65
7	55	289	10–60
8	50	209	10–60
9	55	246	0–50
10	50	257	10–60
11	60	230	10–60
12	50	353	0–60
13	55	324	0–65
14	50	376	10–60
15	60	310	0–50
16	55	356	0–65

[a]Annealing temperature °C

Table 5
DGGE density gel solutions

Gel (%)[a]	0% Denaturant solution (mL)	100% Denaturant solution (mL)
0	30.0	0.0
10	27.0	3.0
20	24.0	6.0
28	21.6	8.4
45	16.5	13.5
50	15.0	15.0
60	12.0	18.0
65	10.5	19.5
80	6.0	24.0

[a]Percentage denaturation of DGGE gel

3.4. DNA Sequencing Reactions

1. For PCR products that show abnormal bands on the DGGE gel, reamplify with the relevant primer pair specific for that exon/fragment (see Note 11).
2. Following the manufacturers' instructions, perform sequencing reactions with ABI PRISM BigDye terminator cycle sequencing ready reaction kit with Ampli*Taq* DNA polymerase in the ABI PRISM model 377 (Perkin Elmer) (see Note 12).

4. Notes

1. The 40 bp GC-clamp that was originally described by Sheffield et al. (15) has the following sequence: 5'-CGCCCGCC GCGCCCCGCGCCCGTCCCGCCGCCCCGCCCC-3' and should be attached to the 5' end of either the forward or reverse primer. The GC-clamp serves as a high TM domain and prevents complete denaturation of the amplified PCR fragment, therefore improving the mutation detection rate close to 100%. We had to split exon 13 of hMLH1 in two overlapped fragments due to more than one T_m domain.
2. To deionize formamide, add 3 g of mixed bed resin to 100 mL formamide and mix for 30 min (in a fume hood). Filter through Whatman paper (again in a fume hood) and store in a dark bottle at 4°C.
3. For exons 4, 7, 8. 14, 16 and 18 of hMLH1, 2.0 mM MgCl were used to improve efficiency of the amplification.
4. For exons 1 and 4 of the gene hMLH1, annealing condition used for PCR are 57 and 50°C, respectively; while optimal annealing temperature for exons 1, 3, 11 and 15 of the gene hMSH2 is 60°C, and for exons 8, 10 and 12 is 50°C.
5. The protocol is based on the HOEFER SE 620 (San Francisco, CA) gel electrophoresis system.
6. A proper plug is important to prevent leakage when the gradient gel is cast.
7. The temperature of the running buffer is very important, and it must not be allowed to deviate from 60°C, as this is an important characteristic of the denaturing gradient. If the temperature is too high, DNA fragments may not migrate far enough into the gel, and if it is too low, migration may be too far.
8. It was difficult to obtain conclusive results with DGGE for exon 5 of the hMSH2, therefore constant denaturant gel electrophoresis (CDGE) was performed as described previously [16].
9. In case of a high background observed, an additional 15 min destaining step can be used to improve visualization.

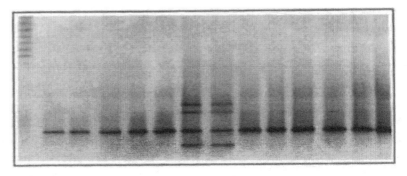

Fig. 1. Mutation detection in the MMR gene, hMLH1. DGGE showing aberrant bands of exon 7 of hMLH1 in two affected individuals from a HNPCC family.

10. Figure 1 shows typical silver stained DGGE gel for a splice site variation in hMLH1. It is a substitution of A→G at position-2 of the splice acceptor site upstream of exon 7. This mutation would cause skipping of exon 7, resulting in an out-frame deletion that would lead to premature translation at downstream stop codon. Two affected family members shared this mutation indicating that it is most likely to be a disease causing mutation.
11. In this case, samples are amplified using the non-GC-clamp primer and sequenced directly.
12. Other optional sequencing methods can be applied.

Acknowledgements

The author would like to thank Professor Annika Lindblom for her advice and encouragement. This work was supported by Swedish Cancer Society.

References

1. Lynch, H.T., and de la Chapelle, A. (1999) Genetic susceptibility to non-polyposis colorectal cancer. *J. Med. Genet.* **36**, 801–818
2. Wijnen, J., Vasen, H., Khan, P. M., Menko, F.H., van der Klift, H., van Leeuwen, C., et al. (1995) Seven new mutations in hMSH2, an HNPCC gene, identified by denaturing gradient-gel electrophoresis. *Am. J. Hum. Genet.* **56**, 1060–1066
3. Han, H.J., Maruyama, M., Baba, S., Park, J.G., and Nakamura, Y. (1995) Genomic structure of human mismatch repair gene, hMLH1, and its mutation analysis in patients with hereditary non-polyposis colorectal cancer (HNPCC). *Hum. Mol. Genet.* **4**, 237–242
4. Froggatt, N.J., Brassett, C., Koch, D.J., Evans, D.G., Hodgson, S.V., Ponder, B.A., et al. (1996) Mutation screening of MSH2 and MLH1 mRNA in hereditary non-polyposis colon cancer syndrome. *J. Med. Genet.* **33**, 726–730
5. Luce, M.C., Binnie, C.G., Cayouette, M.C., and Kam-Morgan, L.N. (1996) Identification

of DNA mismatch repair gene mutations in hereditary nonpolyposis colon cancer patients. *Int. J. Cancer* **69**, 50–52

6. Wang, Q., Desseigne, F., Lasset, C., Saurin, J. C., Navarro, C., Yagci, T., et al. (1997) Germline hMSH2 and hMLH1 gene mutations in incomplete HNPCC families. *Int. J. Cancer* **73**, 831–836

7. Farrington, S.M., Lin-Goerke, J., Ling, J., Wang, Y., Burczak, J.D., Robbins, D.J., et al. (1998) Systematic analysis of hMSH2 and hMLH1 in young colon cancer patients and controls. *Am. J. Hum. Genet.* **63**, 749–759

8. Papadopoulos, N., Leach, F.S., Kinzler, K.W., and Vogelstein, B. (1995) Monoallelic mutation analysis (MAMA) for identifying germline mutations. *Nat. Genet.* **11**, 99–102

9. http://www.hgmd.cf.ac.uk/ac/index.php

10. Wahlberg, S., Liu, T., Lindblom, P., and Lindblom, A. (1999) Various mutation screening techniques in the DNA mismatch repair genes hMSH2 and hMLH1. *Genet. Test.* **3**, 259–264

11. Fischer, S.G., and Lerman, L.S. (1983) DNA fragments differing by single base-pair substitutions are separated in denaturing gradient gels: correspondence with melting theory. *Proc. Natl. Acad. Sci. USA* **80**, 1579–1583

12. Myers, R.M., Fischer, S.G., Lerman, L.S., and Maniatis, T. (1985) Nearly all single base substitutions in DNA fragments joined to a GC-clamp can be detected by denaturing gradient gel electrophoresis. *Nucleic Acids Res.* **13**, 3131–3145

13. Olschwang, S., Laurent-Puig, P., Groden, J., White, R., and Thomas, G. (1993) Germ-line mutations in the first 14 exons of the adenomatous polyposis coli (APC) gene. *Am. J. Hum. Genet.* **52**, 273–279

14. Olschwang, S., Tiret, A., Laurent-Puig, P., Muleris, M., Parc, R., and Thomas, G. (1993) Restriction of ocular fundus lesions to a specific subgroup of APC mutations in adenomatous polyposis coli patients. *Cell* **75**, 959–968

15. Fodde, R., and Losekoot, M. (1994) Mutation detection by denaturing gradient gel electrophoresis (DGGE). *Hum. Mutat.* **3**, 83–94

16. Sheffield, V.C., Cox, D.R., Lerman, L.S., and Myers, R.M. (1989) Attachment of a 40-basepair G+C-rich sequence (GC-clamp) to genomic DNA fragments by the polymerase chain reaction results in improved detection of single-base changes. *Proc. Natl. Acad. Sci. USA* **86**, 232–236

Chapter 12

s-RT-MELT: A Novel Technology for Mutation Screening

Jin Li and G. Mike Makrigiorgos

Abstract

The fast growing understanding of genetic pathways that mediate cancer etiology, biology, and personalized medicine leads to an increasing need for extensive and reliable mutation screening on a population or on a single patient basis. Here we describe s-RT-MELT, a novel technology that enables expanded-throughput enzymatic mutation scanning in clinical cancer samples for germline or low-level somatic mutations, or for SNP genotyping. GC-clamp-containing PCR products from tumor and normal cells are hybridized to generate mismatches at the positions of mutations over one or multiple sequences in parallel. Mismatches are converted to double strand breaks using a DNA endonuclease (Surveyor™), and poly A oligonucleotide tails are enzymatically attached at the position of the mutations. A novel application of PCR that operates at low denaturation temperatures enables the selective amplification of mutation-containing DNA fragments and high-throughput, closed-tube mutation scanning via melting curve analysis on conventional or nanotechnology real-time PCR platforms. We have applied s-RT-MELT in the screening of TP53 and EGFR mutations in cell lines and clinical samples and demonstrate its advantages for rapid, multiplexed mutation scanning in cancer.

Key words: Cancer, Mutation detection, Low-level somatic mutation, SNP, Surveyor™, Melting curve, Low denaturation temperatures

1. Introduction

Screening for genetic changes to unveil molecular attributes of tumor specimens is important for predicting the outcome of diseases and identifying cancer biomarkers and can affect treatment decisions for individual patients (1–3). For example, mutations in genes like EGFR can profoundly influence EGFR tyrosine kinase inhibitors' response in lung cancer and the response is modulated by mutations in other genes of the same signaling pathway (e.g., K-ras, HER2, ErbB-3) (4–7). Therefore, there is a need for an efficient and high throughput mutation screening of several genes along identified signal transduction pathways in tumor samples.

Because a large portion of cancer-causing mutations remains unknown and can occur in numerous positions along tumor suppressor genes (e.g., TP53, ATM, PTEN), mutation scanning rather than detection of specific mutations is frequently required for molecular cancer profiling (8–10).

Recently, an enzymatic mutation scanning method based on the Surveyor™ (CELI/II) nuclease combined with dHPLC detection was introduced (11–13). This method shows satisfactory selectivity and reliability (1% mutant to wild type alleles is detectable) and also identifies all base substitutions and small deletions that are important to cancer (14, 15). While reliable, the use of dHPLC for examining Surveyor™-generated DNA fragments is a slow endpoint detection method restricted to examining a single DNA fragment at a time and the resulting DNA fragments cannot be sequenced. This limits the analysis of cancer specimens when numerous samples or genetic regions need to be screened.

We recently developed a new approach that enables Surveyor™ to scan for mutations over one or several PCR products simultaneously and selectively amplifies and isolates the mutation-containing DNA fragment(s) via linker-mediated PCR, known as s-RT-MELT (see Fig. 1) (16). By selectively amplifying mutation-containing DNA from wild type fragments, the present approach decouples enzymatic mutation scanning from the endpoint detection step. As a result, following enzymatic action on mismatches, any chosen DNA detection method (real-time PCR, gel/capillary electrophoresis, microarray-based detection) can potentially be used to identify the mutated DNA fragments in a simplex or multiplex fashion. Here we utilize real-time PCR coupled with melting curve analysis to validate the new technology. We demonstrate that this approach increases the mutation scanning throughput by one to two orders of magnitude when several (>100) samples are to be prescanned for mutations, enables mutation scanning over several PCR fragments simultaneously, and mutation-positive samples can be directly sequenced when somatic mutations are at a low-level (~1–10% mutant-to-wild type ratio) in surgical cancer specimens.

The principle of s-RT-MELT is explained in Fig. 1. The s-RT-MELT assay converts PCR fragments generated at positions of mutations by the Surveyor™ enzyme to fully amplifiable sequences that enable selective PCR amplification in a subsequent quantitative PCR detection method. Following denaturation and reannealing of PCR products that leads to the formation of heteroduplexes at the positions of mutations (see Fig. 1a), the sample is exposed to Surveyor™ endonuclease that recognizes base pair mismatches or small loops with high specificity and generates a break on both DNA strands 3′ to the mismatch. The resulting DNA fragments participate in a terminal transferase

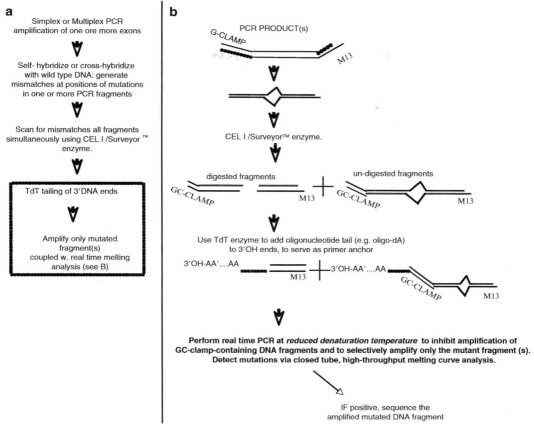

Fig. 1. s-RT-MELT for rapid mutation scanning using enzymatic selection and real-time DNA-melting. (**a**) General outline of the approach. The *dotted line* contains the new steps involved in s-RT-MELT relative to previous approaches. (**b**) Detailed outline of the procedure used to selectively amplify the mutation-containing fragments in s-RT-MELT.

(TdT) reaction, which leads to polynucleotide "tailing" (sequential addition of adenine, polyA-tail) at the 3′ ends. A real-time PCR reaction is subsequently performed using adjusted conditions that enable the selective amplification of the mutant-only fragments, followed by real-time melting curve analysis for the identification of mutations in the presence of SYBR-GREEN™ or LC-GREEN™ DNA dye.

To enable the selective amplification of the mutation-containing fragments in the real-time PCR step, modified primers are employed for the original amplification from genomic DNA (see Fig. 1b). The forward primer contains a region specific to the target gene and a high melting domain (GC-clamp) at the 5′ end, while the reverse primer contains a region specific to the target gene and an M13 tail (or vice versa). Following the TdT tailing reaction, the M13 primer is used for real-time PCR in conjunction with a primer that binds to the polyA tail. The denaturation temperature of the real-time PCR reaction is lowered to enable PCR amplification only for fragments that do not contain GC-clamps. Because the PCR products that escape digestion by Surveyor™ contain GC-clamps (see Fig. 1b), these fragments do not amplify efficiently during PCR, thereby enabling the selective amplification of Surveyor™-selected fragments, that is, an effective "purification" of mutation-containing fragments. The subsequent closed-tube melting curve analysis enables clear separation of true mutant sequences from PCR dimers or other artifacts.

Because s-RT-MELT does not require size separation for the identification of enzymatically generated fragments, more than one sequence can be scanned in parallel for unknown mutations in a single tube reaction of Surveyor™. This simple procedure enables the specificity of the Surveyor™ enzyme to be combined with the throughput and convenience of real-time PCR for rapid mutation scanning. Finally, because the amplified mutated sequences contain defined primers at their ends, direct sequencing of enzymatically selected PCR products is readily possible following the real-time melting step, enabling the sequencing of low-level mutations identified by Surveyor™.

2. Materials

2.1. Samples and DNA Extraction

1. Cancer cell line DNA containing known mutations, for example, SW480 cell line DNA with defined mutations in TP53 exon 8 and 9 (American Type Culture Collection, Manassas, VA).
2. Tumor specimens, for example, surgical colon cancer tumor samples (Massachusetts General Hospital Tumor Bank, Boston, MA).
3. DNeasy™ Tissue Kit for DNA extraction (Qiagen, Valencia, CA).

2.2. PCR with Primers Containing 5'-GC-Clamp and 5'-M13

1. Sequences for the 5'-M13 and GC-clamp portion of the primers as well as the gene-specific portion of the primers used in this investigation are listed in Table 1. The M13f and GC-clamp sequence was added to the 5' end of the forward and reverse gene-specific primers, respectively, or vice versa. Primers are synthesized by IDT (Coralville, IA).
2. PCR reagents: ultra pure distilled water DNAse, RNAse free (Invitrogen, Carlsbad, CA); 10× JumpStart™ buffer with 15 mM $MgCL_2$ and polymerase (Sigma, St. Louis, MO); dNTP, 10 mM each (New England Biolabs, Ipswich, MA).
3. PCR machine: Perkin Elmer 9600 PCR machine (Perkin Elmer, Waltham, MA).

Table 1
Primer sequences used to amplify p53 exon 5–9

	Direction	Sequence (5'→3')
P53-exon-5	Forward	GGGCAGGGCGGCGGGGGCGGGGCC ACTTGTGCCCTGACTTTCAAC
	Reverse	TGTAAAACGACGGCCAGTG CAACCAGCCCTGTCGTCTC
P53-exon-6	Forward	GCGGGCAGGGCGGCGGGGGCGGGGCC GGTTGCCCAGGGTCCCCAG
	Reverse	TGTAAAACGACGGCCAGTG GCCACTGACAACCACCCTTAACC
P53-exon-7	Forward	TGTAAAACGACGGCCAGTG CCACAGGTCTCCCCAAGGC
	Reverse	GCGGGCAGGGCGGCGGGGGCGGGGCC TGGGGCACAGCAGGCCAGTG
P53-exon-8	Forward	TGTAAAACGACGGCCAGTG GACCTGATTTCCTTACTGCC
	Reverse	GGCAGGGCGGCGGGGGCGGGGCC GAATCTGAGGCATAACTGCACC
P53-exon-9	Forward	TGTAAAACGACGGCCAGTG GGTGCAGTTATGCCTCAGATT
	Reverse	GCAGGGCGGCGGGGGCGGGGCC CGGCATTTTGAGTGTTAGACTGG

2.3. Treatment of Heteroduplexes with the Surveyor™ Endonuclease

1. Surveyor™ and Enhancer™ (Transgenomic, Omaha, NE).
2. Qiaquick™ PCR Purification Kit (Qiagen, Valencia, CA).

2.4. Addition of PolyA-Tail on the 3'-End

Reaction buffer-4, $CoCl_2$, dATP, Terminal Transferase (New England Biolabs, Ipswich, MA).

2.5. Real-Time PCR, Melting Curve Analysis, Sequencing, and dHPLC

1. Real-time PCR reagents: Titanium-Taq™ polymerase (Clontech, Mountain View, CA); dNTP, 10 mM each (New England Biolabs, Ipswich, MA); LCGreen™ (Salt Lake City, Utah); m13f primer, oligodT-anchor mix GACCACGCGT ATCGATGTCGACTTTTTTTTTTTTTTTTV (V represents A, C, and G, each oligodT-anchor concentration is 0.067 µM, as per RACE protocol) (synthesized by IDT, Coralville, IA).
2. Real-time PCR machine: SmartCycler™ (Cepheid, Sunnyvale, CA).

3. WAVE™ system (Transgenomic, Omaha, NE).
4. OpenArray™ (BioTrove, Woburn, MA).
5. ExoSAP-IT® (USB, Cleveland, OH).

3. Methods

3.1. Extraction of Genomic DNA

Extract and purify genomic DNA from cell lines and fresh tissues using the DNeasy™ Tissue Kit, according to the manufacturer's instructions (see Note 1).

3.2. Simplex s-RT-MELT

Simplex s-RT-MELT is designed for the detection of mutations in single amplicon with s-RT-MELT method.

3.2.1. PCR with Primers Containing 5'-GC-Clamp and 5'-M13

1. For each sample to test, combine the following reagents in a 20 µL volume reaction (see Note 2).

Components	Final concentration
10× JumpStart buffer (with 15 mM MgCl$_2$)	1× JumpStart buffer (with 1.5 mM MgCl$_2$)
dNTP, 10 mM each	dNTP, 0.2 mM each
Forward primer	0.2 µM
Reverse primer	0.2 µM
JumpStart Taq polymerase	1× JumpStart Taq polymerase
Water	Balance to 20 µL

PCR primer design follows general rules. Here, we use Oligo 6 software to design all the primers (see Note 3). M13 tail: TGTAAAACGACGGCCAGTG and GC clamp tail: GCGGGCAGGGCGGCGGGGGCGGGGCC can be added to 5' end of forward and reverse gene specific primers, respectively, or vice versa. These long primers should be PAGE or HPLC purified by the vendor (see Note 4). In some cases, GC clamp can only be added to one of the two primers to allow specific and robust amplification of the target sequence.

2. Add 5–20 ng of sample template DNA to each tube and mix well. Run the PCR on the Perkin Elmer 9600 PCR machine using the following thermocycling program: 94°C, 90 s; (94°C, 20 s/65°C, 20 s/68°C, 1 min) × 10 cycles, with annealing temperature decreasing 1°C/cycle, touch-down PCR; (94°C, 20 s/55°C, 20 s/68°C, 1 min) × 30 cycles; and 68°C, 5 min (see Note 5). This PCR program was linked to

a program for denaturation and reannealing of the PCR product over 10 min: 94°C, 60 s; 12°C, 60 s with the slope of decreasing temperature defined as 10 min. The PCR product should be checked with agarose gel or dHPLC before moving to the next step.

3.2.2. Treatment of Heteroduplexes with the Surveyor™ Endonuclease

1. 5 µL PCR product (300–500 ng) from Subheading 3.2.1 was mixed with 0.5 µL Enhancer™ and 0.5 µL Surveyor™ and incubated at 42°C for 20 min followed by adding 1 µL stop-solution, as per manufacturer's protocol (see Note 6).

2. The inactivated Surveyor™-digested product was purified using a QiaQuick™ PCR purification kit and eluted in 35 µL water.

3.2.3. Addition of PolyA-Tail on the 3'-End

Following the purification of the Surveyor™-treated sample, Poly-adenine tail was added to the 3' ends of DNA fragments (see Note 7). For each reaction, we added 5 µL: purified surveyor-digested PCR product to a final volume of 20 µL with final concentration of 1× reaction buffer-4, 1× $CoCl_2$, 0.2 mM dATP, and 4 U Terminal Transferase. The reaction was incubated at 37°C for 10 min and inactivated by heating at 75°C for 10 min.

3.2.4. Real-Time PCR to Selectively Amplify Mutant Fragment

1. For each sample to test, combine the following reagents in a 20 µL volume reaction (see Note 8).

Components	Final concentration
10× Titanium buffer	1× Titanium buffer
dNTP, 10 mM each	dNTP, 0.2 mM each
M13f	0.2 µM
OligodT-anchor mix	0.2 µM total, each 0.067 µM
10× LCGreen	0.1× LCGreen
PolyA-tailed DNA	0.5 µL
50× Titanium Taq polymerase	1× Titanium Taq polymerase
Water	Balance to 20 µL

2. The real-time PCR amplification was performed in a Smart Cycler real-time PCR machine (see Note 9). The thermocycling program was as follows: 1 cycle of 94°C for 2 min, 25 cycles of denaturation temperature for 15 s, 55°C for 20 s and 68°C for 30 s for reading fluorescence. Denaturation temperatures were from 94 to 82°C (decreasing 1°C with each reaction) to experimentally determine conditions that selectively enable mutation-containing fragments to amplify (see Note 10).

3.2.5. Down-Stream Assays for Mutant Detection

1. Melting curve analysis: The real-time PCR step was immediately followed by real-time differential melting curve analysis using the SmartCycler™ machine. Samples were heated from 70 to 95°C at a rate of 0.1°C/s. Differential fluorescent intensity curves (–dF/dT) were smoothed and used for the identification of melting peak(s).

2. dHPLC: the s-RT-melt product and original Surveyor digested PCR product can be run on dHPLC to observe the enrichment of the mutant fragment and inhibition of the full-length PCR product with the GC clamp (see Note 11).

   dHPLC running gradients:

Gradient name	Time (min)	Buffer A (%)	Buffer B (%)
Loading	0	65	35
Starting gradient	0.5	60	40
Stop gradient	9.5	35	65
Start clean	9.6	0	100
Stop clean	10.1	0	100
Start equilibration	10.2	65	35
Stop equilibration	11.1	65	35

   This program is designed for amplicons of 100–350 bp.

3. Sanger sequencing: PCR product from s-RT-melt can be cleaned up with ExoSAP-IT®, which contains Exonuclease I and Shrimp Alkaline Phosphotase to degrade primers and dephosphorylate dNTP. The conditions follow the protocol described in the manufacturer's instructions. M13f primer will be used as a sequencing primer (see Note 12).

4. Expected results: To provide initial proof of principle for unknown mutation scanning using s-RT-MELT, we utilized cell lines containing known mutations at several positions of TP53 exon 8. Figure 2a depicts dHPLC chromatograms of the products obtained using a sample containing a TP53 exon 8 G>A mutation or a wild type sample. The standard Surveyor™-dHPLC approach was first employed to identify the mutation following PCR amplification of exon 8 from genomic DNA. The resulting dHPLC traces contain a single product for the wild type and two products for the mutation-containing sequences (see Fig. 2a, curves 1 and 2, respectively). Next, s-RT-MELT was used to screen the same TP53 exon 8 sequence. Following PCR amplification with GC/M13-modified primers, we heteroduplexed PCR products and exposed them to Surveyor™ and TdT tailing. The subsequent real-time PCR was run at different denaturation temperatures and the products were examined either via dHPLC

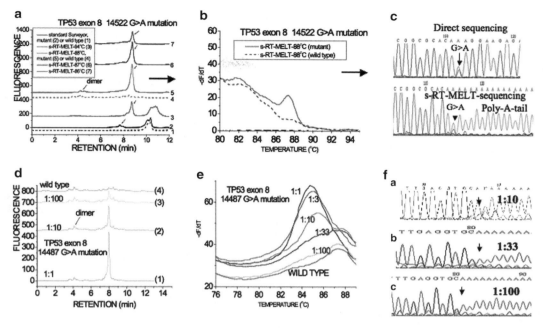

Fig. 2. Detection of TP53 exon 8 mutations using s-RT-MELT. (**a**) dHPLC chromatograms of the products obtained using CT5 containing a TP53 exon 8 G>A mutation or a wild type sample with gradient denaturing temperature. (**b**) Real-time differential melting curves for the PCR of the CT5 reaction run at 88°C. (**c**) Sequencing of the s-RT-MELT-generated PCR fragment and the direct sequencing of the PCR product of TP53 exon 8 from genomic DNA of CT5. The *arrow* indicates the mutation. (**d**) dHPLC chromatograms of the PCR products obtained using serial dilution of SW480 in wild type DNA at a denaturing temperature of 88°C. (**e**) Melting curve analysis of the PCR products obtained using serial dilution of SW480 in wild type DNA at a denaturing temperature of 88°C. (**f**) s-RT-MELT-sequencing of PCR products obtained using serial dilution of SW480 in wild type DNA at a denaturing temperature of 88°C. The *arrow* indicates the mutation.

or via real-time melting-curve analysis. At the standard denaturation temperature of 94°C, the mutation-containing sample contains two peaks, corresponding to the anticipated amplification of both Surveyor™-digested and undigested fragments (see Fig. 2a, curve 3). However, when the PCR denaturation temperature is lowered (e.g., 86–88°C) (see Note 13), a single PCR product is generated for the mutant sample, while the wild type sample demonstrates no product (see Fig. 2a, curves 4–7). In Fig. 2b, real-time differential melting curves for the PCR reaction run at 88°C are depicted. A peak corresponding to the PCR product from the mutant sample is again clearly evident, which is absent in the wild type sample. Finally, Fig. 2c depicts the sequencing of the s-RT-MELT-generated PCR fragment, as well as the direct sequencing from genomic DNA. The G>A mutation is evident in both samples. In the s-RT-MELT product, the anticipated addition of the polyA tail at the 3′-position next to the mutation is illustrated.

To examine the selectivity of s-RT-MELT, dilutions of mutant to wild type DNA were performed using DNA from SW480 cells that harbor a TP53 exon 8 14487 G>A homozygous mutation. The real-time PCR reaction was again performed at 88°C and mutant-to-wild type ratios down to 1% were distinguished from the wild type using either dHPLC (see Fig. 2d) or melting curve analysis (see Fig. 2e). s-RT-MELT products, including the 1% sample were successfully sequenced (see Fig. 2f). Direct di-deoxy-sequencing could not identify a mutation if the ratio of mutant to wild type was less than ~25% (not shown) (see Notes 14 and 15).

3.3. Multiplex s-RT-MELT

Multiple PCR products amplified from different exons are mixed together at equimolar concentrations and digested with Surveyor, followed by poly A tailing and real-time PCR enrichment. The denaturing temperature is determined as the highest temperature to allow the inhibition of the amplification of all the GC-tailed amplicons (see Note 13 and 16). An example of the results produced is shown in Fig. 3a.

3.4. s-RT-MELT on OpenArray™ Platform

The OpenArray™ high throughput, massively parallel real-time PCR platform (BioTrove) was adopted for increasing the throughput of simplex s-RT-MELT. The real-time PCR was done with LightCycler FastStart DNA Master SYBR Green I (Roche) with 0.2 µM m13f primer, 0.2 µM oligodT-anchor mix and polyA-tailed DNA as template in OpenArray platform. The cycling condition is as follows: 1 cycle of 94°C for 2 min, 25 cycles of 90°C for 15 s, 55°C for 20 s, and 68°C for 30 s for reading fluorescence. The real-time PCR step was immediately followed by real-time

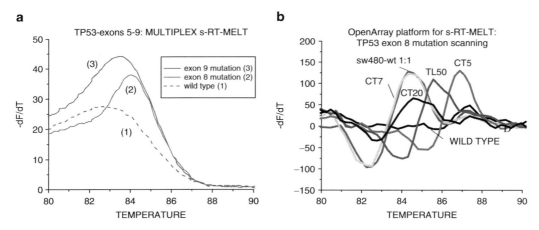

Fig. 3. Multiplex s-RT-MELT or OpenArray™-based s-RT-MELT. (**a**) Melting curves obtained following Multiplex s-RT-MELT of TP53 exon 5–9 for an exon 8 mutation (1:1 mixture of DNA from SW480 and wild type) and an exon 9 mutation (1:1 mixture of DNA from SW480 and wild type) and wild type. (**b**) Melting curves obtained following OpenArray based s-RT-MELT of TP53 exon 8 with lung and colon tumor samples.

differential melting curve analysis. Data were exported and analyzed in Origin. An example of the results produced is shown in Fig. 3b.

4. Notes

1. Other genomic DNA extraction kits could alternatively be used.
2. Other PCR kits could alternatively be used.
3. Other PCR primer design software could alternatively be used.
4. The aim of the purification of long primers is to prevent truncated primers from interfering with the inhibition effect of full length GC clamp on undigested amplicons by Surveyor.
5. Touchdown PCR is used for acquiring specific amplification of target sequence with less effort to optimize the PCR condition.
6. It is not necessary to purify PCR products before Surveyor digestion. The incubation should not be longer than 20 min because the enzymes may start digesting the end of the DNA, which will result in the loss of the GC clamp. It is therefore important to add STOP solution (EDTA) into the reaction immediately following the incubation. In some experiments, the PCR product was mixed with an approximately equal amount of PCR product from wild type DNA prior to forming heteroduplexes, to facilitate the detection of homozygous mutations.
7. dCTP, dGTP, or dTTP can be used for tailing instead of dATP. Thus, the corresponding complementary oligo-anchor primer needs to be used in the PCR (e.g., for poly T tail, oligodA-anchor mix 5′-GACCACGCGTATCGATGTCGA CAAAAAAAAAAAAAAAA<u>V</u>-3′ <u>V</u> represents T, C, and G, each oligodA-anchor concentration is 0.067 µM).
8. Other Taq polymerases can be used except proof-reading Taq polymerase because a proof-reading enzyme will destroy the allele specificity of the oligodT-anchor primer. The final concentration of LCGreen can be 1× here.
9. Other types of PCR machine can be used.
10. A temperature window, which is able to inhibit the amplification of DNA containing a GC clamp, but allows the amplification of DNA without GC clamp, can be found experimentally by applying multiple reactions in parallel with decreasing denaturing temperature. The width of the window is usually

2–6°C. If the final concentration of LCGreen is increased to 1×, it will increase the temperature window by approximately 1°C.

11. A 2% agarose gel can be used to substitute for dHPLC, with less discrimination ability, however.

12. If the PCR product is larger than 100 bp, commercialized PCR purification kits such as the Qiaquick™ PCR Purification Kit can be used instead of the Exo-SAP. When nonspecific PCR products are present, the specific band can be cut from the agarose gel, followed by sequencing.

13. The temperature window is defined as temperatures to allow the enrichment of the mutant peak and full inhibition of GC-tailed amplicon. Different amplicons may have different ranges, for example, the window of exon 8 is 84–88°C and the window of exon 9 is 83–84°C. Therefore, the denaturing temperature for the multiplex s-RT-MELT of these two amplicons should be 84°C.

14. sRT-MELT sequencing generated traces with polyA tails depicting the presence and the position of the mutation, although the exact nucleotide change was less clear than the one in Fig. 2c (i.e., the position ±1 base from the mutation might also be confused to be a mutation). The reason for this ±1 base ambiguity of the exact position of the mutation can probably be understood. The PCR performed following polyA tail addition contains an equimolar mixture of three reverse primers (3′ ending in V = G, A or C). Depending on the exact nucleotide at the mutation, the correct primer should in theory be preferred, while the other two primers should not allow efficient polymerase extension due to the mismatched 3′-end. However, in practice, this "allele-specific PCR" step occasionally allows 3′-mismatched primer extension, enabling more than one version of the primer to amplify over the position of the mutation, or alternatively the incorporation of the polyA tail may occur ±1 base from the exact position of the mutation. We conclude that in certain cases, s-RT-MELT indicates the position of the mutation to within 1 base, while in others (e.g., TP53 exon 5), it indicates the position and the actual nucleotide change.

15. Yet in the case of ambiguous sequencing by s-RT-MELT, the position of the mutation can be defined and the restriction site mutation method can be applied to confirm the mutation.

16. The overlapped temperature among the denaturation temperature windows of different amplicons will be used for denaturing in the multiplex application.

References

1. Simpson, A.J. (2009) Sequence-based advances in the definition of cancer-associated gene mutations. *Curr. Opin. Oncol.* **21**, 47–52.
2. Chan, T.A., Glockner, S., Yi, J.M., Chen, W., Van Neste, L., Cope, L., et al. (2008) Convergence of mutation and epigenetic alterations identifies common genes in cancer that predict for poor prognosis. *PLoS Med.* **5**, e114.
3. Herbst, R.S., Heymach, J.V., and Lippman, S.M. (2008) Lung cancer. *N. Engl. J. Med.* **359**, 1367–1380.
4. Paez, J.G., Janne, P.A., Lee, J.C., Tracy, S., Greulich, H., Gabriel, S., et al. (2004) EGFR mutations in lung cancer: correlation with clinical response to gefitinib therapy. *Science* **304**, 1497–1500.
5. Baselga, J. (2006) Targeting tyrosine kinases in cancer: the second wave. *Science* **312**, 1175–1178.
6. Kobayashi, S., Boggon, T.J., Dayaram, T., Janne, P.A., Kocher, O., Meyerson, M., et al. (2005) EGFR mutation and resistance of non-small-cell lung cancer to gefitinib. *N. Engl. J. Med.* **352**, 786–792.
7. Engelman, J.A., and Janne, P.A. (2008) Mechanisms of acquired resistance to epidermal growth factor receptor tyrosine kinase inhibitors in non-small cell lung cancer. *Clin. Cancer Res.* **14**, 2895–2899.
8. Ding, L., Getz, G., Wheeler, D.A., Mardis, E.R., McLellan, M.D., Cibulskis, K., et al. (2008) Somatic mutations affect key pathways in lung adenocarcinoma. *Nature* **455**, 1069–1075.
9. Jones, S., Zhang, X., Parsons, D.W., Lin, J.C., Leary, R.J., Angenendt, P., et al. (2008) Core signaling pathways in human pancreatic cancers revealed by global genomic analyses. *Science* **321**, 1801–1806.
10. Parsons, D.W., Jones, S., Zhang, X., Lin, J.C., Leary, R.J., Angenendt, P., et al. (2008) An integrated genomic analysis of human glioblastoma multiforme. *Science* **321**, 1807–1812.
11. Oleykowski, C.A., Bronson Mullins, C.R., Godwin, A.K., and Yeung, A.T. (1998) Mutation detection using a novel plant endonuclease. *Nucleic Acids Res.* **26**, 4597–4602.
12. Yeung, A.T., Hattangadi, D., Blakesley, L., and Nicolas, E. (2005) Enzymatic mutation detection technologies. *Biotechniques* **38**, 749–758.
13. Yang, B., Wen, X., Kodali, N.S., Oleykowski, C.A., Miller, C.G., Kulinski, J., et al. (2000) Purification, cloning, and characterization of the CEL I nuclease. *Biochemistry* **39**, 3533–3541.
14. Janne, P.A., Borras, A.M., Kuang, Y., Rogers, A.M., Joshi, V.A., Liyanage, H., et al. (2006) A rapid and sensitive enzymatic method for epidermal growth factor receptor mutation screening. *Clin. Cancer Res.* **12**, 751–758.
15. Poeta, M.L., Manola, J., Goldwasser, M.A., Forastiere, A., Benoit, N., Califano, J.A., et al. (2007) TP53 mutations and survival in squamous-cell carcinoma of the head and neck. *N. Engl. J. Med.* **357**, 2552–2561.
16. Li, J., Berbeco, R., Distel, R.J., Janne, P.A., Wang, L., and Makrigiorgos, G.M. (2007) s-RT-MELT for rapid mutation scanning using enzymatic selection and real time DNA-melting: new potential for multiplex genetic analysis. *Nucleic Acids Res.* **35**, e84.

Chapter 13

Zoom-In Array Comparative Genomic Hybridization (aCGH) to Detect Germline Rearrangements in Cancer Susceptibility Genes

Johan Staaf and Åke Borg

Abstract

Disease predisposing germline mutations in cancer susceptibility genes may consist of large genomic rearrangements, including deletions or duplications that are challenging, to detect and characterize using standard PCR-based mutation screening methods. Such rearrangements range from single exons up to hundreds of kilobases of sequence in size. Array-based comparative genomic hybridization (aCGH) has evolved as a powerful technique to detect copy number alterations on a genome-wide scale. However, the conventional genome-wide approach of aCGH still provides only limited information about copy number status for individual exons. Custom-designed aCGH arrays focused on only a few target regions (zoom-in aCGH) may circumvent this drawback. Benefits of zoom-in aCGH include the possibility to target almost any region in the genome, and an unbiased coverage of exonic and intronic sequence facilitating convenient design of primers for sequence determination of the breakpoints. Furthermore, zoom-in aCGH can be streamlined for a particular application, for example, focusing on breast cancer susceptibility genes, with increased capacity using multiformat design.

Key words: BRCA1, BRCA2, MSH2, MLH1, Germline mutation, Large rearrangement, Array CGH

1. Introduction

Germline mutations in cancer susceptibility genes, such as the breast–ovarian cancer genes *BRCA1* and *BRCA2*, and the hereditary nonpolyposis colorectal cancer (HNPCC) genes *MSH2* and *MLH1* (among other mismatch repair genes), are highly penetrant and confer a high lifetime risk of developing disease (1, 2). Most deleterious mutations constitute either small frameshift insertions/deletions or nonsense mutations that give rise to premature stop codons, missense mutations in conserved and functionally important domains, or splice site mutations resulting in aberrant transcript processing (3, 4). Mutations may also comprise more complex rearrangements, including deletions and duplications of larger genomic regions, that may escape detection using traditional nonquantitative PCR-based mutation screening and sequencing of DNA templates due to the removal of primer sites (5). Screening of hereditary cancer susceptibility genes is important for genetic counseling in affected families and for early diagnosis or disease prevention in carriers.

Several DNA-based assays suitable as clinical screening tools exist for the detection of exon-sized deletions or duplications in cancer susceptibility genes, for example, Southern blot, color bar coding, quantitative multiplex PCR of short fluorescent fragments (QMPSF), semi-quantitative multiplex PCR, and multiplex ligation-dependent probe amplification (MLPA) (6–10). Although many techniques provide information as to whether specific exons are deleted or duplicated, mutation verification using PCR and sequencing is often a tedious step-wise approach as only limited or no information is provided about the location of the genomic breakpoints. During recent years, array comparative genomic hybridization (aCGH) has evolved as a powerful technique to detect and delineate genomic alterations originating from copy number gain or loss, either as somatic events in tumors (11) or germline events as highlighted for different congenital disorders (12). Conventional aCGH has been useful in detecting genomic alterations on a genome-wide scale while providing only limited information on alterations in individual genes at the exonic and intronic level. Custom-designed focused oligonucleotide-based aCGH (zoom-in aCGH) has recently been successfully applied for the detection and precise mapping of exon-sized deletions and duplications both for somatic rearrangements in tumors (13) and for germline rearrangements in cancer susceptibility genes (14, 15).

2. Design of a Zoom-In aCGH Platform for Detection of Exon Sized Copy Number Alterations

Conventional aCGH is based on a competitive hybridization between test DNA and reference DNA (labeled with different fluorescent dyes) to a microarray surface populated with a large number of precisely positioned spots containing unique DNA fragments (probes). After the removal of unbound DNA, the fluorescent intensity signals for the remaining test and reference DNAs that hybridized to the array are recorded separately for each probe. A comparative measurement of the amount of DNA in the sample compared to the reference for each probe is obtained by calculating intensity ratios (test/reference). In aCGH, the reference sample is conventionally selected as being DNA from blood cells of a healthy individual, or from a pool of individuals having an expected diploid representation of DNA at any given genomic locus. Reference pools are commonly employed to reduce the impact of individual copy number variations (CNVs). The intensity ratio for a probe thus reflects a quantitative estimate of genetic material in the test sample compared to an expected amount in the reference sample (copy number estimate) for a unique position in the investigated genome. Recently SNP-CGH (16), based on the analysis of single nucleotide polymorphisms (SNP) loci in a microarray format, has become increasingly popular as it offers both detection of copy number alterations and allele-specific changes such as allele imbalances and loss of heterozygosity (LOH). In SNP-CGH, only the test DNA sample is hybridized to the array. Copy number estimates for each SNP locus are formed by using bioinformatic algorithms to compare test sample (allele-specific) signal intensities to those of a predetermined set of reference samples processed identically.

Ordering of intensity ratios based on each probe's or SNP's unique genomic position generates a genomic profile of copy number estimates. On the basis of this genomic profile, regions of copy number gain, loss, or neutral status can be identified. The distance in base pairs between ordered probes in the genome determines the resolution of the analysis, that is, the level of detail on which a genomic alteration may be defined. Conventional aCGH and SNP-CGH analysis has primarily been focused on providing a genome-wide coverage, that is, having essentially equidistant spacing between probes throughout the entire genome. This approach is often unsuitable for the detection and precise mapping of very small genomic alterations, for example, of the size of one or a few exons in cancer susceptibility genes, due to the scarcity of probes in these small genomic regions. The insufficiency of conventional aCGH can be circumvented using custom-designed aCGH assays targeting only a few well-defined genomic regions. Focusing on only a limited number of defined genomic regions combined with the maximization of the number of probes in these regions, irrespective of association to coding or intronic sequences, allows for a significant increase in resolution and thus the possibility to precisely delineate very small genomic alterations. The benefits of zoom-in aCGH include the possibility of tailoring the assay to cover almost any region of the genome at high resolution as well as the redundancy of array probes, which makes the technique insensitive to sequence variants in probe binding sites and to problems that compromise assays such as MLPA. A high number of array probes covering both exonic and intronic regions allow zoom-in aCGH to detect genomic alterations affecting only parts of exons, as well as alterations located entirely within intronic regions and not previously recognized. Importantly, zoom-in aCGH can pinpoint breakpoints with great accuracy to facilitate primer design for mutation verification, thereby reducing the tedious step-wise PCR approach.

2.1. Choice of aCGH Platform

Zoom-in aCGH may be performed using a variety of either custom-designed commercial or in-house developed microarray platforms. Microarray platforms based on short oligonucleotide probes appear as the ideal choice for zoom-in aCGH since such probes can be designed bioinformatically to have similar hybridization properties and to avoid repetitive sequences, and are easily reproducibly manufactured on a large scale. Today, several commercial alternatives exist. Both Agilent Technologies (http://www.agilent.com) and Nimblegen (http://www.nimblegen.com) allow researchers to create custom-designed aCGH assays based on longer oligonucleotide probes (60–85 mers), while Affymetrix (http://www.affymetrix.com) and Illumina (http://www.illumina.com) offer the possibility to create custom-designed SNP assays. A major advantage of selecting commercially available platforms is that manufacturers often have precompiled databases consisting of millions of array probes to select from. These probe libraries are often designed to create a near to tiling path of probes throughout a genome, and to offer the best chance of success with standardized experimental protocols. Importantly, probes in these libraries have been designed to avoid repetitive regions in the genome consisting of short interspersed nuclear elements (SINEs), including Alu repeats, long interspersed nuclear elements (LINEs) or simple repeat sequences as exemplified in Fig. 1a. Unequal homologous recombination of such repetitive regions has been found to be the basis of many genomic rearrangements in cancer susceptibility genes (17, 18).

Due to different manufacturing technologies, suppliers offer different array formats (number and density of probes per sample) and possibilities to analyze several samples on a single microarray slide/chip for reduced experimental cost and increased throughput. For the experimental procedures described here, the Agilent Technologies oligonucleotide aCGH platform, based on inkjet synthesis of 60 mer oligonucleotide probes, was selected due to the simplicity of design, a reported high probe signal dynamic range in response to copy number alterations (19, 20), and the possibility to multiplex four samples with a high probe density (44,000 probes per sample) on each microarray slide (4 × 44 K microarrays).

2.2. Design Decisions Associated with Zoom-In aCGH

The main objective of zoom-in aCGH is to provide maximal probe coverage within predefined genomic regions of limited size. Relevant decisions for a zoom-in aCGH design include: (1) platform selection as discussed in Subheading 2.1, (2) format of the microarray

Zoom-In aCGH to Detect Germline Rearrangements in Cancer Susceptibility Genes 225

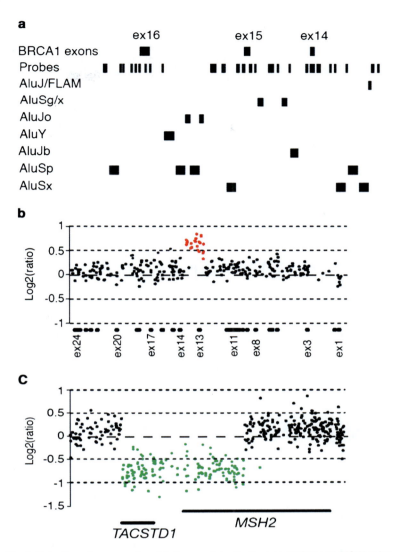

Fig. 1. Detection of copy number deletions and duplications in *BRCA1* and *MSH2* using zoom-in aCGH. Exonic structure is based on RefSeq NM_007294.2 for *BRCA1* and NM_000251.1 for *MSH2*. (**a**) A 9,153 bp window (chr17:38,475,250–38,484,603), including *BRCA1* exons 14–16, illustrating the position of zoom-in array probes compared to surrounding repetitive Alu elements. (**b**) Duplication of *BRCA1* exon 13 in sample L2089 from Staaf et al. (14). Array probes identified as duplicated by aCGH analysis is highlighted in *red*. (**c**) Deletion of *MSH2* exons 1–7 in Kl347 from Staaf et al. (14). Addition of 200 kbp flanking regions 3′ and 5′ of the *MSH2* gene greatly facilitates the complete characterization of the hemizygous deletion. Array probes identified as subjected to deletion by aCGH analysis is highlighted in *green*. Reprinted and adapted with permission from ref. 14. ©2008 Wiley Interscience.

layout, and (3) defining genomic coordinates in order to select probes. Deciding on layout corresponds to fixating the number of probes per sample and number of samples per microarray slide/chip. As discussed in Subheading 2.1, several microarray manufacturers offer the possibility to simultaneously analyze several samples on a single slide/chip at the expense of a lower number of probes per sample. Sample multiplexing using multiformat arrays is often the most efficient way of reducing the experimental cost per sample. Agilent Technologies, for instance, offers microarray formats of 1×244 K (number of samples × number of probes per sample), 4×44 K and 8×15 K for aCGH applications. Multiformat arrays can be suitable for applications where only a few small target regions are of interest, for example, highly focused arrays for the clinical analysis of specific disorders such as cancer syndromes including the screening of the *BRCA1* and *BRCA2*, or mismatch repair genes. Using zoom-in aCGH in a more discovery-based setting, for example, in the investigation of a larger number of genomic regions for somatic rearrangements in tumors, often requires more probes per sample leading to reduced sample multiplexing.

The task of deciding on the genomic regions of interest includes fixating the genomic coordinates in base pairs in order to identify suitable array probes. Additional design decisions related to this step include selecting whether or not to have an unbiased coverage of exonic and intronic sequence, to include flanking regions before and after the target region, as well as decisions on the degree of probe replication. The addition of high-density coverage of 5′ and 3′ flanking regions to each target region makes the zoom-in aCGH platform ideal for mapping alterations that extend in either direction outside the original region, which can greatly facilitate breakpoint validation. Importantly, using predefined probe libraries that are designed to avoid repetitive regions in the genome for probe selection alleviates the need for the individual researcher to perform probe design and sequence repeat masking, which is otherwise a crucial step in the process. Finally, all of these decisions need to be matched to the space and number of probes possible to apply for the array layout chosen. Care needs to be taken to avoid generating highly unbalanced aCGH profiles that will create skewed two-color signals and introduce bias in data centering and normalization, as underlined by recent reports (21, 22). To circumvent this, additional probes outside zoom-in regions may be required.

2.3. Specific Design Criteria for Agilent Zoom-In aCGH Design 015562

In this section, we aim to comprehensively describe the strategy and design selections behind the zoom-in aCGH platform used by Staaf et al. (14) for the detection of germline rearrangements and somatic copy number alterations in six cancer susceptibility genes. The purpose of the zoom-in design used by Staaf et al. (Agilent design identifier: 015562) was to investigate germline rearrangements in *BRCA1*, *BRCA2*, *PTEN*, *CDKN2A*, *MLH1*, and *MSH2* at high resolution in blood samples from patients referred to oncogenetic counseling, as well as to analyze the presence of somatic alterations in breast tumor tissue. The selection of these genes allowed arrays to be used in the screening of several genetic syndromes such as familial breast cancer, familial malignant melanoma, and HNPCC. Array format was set to 4 × 44 K creating four identical 44 K arrays on a single slide in order to reduce the experimental cost and increase sample throughput.

A zoom-in region was defined for each gene as the genomic sequence of the gene itself plus 200 kbp flanking regions (300 kbp for *BRCA1* and *BRCA2*) 3′ and 5′ of the gene, respectively. The usefulness of flanking regions for mutation characterization can be exemplified by the recurrent deletions of the promoter region and first exon of *MSH2* in HNPCC families (14, 23). Genomic coordinates for each zoom-in region were generated using the high-density probe search function in the Agilent ver 4.5 eArray web-based software (http://earray.chem.agilent.com/earray/). The eArray web-based software contains a precompiled 60 mer probe database consisting of a vast number of aCGH probes designed to have a balanced GC-content and sequence avoiding repetitive regions and other means of cross-hybridization in the human genome. All identified probes for each zoom-in region were selected to obtain the highest unbiased coverage of exonic and intronic sequences. This selection corresponded to 1,367 probes (covering 680,496 bp) for *BRCA1*, 2,483 probes (683,529 bp) for *BRCA2*, 1,463 probes (456,451 bp) for *MLH1*, 1,296 probes (478,238 bp) for *MSH2*, 1,747 probes (502,924 bp) for *PTEN*, and 1,256 probes (425,103 bp) for *CDKN2A*. The median nonoverlapping distance between selected probes was between 150 and 300 bp for the six genes. The inter-probe distance varied between genes according to the presence of repetitive elements in the zoom-in regions. In this aspect, *BRCA1* stood out with the lowest number of probes for the second largest base pair region. The reason is the high presence of repetitive sequence in the *BRCA1* zoom-in region, for example, more than 40% of the 81 kbp *BRCA1* gene region consists of Alu repetitive DNA (24). To facilitate the usage of the zoom-in design with complex tumor samples, oligonucleotide probes from the Agilent Technologies CGH 44B probe set covering chromosomes 2, 3, 8, 9, 10, 11, 12, 13, 17, 22 ($n = 19{,}983$) were added. The purpose of these probes was to assist in normalization and data centering. Furthermore, aberrations observed on these chromosomes could be correlated to preexisting data on analyzed samples. A high level of probe replication in zoom-in regions was chosen to avoid loss of data due to experimental artifacts. Oligonucleotide probes within gene boundaries were replicated four times, while probes within flanking regions were replicated twice. Remaining probes were not replicated. Finally, Agilent control probes ($n = 2{,}118$) were added to finalize the design.

3. Experimental Usage of a Zoom-In aCGH Platform

This section serves as an overview of the different steps involved in processing a custom-designed Agilent aCGH microarray.

3.1. Extraction of DNA Used as Template for aCGH Analysis

DNA suitable for aCGH analysis may be extracted using a variety of methods. Of importance is to obtain high quality intact genomic DNA, free of contaminants such us carbohydrates, proteins, and traces of organic solvents. Successful studies have used, for example, the DNeasy Tissue kit (Qiagen, Hilden, Germany), PUREGENE Cell and Tissue Kit (Qiagen), or the Wizard Genomic DNA Purification System (Promega, Madison, WI). Extracted DNA may be stored in nuclease-free water or elution buffers from extraction kits at 4°C or at −80°C for extended periods. Reference DNA used for analysis may be selected differently based on experiment setup, for example, using sex-based references. Commercially available reference DNA containing pooled DNA aliquots from several individuals (male or females) is available (Promega). DNA concentration should be established with care, for example, by using the NanoDrop ND-1000 UV-VIS spectrophotometer or fluorescent nucleic acid assays such as the Quant-iT PicoGreen dsDNA Assay kit (Invitrogen, Carlsbad, CA). High quality DNA typically exhibits an A_{260}/A_{280} ratio of 1.8–2.0 and an A_{260}/A_{230} ratio above 2.0. DNA integrity may be investigated using agarose gel electrophoreses, where intact genomic DNA should appear as a compact, high-molecular weight band with no lower molecular weight smear. The amount of DNA used as input in labeling reactions varies between platforms. SNP platforms usually require a strict input amount, while for the Agilent 4×44 K arrays, DNA input may be varied from 0.5 to 1.5 µg. A good starting point is to use equal amounts of sample and reference DNA for labeling.

3.2. aCGH Experimentation

The processing of custom-designed Agilent 60-mer zoom-in aCGH arrays described here reflects the usage of the Agilent CGH protocol ver 4.0 from June 2006 (available at http://www.agilent.com) using direct labeling of template DNA without prior DNA amplification. In order to obtain high quality copy number estimates it is important to use high quality DNA as input for both sample and reference and to ensure a clean and contamination-free working environment (see Notes 1 and 2). Technical replicates, in the form of dye swap experiments can be used to increase data quality. In a dye-swap experiment, the dyes used for labeling have been reversed for the sample and reference compared to the original experiment. Dye assignment for studies without dye swap experiments is a matter of experimental choice.

Briefly, the experimental protocol consists of five steps. The first step is a 2 h enzyme-based digestion of the template DNA using the *Alu*I and *Rsa*I restriction enzymes at 37°C. After the digestion, the majority of digested products should be between 200 and 500 bp in size (can be verified by agarose gel electrophoreses). Step two consists of the incorporation of fluorescently labeled Cy3- and Cy5-dUTP nucleotides by using random primers and the exo-Klenow fragment in a 2-h reaction at 37°C. Cy3 and Cy5 dyes are sensitive to different factors (see Note 3) and should be handled with appropriate care to avoid degradation. In the third step, the labeling reaction is purified from unincorporated nucleotides using spin columns. The fourth step consists of preparing a hybridization solution of the purified labeled DNA, assembling the microarray hybridization chamber followed by 24-h hybridization at 65°C (24 h is specific for 4×44 K arrays) in a rotating oven. In step five, microarrays are washed in a three-step protocol to remove unbound DNA, dried and scanned using a laser scanner to record fluorescence.

3.3. aCGH Image Analysis

Conventional output from a microarray scanner is a TIFF image of the microarray surface. The TIFF image consists of a vast number of elements, pixels, with associated intensity values representing the amount of recorded fluorescence for each channel (dye). A probe is observed as a usually brightly shining spot in the TIFF image, consisting of several pixels. Image analysis software is required to associate pixels to a specific spot (probe). The image analysis requires, besides the TIFF image, information about probe positioning on the microarray. This information is usually contained in a design file specific for an aCGH design. For Agilent aCGH arrays, image analysis is conveniently performed using the Feature Extraction Software (Agilent Technologies, Santa Clara, CA) as extensively described in the Agilent Feature Extraction Software Reference Guide (http://www.agilent.com). Although user input may be required to identify parts of the microarray surface affected by experimental artifacts, image analysis of high-density microarrays is becoming highly automated due to the vast number of probes. Primary output from the image analysis consists of signal and background intensity estimates for each dye and probe. Output from the Agilent Feature Extraction Software contains both raw signal and background intensities, as well as background corrected and dye normalized intensities for each probe (see the Agilent Feature Extraction Software Reference Guide for details, and Note 4). The intensity ratio for a probe is often formed from background corrected intensities and is subsequently $\log_2$ transformed ($\log_2$ratio). Experimental variation due to different properties of the used dyes, as well as DNA quality, can introduce bias in recorded intensities within and between hybridizations. Consequently, $\log_2$ratios are commonly normalized in order to facilitate cross array comparisons. Normalization can be performed in a variety of ways using different algorithms and software packages. The main purpose of normalization is to shift $\log_2$ratios for a hybridization toward an expected baseline, commonly selected to be equal to the amount of genetic material in the test and reference sample (intensity ratio = 1, $\log_2$ratio = 0). A doubling of genetic material in the test sample then corresponds to a theoretical $\log_2$ratio of 1, and a decrease of genetic material by half (loss of one allele) corresponds to a $\log_2$ratio of −1. A duplication of one allele in the test sample corresponds to a theoretical $\log_2$ratio of 0.58 ($\log_2(3/2)$).

3.4. Initial aCGH Data Analysis

The aim of the initial data analysis described here is to rapidly identify breakpoints of copy number alterations detected by zoom-in aCGH in order to provide regions suitable for primer design, PCR and sequence characterization. Prior to breakpoint analysis, aCGH data needs to be normalized and probes ordered according to their genomic position. Here, normalized and background corrected intensities from the Agilent Feature Extraction Software (see Note 4) are used to calculate $\log_2$ratios for each probe. Deletions and duplications can now be visualized by plotting the genomic position for each probe versus its $\log_2$ratio (Fig. 1b, c). The identification of breakpoints for genomic alterations can be performed using a variety of algorithms. In the simplest way, we identify breakpoints by applying a threshold to normalized and ordered $\log_2$ratios. If a probe has a $\log_2$ratio below the threshold, we identify it as subjected to copy number loss, and if above the threshold as copy number gain. The breakpoints will then correspond to the first (n_{first}) and last probe (n_{last}) in a consecutive series of gain/loss calls for a particular genomic alteration. The true breakpoints are then expected to be between ($n_{first-1}$, n_{first}) and (n_{last}, n_{last+1}). To extract initial regions for primer design, we use the genomic regions defined by ($n_{first-2}$, n_{first}) and (n_{last}, n_{last+2}). Depending on the underlying genomic sequence, these initial regions may have to be expanded for successful primer design. This analysis approach is mainly applicable when analyzing high quality samples with germline rearrangements. Germline rearrangements are expected to be present in all analyzed sample cells and consequently the $\log_2$ratio response to a copy number alteration is expected to be the largest obtainable. The observed $\log_2$ratio of a probe subjected to deletion is then expected to be close to the theoretical value of −1. Similarly, for a duplication of one allele in the test sample, the observed $\log_2$ratio should be close to the theoretical value. For the example given in Subheading 3.5, we will use a threshold of 0.45 to detect copy number gain and −0.45 to detect copy number loss applied to background corrected, normalized, and ordered $\log_2$ratios obtained from the Agilent Feature Extraction software.

3.5. Verification of Germline Rearrangements Delineated by Zoom-In aCGH Using PCR and Sequencing

This section serves as an example on how a germline deletion of exon 8–11 in BRCA2 (sample L2227 from Staaf et al. (14)) delineated by zoom-in aCGH can be completely characterized using PCR and sequencing.

3.5.1. Extraction of Regions for Primer Design from Zoom-In aCGH Data

Regions for primer design were first extracted as described in Subheading 3.4 corresponding to base pairs ($n_{first-2} = 31,799,181$, $n_{first} = 31,800,267$) and ($n_{last} = 31,809,916$, $n_{last+2} = 31,810,346$). PCR primers in extracted regions were designed using the primer3 software (http://primer3.sourceforge.net/) (25) (Fig. 2a). For the forward 5′ primer, the region for primer design was extended to include ($n_{first-5} = 31,798,447$, $n_{first} = 31,800,267$) for the identification of a suitable sequence. Primer sequences were as follows:

Forward 5′ CCTTAATGATCAGGGCATTTC *BRCA2* 7F, cDNA pos: 745-53

Reverse 5′ GCTGCTGTCTACCTGACCAA *BRCA2* 11HR, cDNA pos: 3,765

3.5.2. PCR and Sequencing

PCR, using 150 ng of genomic DNA as template was performed according to the following protocol (see Note 5):

1. Reaction mix (final concentrations in 25 μL reaction volume):

   150 ng DNA

   2.5 mM Mg^{2+}

   0.2 μM of each primer

   0.4 mM dNTP (all four primers together)

   0.5 U AmpliTaq Gold (Applied Biosystems)

2. PCR protocol:

   Annealing 61–54°C, 2 min 30 s, 37 cycles (touchdown: first cycle 61°C annealing, next 60.5°C, etc., for 15 cycles down to 54°C followed by 22 cycles at 54°C).

3. PCR verification and purification:

   PCR products were visualized by gel electrophoreses using 7.5% polyacrylamide gel. PCR products were purified using Multiscreen$_{HTS}$ PCR filter plates (Millipore, Billerica, MA).

4. Sequencing:

   Sequencing of the purified PCR product was performed using the BigDye Terminators v1.1 Cycle Sequencing Kit (Applied Biosystems, Foster City, CA) in an ABI3130 (Applied Biosystems) system according to the manufacturer's instructions. Sequence results were evaluated manually using

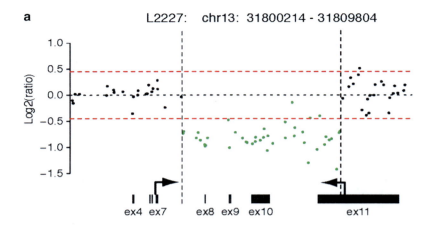

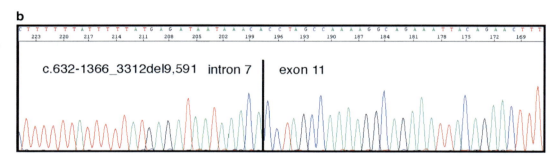

Fig. 2. Example of sequence characterization using zoom-in aCGH for the delineation of a germline deletion of BRCA2 exons 8–11 in sample L2227 from Staaf et al. (14). Exonic mapping for BRCA2 was based on RefSeq NM_000059.2. (a) Log$_2$ratios of array probes in the region covering BRCA2 exons 4–11 (chr13:31,794,212–31,813,333). Array probes identified as deleted are highlighted in *green*. *Arrows* indicate forward and reverse primer start positions. *Vertical dashed lines* indicate the genomic position of the sequenced verified breakpoints. *Red horizontal dashed lines* indicate log$_2$ratio thresholds (±0.45) for detection copy number gain and loss. (b) Sequence verification, showing the merging of intron 7 and remaining part of exon 11. Reprinted and adapted with permission from ref. 14. ©2008 Wiley Interscience.

Sequencher ver 4.5 (Gene Codes Corporation, Ann Arbor, MI) in order to define the exact base pair breakpoints (Fig. 2b). The mutation was characterized as c.632-1366_3312del9591.

4. Notes

1. When handling genomic DNA, avoid repeated freeze-thaw cycles, instead prepare aliquots for multiple usage. Avoid vortexing of solutions containing genomic DNA. Instead, use gentle mixing by hand or pipette.

2. When processing microarrays, it is important to maintain a clean working environment to avoid the contamination of

arrays and reagents. The usage of powder-free laboratory gloves, and designated pipettes with nuclease-free tips is required to ensure that there is no contamination of reagents. When handling microarrays, avoid touching the active side and handle slides by their edges.

3. Fluorescent dyes (Cy3 and Cy5) are light sensitive and should be handled in a way to minimize light exposure. Furthermore, Cy3 and Cy5 are sensitive to repeated freeze-thaw cycles and Cy5 is especially sensitive to ozone degradation. Special measures may be required to avoid ozone degradation, such as the use of a protective surface coating of processed arrays, or the establishment of an ozone-free working environment by, for example, air filtration.

4. In the Agilent Feature Extraction (FE) ver 9.5 text output files, the Features Table contains the following data columns referred to in Subheading 3.4 (see the Agilent Feature Extraction Software (ver 9.5) Reference Guide for more detailed information):

    - ProbeName: Agilent identifier for probes synthesized on the microarray.
    - Probe_mapping: Genomic mapping in base pairs for probes, given as, for example, chr17:356-426. This information can be parsed by, for example, Microsoft Excel into separate columns usable for sorting and subsequent plotting.
    - gProcessedSignal: The processed FE signal for the green channel (Cy3). Background corrected and normalized.
    - rProcessedSignal: The processed FE signal for the red channel (Cy5). Background corrected and normalized.

    The intensity ratio is formed as test/reference, equaling gProcessedSignal/rProcessedSignal for experiments where the test DNA is labeled with Cy3 and reference DNA with Cy5. Intensity ratios are subsequently $\log_2$ transformed. $\log_2$ ratios are ordered based on chromosome and start position for each probe using parsed information from the Probe Mapping column. If replicated probes exist in the zoom-in design, these are preferably merged by, for example, taking the mean/median of all replicates.

5. The presented PCR protocol is intended to serve as an example. In a successful experiment, a single strong band should be observed when PCR products are analyzed using gel electrophoresis. Based on the outcome of the PCR reaction, a number of different changes are conceivable:

    - No bands observed due to high stringency in the PCR reaction. Lowering the annealing temperature, and/or raising the Mg^{2+} concentration lowers the stringency of the PCR reaction.

- Several bands observed due to low stringency in the PCR reaction. Raising the annealing temperature, and/or lowering the Mg^{2+} concentration raises the stringency of the PCR reaction.
- High GC content of PCR products. Addition of DMSO to the PCR reaction (e.g., 5% DMSO as final concentration) can potentially address problems with a high GC content. Furthermore, specific PCR enzymes that are more suited to amplify GC-rich regions exist.

Acknowledgments

This work was supported by grants from the Swedish Cancer Society, the Swedish Research Council, the Mrs. Berta Kamprad Foundation, the Gunnar Nilsson Cancer Foundation, and the Swedish Foundation for Strategic Research. The authors acknowledge the contribution by Therese Törngren, Department of Oncology, Lund University.

References

1. Nathanson, K.L., Wooster, R., and Weber, B.L. (2001) Breast cancer genetics: what we know and what we need. *Nat. Med.* 7, 552–556.
2. Peltomaki, P. (2005) Lynch syndrome genes. *Fam. Cancer* 4, 227–232.
3. Szabo, C.I., Worley, T., and Monteiro, A.N. (2004) Understanding germ-line mutations in BRCA1. *Cancer Biol. Ther.* 3, 515–520.
4. Wang, Y., Friedl, W., Lamberti, C., Jungck, M., Mathiak, M., Pagenstecher, C., et al. (2003) Hereditary nonpolyposis colorectal cancer: frequent occurrence of large genomic deletions in MSH2 and MLH1 genes. *Int. J. Cancer* 103, 636–641.
5. Mazoyer, S. (2005) Genomic rearrangements in the BRCA1 and BRCA2 genes. *Hum. Mutat.* 25, 415–422.
6. Swensen, J., Hoffman, M., Skolnick, M.H., and Neuhausen, S.L. (1997) Identification of a 14 kb deletion involving the promoter region of BRCA1 in a breast cancer family. *Hum. Mol. Genet.* 6, 1513–1517.
7. Schouten, J.P., McElgunn, C.J., Waaijer, R., Zwijnenburg, D., Diepvens, F., and Pals, G. (2002) Relative quantification of 40 nucleic acid sequences by multiplex ligation-dependent probe amplification. *Nucl. Acids Res.* 30, e57.
8. Hofmann, W., Gorgens, H., John, A., Horn, D., Huttner, C., Arnold, N., et al. (2003) Screening for large rearrangements of the BRCA1 gene in German breast or ovarian cancer families using semi-quantitative multiplex PCR method. *Hum. Mutat.* 22, 103–104.
9. Gad, S., Aurias, A., Puget, N., Mairal, A., Schurra, C., Montagna, M., et al. (2001) Color bar coding the BRCA1 gene on combed DNA: a useful strategy for detecting large gene rearrangements. *Genes Chromosomes Cancer* 31, 75–84.
10. Casilli, F., Di Rocco, Z.C., Gad, S., Tournier, I., Stoppa-Lyonnet, D., Frebourg, T., et al. (2002) Rapid detection of novel BRCA1 rearrangements in high-risk breast-ovarian cancer families using multiplex PCR of short fluorescent fragments. *Hum. Mutat.* 20, 218–226.
11. Albertson, D.G., and Pinkel, D. (2003) Genomic microarrays in human genetic disease and cancer. *Hum. Mol. Genet.* 12 Spec No. 2, R145–R152.

12. Vissers, L.E., Veltman, J.A., van Kessel, A.G., and Brunner, H.G. (2005) Identification of disease genes by whole genome CGH arrays. *Hum. Mol. Genet.* **14 Spec No. 2**, R215–R223.

13. Saal, L.H., Gruvberger-Saal, S.K., Persson, C., Lovgren, K., Jumppanen, M., Staaf, J., et al. (2008) Recurrent gross mutations of the PTEN tumor suppressor gene in breast cancers with deficient DSB repair. *Nat. Genet.* **40**, 102–107.

14. Staaf, J., Torngren, T., Rambech, E., Johansson, U., Persson, C., Sellberg, G., et al. (2008) Detection and precise mapping of germline rearrangements in BRCA1, BRCA2, MSH2, and MLH1 using zoom-in array comparative genomic hybridization (aCGH). *Hum. Mutat.* **29**, 555–564.

15. Rouleau, E., Lefol, C., Tozlu, S., Andrieu, C., Guy, C., Copigny, F., et al. (2007) High-resolution oligonucleotide array-CGH applied to the detection and characterization of large rearrangements in the hereditary breast cancer gene BRCA1. *Clin. Genet.* **72**, 199–207.

16. Peiffer, D.A., Le, J.M., Steemers, F.J., Chang, W., Jenniges, T., Garcia, F., et al. (2006) High-resolution genomic profiling of chromosomal aberrations using Infinium whole-genome genotyping. *Genome Res.* **16**, 1136–1148.

17. Deininger, P.L., and Batzer, M.A. (1999) Alu repeats and human disease. *Mol. Genet. Metab.* **67**, 183–193.

18. van der Klift, H., Wijnen, J., Wagner, A., Verkuilen, P., Tops, C., Otway, R., et al. (2005) Molecular characterization of the spectrum of genomic deletions in the mismatch repair genes MSH2, MLH1, MSH6, and PMS2 responsible for hereditary nonpolyposis colorectal cancer (HNPCC). *Genes Chromosomes Cancer* **44**, 123–138.

19. Gunnarsson, R., Staaf, J., Jansson, M., Ottesen, A.M., Goransson, H., Liljedahl, U., et al. (2008) Screening for copy-number alterations and loss of heterozygosity in chronic lymphocytic leukemia-A comparative study of four differently designed, high resolution microarray platforms. *Genes Chromosomes Cancer* **8**, 697–711.

20. Greshock, J., Feng, B., Nogueira, C., Ivanova, E., Perna, I., Nathanson, K., et al. (2007) A comparison of DNA copy number profiling platforms. *Cancer Res.* **67**, 10173–10180.

21. Staaf, J., Jonsson, G., Ringner, M., and Vallon-Christersson, J. (2007) Normalization of array-CGH data: influence of copy number imbalances. *BMC Genomics* **8**, 382.

22. Chen, H.I., Hsu, F.H., Jiang, Y., Tsai, M.H., Yang, P.C., Meltzer, P.S., et al. (2008) A probe-density-based analysis method for array CGH data: simulation, normalization and centralization. *Bioinformatics* **24**, 1749–1756.

23. Charbonnier, F., Olschwang, S., Wang, Q., Boisson, C., Martin, C., Buisine, M.P., et al. (2002) MSH2 in contrast to MLH1 and MSH6 is frequently inactivated by exonic and promoter rearrangements in hereditary nonpolyposis colorectal cancer. *Cancer Res.* **62**, 848–853.

24. Smith, T.M., Lee, M.K., Szabo, C.I., Jerome, N., McEuen, M., Taylor, M., et al. (1996) Complete genomic sequence and analysis of 117 kb of human DNA containing the gene BRCA1. *Genome Res.* **6**, 1029–1049.

25. Rozen, S., and Skaletsky, H. (2000) Primer3 on the WWW for general users and for biologist programmers. *Methods Mol. Biol.* **132**, 365–386.

Chapter 14

Development of a Scoring System to Screen for BRCA1/2 Mutations

Gareth R. Evans and Fiona Lalloo

Abstract

Selection for genetic testing for pathogenic mutations in *BRCA1* and *BRCA2* is an important area of healthcare. While testing costs for mutational analysis are falling, costs of tests in North America remain in excess of $3,000. Most countries state that there should be at least a 10–20% likelihood of detecting a mutation in *BRCA1* or *BRCA2* within a family before mutational analysis is performed. A number of computer-based models have been developed to assess this likelihood, and these continue to be improved to incorporate mutation frequencies, breast cancer incidence and tumour histology. However, these can be time-consuming and difficult to use in a busy clinic. The Manchester scoring system was developed in 2003, and we have continued to validate its use in Western populations. The scoring system discriminates well at both the 10 and 20% threshold for testing and compares very well with more complex computer-based models. However, it should not be used in its current form in founder populations or populations with low incidence of breast cancer, although a lower points threshold could be used to determine an appropriate cut off. The development of the Manchester score and its comparison with other models will be described in this chapter.

Key words: BRCA1, BRCA2, Manchester score, BOADICEA, BRCAPRO, Myriad, Sensitivity, Threshold, Breast cancer, Ovarian cancer

1. Introduction

Breast cancer is the most common form of cancer affecting women. One in 9–12 women will develop the disease in their lifetime in the developed world. Every year, 44,000 women develop the disease in England and Wales (population 55 million) and as a result, 12,000 will die (1).

The presence of a significant family history is the greatest risk factor for the development of breast cancer. Even at extremes of age, the presence of a *BRCA1* mutation will confer higher risks.

For example, a 25-year-old woman who carries a mutation in *BRCA1* has a greater risk in the next decade than a woman aged 70 years from the general population. Approximately 4–5% of breast cancer is thought to be due to the inheritance of a dominant cancer predisposing gene (2, 3). While hereditary factors are highly likely to play a part in a high proportion of the rest, these are harder to evaluate at present. Genome-wide association studies may unravel these in the next 10 years (4, 5). Apart from rare cases such as Cowden's disease (6), there are no phenotypic clues that assist in the identification of those who carry pathogenic mutations in breast cancer-predisposing genes. The evaluation of the family history therefore remains necessary to assess the likelihood that a mutation in a predisposing gene is present within a family. Inheritance of a germ line mutation or deletion in a predisposing gene results in early-onset and frequently bilateral breast cancer. Mutations in certain genes also confer an increased susceptibility to other malignancies, such as epithelial ovarian, prostate and pancreatic cancer (7, 8), or more rarely gliomas and sarcomas (9). Multiple primary cancers in one individual or related early-onset cancers in a pedigree are highly suggestive of a predisposing gene. Indeed, we have shown that at least 20% of breast cancers aged 30 years and younger are due to mutations in the known high-risk genes *BRCA1*, *BRCA2* and *TP53* (10).

There are two main types of risk which need to be assessed

- The probability of developing breast cancer over a given timespan or lifetime risk (aged 40 years)
- The probability of a mutation in a known high-risk gene such as *BRCA1* or *BRCA2*

While some risk assessment models are aimed primarily at solving one of the questions, many also have an output for the other. For example, BRCAPRO is primarily aimed at assessing the probability of a mutation but can have an output to assess breast cancer risk over time. The Tyrer–Cuzick model was developed to assess breast cancer risk over time but does generate a probability of a mutation in *BRCA1/2* for the individual.

In order to assess breast cancer risks over time as accurately as possible all known risk factors for breast cancer need to be assessed.

A number of models/scoring systems have been derived to assess the probability of a *BRCA1* or *BRCA2* mutation in a given individual dependant on their family history.

Some of the earlier models such as the Couch (11) and Shattuck-Eidens models (12) were derived before widespread genetic testing had been performed.

Two tabular scoring systems have been derived from the Myriad laboratories genetic testing programme (13, 14) with the second based on testing in over 10,000 individuals (14).

The most widely used and validated model is BRCAPRO (15–17), which requires computer entry of the family history information.

In 2002, we developed a scoring system to facilitate more accurate selection of families for *BRCA1/2* testing. This was undertaken primarily because these existing systems were either labourious or had had little validation.

2. Development of Scoring System

2.1. Initial (Developmental) Set of Samples

1. A set of 420 families were tested for mutations in *BRCA1* and 324 were tested for mutations in *BRCA2* which included:

   99 breast cancer patients diagnosed aged 30 years or less (10).

   34 families containing a proven male breast cancer case.

2. All cancers in the most significant blood line were assessed for the presence of cancers known to be associated with increased risk with *BRCA1/2* mutations, that is, breast, ovarian, prostate and pancreas. The age at onset and type of cancer was verified from hospital records, cancer registries or death certification.

3. A weighted score for each cancer in the bloodline was developed such that a total score of 10 points for each gene equated to a 10% probability of a pathogenic mutation in that gene.

4. Scoring was initially based on sequential testing of the two genes rather than simultaneous testing.

2.2. Mutation Screening

1. Mutation screening in this and all subsequent datasets was of a living affected individual with a relevant cancer, or an assumed obligate gene carrier.

2. Mutation screening of both genes was undertaken with a whole gene approach using SSCP (single strand conformation polymorphism) of all small exons and PTT (protein truncation test) of exon 11 in *BRCA1*, and of exons 10 and 11 in *BRCA2*. All mutations were confirmed by sequencing. Fifteen families were referred, without such testing, to direct sequencing of both genes by Myriad Genetics.

3. As *BRCA1* testing was established earlier, a larger number of families had mutation screening for *BRCA1* than for *BRCA2*.

4. Those families with male breast cancer were screened for mutations in *BRCA2* before screening for mutations in *BRCA1*.

5. Families with ovarian cancer were always screened for mutations in *BRCA1* before *BRCA2* unless male breast cancer was present.

2.3. The Scoring System

1. The scoring system was developed using parameters in Table 1 with age ranges being used for simplicity (see Table 2).
2. Using the data from population studies and the developmental set of families, no sporadic cancer reached a 10% likelihood of having a *BRCA1/2* mutation; therefore, no individual cancer without a family history obtained a score of 10. For example, sporadic breast cancer aged <31 in our series resulted in only one BRCA1 and one BRCA2 mutation in 65 cases (10).
3. A maximum score of 8 points was given to early onset ovarian and male breast cancer for *BRCA1* and *BRCA2*, respectively.
4. The relative risk of prostatic and pancreatic cancers associated with mutations in *BRCA1* was not considered high enough to warrant a score.

Table 1
Possible parameters to be used in algorithms and scoring systems for the identification of mutations

Item	Increase chances *BRCA1*	Increase chances *BRCA2*	Decrease chances Both
Breast cancer			
Early onset	+++	++	
Bilaterality	+++	+++	
ER negative	+++	+	
High grade	+++	++	
Lobular	−	+	
Ovarian cancer			
Early onset	+++	++	
Epithelial non-mucinous	+++	+++	
Mucinous	−	−	
Germ cell	−	−	
Pancreatic cancer	+	++	
Prostate	+	++	
Early onset	+	+++	
Number of unaffected females in pedigree			++
Intervening unaffected females			++

Table 2
Manchester scoring system

Age	BRCA1	BRCA2
FBC <30	6	5
FBC 30–39	4	4
FBC 40–49	3	3
FBC 50–59	2	2
FBC >59	1	1
MBC <60	5 (if *BRCA2* tested)	8
MBC >59	5 (if *BRCA2* tested)	5
Ovarian cancer <60	8	5 (if *BRCA1* tested)
Ovarian cancer >59	5	5 (if *BRCA1* tested)
Pancreatic cancer	0	1
Prostate cancer <60	0	2
Prostate cancer >59	0	1

FBC female breast cancer, *MBC* male breast cancer
Scores are added for each cancer in a direct lineage

5. The scoring system (see Table 2) was developed using multiple applications of different scores within the developmental set.

6. Application of this scoring system in the 420 developmental patients allowed a good discrimination between 10–11 points and 8–9 points in identifying a sample with at least a 10% likelihood of a mutation in either *BRCA1* or *BRCA2* and was supported by data from the validation set.

7. In the combined set, for *BRCA1*, the 10–11 point cut-off identified mutations in 9/76 samples (11.5%) versus 4/104 (3.8%) for 8–9 point cut-off while for BRCA2, the 10–11 point identified mutations in 10/64 samples (15.6%) versus 3/70 (4.3%) for the 8–9 point cut-off.

2.4. Validating the Scoring System

Most countries in Europe and North America have determined thresholds of between 10 and 20% for undertaking mutation analysis in a family. In England and Wales, the threshold is currently set at 20% (18). The efficacy of the Manchester scoring system at 20% threshold level on 921 samples was published in 2005 (19). The combined score of 20 points (adding the individual score for BRCA1 and BRCA2) had good discrimination. At 20–24 points, 27% (39/143) of samples tested positive for mutations in BRCA1/2, whereas with scores of 15–19 points, 17% (33/199) tested positive. A 15-point threshold was useful for a combined 10% discrimination as 12/14 points resulted in only 3.5% (6/165) samples testing positive.

1. The sample set has now increased to 2,075 samples fully tested for *BRCA1* and *BRCA2* mutations (see Table 3).
2. All families were tested with a whole gene testing technique.
3. 650 families were tested by direct sequencing of all exons of both genes.
4. Multiple Ligation dependent Probe Amplification (MLPA) was carried out on all negative samples to detect single or multiple exon deletions or duplications.
5. Families were divided into those containing an ovarian cancer, male breast cancer or neither.
6. All families were scored using the developed Manchester scoring system.
7. A 20-point threshold worked well across all types of families including those containing ovarian cancer, male breast cancer or neither. The 15-point threshold again defines a cut off at the 10% level.

Table 3
Proportion of families with mutations using the combined *BRCA1/2* score

Score	Ovarian	Male breast	All families
40+	70/88 (80%) 58/65 (89%)[a]	9/11 (81%)	81/107 (76%)[b]
35–39	23/39 (59%)	3/4 (75%)	34/61 (55%)
30–34	29/62 (48%)	4/9 (45%)	51/113 (45%)
25–29	34/115 (29%)	4/12 (33%)	67/221 (30%)
20–24	28/119 (24%)	2/10 (20%)	74/341 (22%)
20+			
15–19	9/89 (10%)	1/16 (7%)	44/430 (10%)
12–14	2/38 (5%)	0/7 (0%)	19/407 (5%)
<12	0/0	0/3	16/584 (2.5%)
Total	195/550 (35%)	23/72 (32%)	363/2,075 (18%)

[a] All ovarian cancer contributing to the score were confirmed as non-mucinous epithelial cancer
[b] Eight families achieved a score of 40+ without an ovarian or male breast cancer case

8. The mutation detection rate of 89% in families with 40+ points due to cases of ovarian cancer, which have been confirmed as an epithelial non-mucinous cancer, indicates that nearly all these families have mutations. Given that there is at least a 6% loss of sensitivity due to testing a phenocopy (a case without the family mutation) (20), this 89% detection suggests a 95% sensitivity for full exon scanning and MLPA.

3. Comparison of Models

258 samples from the North West region that were predominantly at a lower risk of breast cancer were screened in a separate research laboratory using whole gene screening techniques. Nine percent (23/258) of families had mutations in both genes. Comparisons between the Manchester score, myriad tables, Couch and BRCAPRO models were undertaken (21).

1. The predicted likelihood of a mutation varied widely between the three other manual methods, even between the two derived from the Myriad dataset (13, 14). In particular, the models did not take account of all the factors that could influence the presence of a mutation.
2. Scores could not be derived from the Frank1 model (13) in 83 patients because the tested individual did not have breast cancer at <50 years of age; three of these families had a *BRCA2* mutation.
3. The six bilateral breast cancers could not be scored in the Frank2 model (14).
4. The Couch model could not derive a score for the families containing only ovarian cancer (11).
5. The Manchester scoring system outperformed all other models, especially in the combined group of both *BRCA1* and *BRCA2*. The area under the ROC curve (C-statistic) was highest for the Manchester score (21).

4. Notes

1. A simple scoring system to assess the likelihood of identifying a *BRCA1* or *BRCA2* mutation in an affected individual within a family has been developed. The scoring system continues to discriminate well at both the 10 and 20% threshold.

2. While simple tabular or scoring systems are easy to use and generate probabilities in 1–2 min, computer-based programmes take 10–20 min to input. The Manchester score is therefore ideal in a busy surgical or oncology clinic when assessing whether a patient is likely to qualify for testing. This will avoid the possibility that an individual will be given the false impression that they will be tested once referred to a specialist clinic if they fall well below a national threshold. Nonetheless, in specialist clinics computer-based assessments may well be carried out in order to generate pedigrees and store family information.

3. Model-based approaches are able to take into account unaffected relatives and can be developed to include details such as histology which may increase the likelihood in particular of a BRCA mutation (see Table 1). Such detail has been deliberately excluded from the Manchester score as it would make it cumbersome and difficult to use given the need for multiple extra additions and reductions. All assessment tools will need to take into account the population frequency of mutations and the incidence of breast cancer in that population. This is a relatively straight forward adjustment in a computer programme. However, for a manual scoring system the points thresholds will need to be reduced if there are founder effects such as in the Jewish population (22) or the incidence of breast cancer is substantially less than in the UK such as in Asia (23).

4. It is not appropriate to combine groups for analysis using the Manchester score, for instance, Jewish families and other founder populations should be dealt with separately when comparing the Manchester score with other models. This mistake may erroneously reduce the threshold discrimination of the Manchester score whereas computer models will automatically adjust for Ashkenazi heritage (20, 24).

5. Validation studies for the BRCA1/2 risk estimation models are much more widespread than for breast cancer risk over time (16, 17, 21, 23–31). Perhaps the most useful aspect of these is the development of a cut off for the intervention of a genetic test at the 10 or 20% level.

6. An assessment of this cut off for several of the models is presented in Table 4.

7. In practice, most genetic testing has been carried out on high-risk families. While a pre-testing assessment of the chances of *BRCA1/2* involvement is useful, it does not alter the decision making of whether or not to test a family member if there is a difference between a 20 and 60% chance of a mutation.

8. With genetic testing for BRCA1/2 costing around $3,000, insurance companies and health care systems require a threshold for test use.

Table 4
***BRCA1/2* mutation in non-Ashkenazi Jewish families for four models/scoring systems based on three validation studies**

Study (numbers – mutation positive)	Barcenas Sensitivity (472 – 96)	Barcenas Specificity	Amir Sensitivity (258 – 23)	Amir Specificity	James Sensitivity (209 – 51)	James Specificity
BOADICEA Both	73	67				
BRCAPRO Both	73	67	61	44	81	66
Myriad 2 Both	68	63	87	33	97	23
Manchester scoring Both	93	41	87	66	81	58
BOADICEA BRCA1	61	84				
BRCAPRO BRCA1	75	71	67	56	88	66
Myriad 1 BRCA1	72	60	100	0	100	23
Manchester scoring BRCA1	83	55	67	17	91	60
BOADICEA BRCA2	48	78				
BRCAPRO BRCA2	40	85	6	83	74	66
Myriad 1 BRCA2	40	89	79	11	94	23
Manchester scoring BRCA2	84	58	82	75	71	60

9. In the UK, this is set at 20% mutation probability (19) but in most of the rest of Europe and North America this is 10%. In order to adequately assess the models at a 10% threshold, a range of families is necessary to test around the threshold. Ideally only around 10% of the samples should be mutation positive.

10. As can be seen in Table 2, apart from our own study (21), the remainder had detection rates above 20% (24, 28).

11. None of the models, tables or scoring systems work perfectly and all need to be adjusted for new information such as the triple negative grade 3 breast cancer histology associated with *BRCA1*.

12. With improvements in the computer models such as BOADICEA, we will hopefully achieve a more accurate and discriminatory cut off (32).

13. Despite the complexity of computer systems, the Manchester score still compares well with newer models such as BOADICEA (29–31) and even with modified updated versions of BRCAPRO (24, 30, 31).

14. In 1934 UK families, the area under the receiver operating characteristic curve gave a C statistic of 0.77 for BOADICEA, 0.76 for BRCAPRO, 0.75 for Manchester score and 0.72 for Myriad tables (14, 30).

15. For a simple first line test in clinic, using a scoring system or table will at least give a guide as to whether a family will qualify for testing.

References

1. CR-UK, *CancerStats Incidence – UK*. Cancer Research UK 2005/6, www.cancerresearchuk.org, 2008.
2. Claus, E.B., Risch, N., and Thompson, D. (1994) Autosomal dominant inheritance of early onset breast cancer. *Cancer* 73, 643–651.
3. Newman, B., Austin, M.A., Lee, M., and King, M. (1988) Inheritance of human breast cancer: evidence for autosomal dominant transmission in high risk families. *Proc. Natl. Acad. Sci. USA* 85, 3044–3048.
4. Easton, D.F., Pharoah, P.D.P., Dunning, A.M., Pooley, K., Cox, D.R., Ballinger, D., et al. (2007) A genome-wide association study in Breast Cancer. *Nat. Genet.* 447, 1087–1093.
5. Stacey, S.N., Manolescu, A., Sulem, P., Thorlacius, S., Gudjonsson, S.A., Jonsson, G.F., et al. (2008) Common variants on chromosome 5p12 confer susceptibility to estrogen receptor-positive breast cancer. *Nat. Genet.* 40, 703–706.
6. Liaw, D., Marsh, D.J., Li, J., Dahia, P.L., Wang, S.I., Zheng, Z., et al. (1997) Germline mutations of the PTEN gene in Cowden disease, an inherited breast and thyroid cancer syndrome. *Nat. Genet.* 16, 64–67.
7. Malkin, D., Li, F.P., Strong, L.C., Fraumeni, J.F. Jr., Nelson, C.E., Kim, D.H., et al. (1990) Germline *TP53* mutations in cancer families. *Science* 250, 1233–1238.
8. Miki, Y., Swensen, J., Shattuck-Eidens, D., Futreal, P.A., Harshman, K., Tavtigian, S., et al. (1994) A strong candidate for the breast and ovarian cancer susceptibility gene BRCA1. *Science* 266, 120–122.
9. Wooster, R., Bignell, G., Lancaster, J., Swift, S., Seal, S., Mangion, J., et al. (1995) Identification of the breast cancer susceptibility gene BRCA2. *Nature* 378, 789–792.
10. Lalloo, F., Varley, J., Ellis, D., O'Dair, L., Pharoah, P., Evans, D.G.R., and the early onset breast cancer study Group. (2003) Family history is predictive of pathogenic mutations in BRCA1, BRCA2 and TP53 with high penetrance in a population based study of very early onset breast cancer. *Lancet* 361, 1011–1012.
11. Couch, F.J., DeShano, M.L., Blackwood, A., Calzone, K., Stopfer, J., Campeau, L., et al. (1997) BRCA1 mutations in women attending clinics that evaluate breast cancer risk. *N. Engl. J. Med.* 336, 1409–1415.
12. Shattuck-Eidens, D., Oliphant, A., McClure, M., McBride, C., Gupte, J., Rubano, T., et al. (1997) BRCA1 sequence analysis in women at high risk for susceptibility mutations: risk factor analysis and implications for genetic testing. *JAMA* 278, 1242–1250.
13. Frank, T.S., Manley, S.A., Olopade, O.I., Cummings, S., Garber, J.E., Bernhardt, B., et al. (1998) Sequence analysis of BRCA1 and BRCA2: correlation of mutations with family history and ovarian cancer risk. *J. Clin. Oncol.* 16, 2417–2425.
14. Frank, T.S., Deffenbaugh, A.M., Reid, J.E., Hulick, M., Ward, B.E., Lingenfelter, B., et al. (2002) Clinical characteristics of individuals with germline mutations in BRCA1 and BRCA2: analysis of 10,000 individuals. *J. Clin. Oncol.* 20, 1480–1490.
15. Parmigiani, G., Berry, D.A., and Aquilar, O. (1998) Determining carrier probabilities for breast cancer susceptibility genes BRCA1 and BRCA2. *Am. J. Hum. Genet.* 62, 145–148.
16. Berry, D.A., Iversen, E.S. Jr., Gudbjartsson, D.F., Hiller, E.H., Garber, J.E., Peshkin, B.N., et al. (2002) BRCAPRO validation, sensitivity of genetic testing of BRCA1/BRCA2, and

prevalence of other breast cancer susceptibility genes. *J. Clin. Oncol.* **20**, 2701–2712.

17. Euhus, D.M., Smith, K.C., Robinson, L., Stucky, A., Olopade, O.I., Cummings, S., et al. (2002) Pretest prediction of BRCA1 or BRCA2 mutation by risk counselors and the computer model BRCAPRO. *J. Natl. Cancer Inst.* **94**, 844–851.

18. McIntosh, A., Shaw, C., Evans, G., Turnbull, N., Bahar, N., Barclay, M., et al. (2004) *Clinical Guidelines and Evidence Review for the Classification and Care of Women at Risk of Familial Breast Cancer.* London: National Collaborating Centre for Primary Care/University of Sheffield. NICE guideline CG014. www.nice.org.uk

19. Evans, D.G.R., Lalloo, F., Wallace, A., and Rahman, N. (2005) Update on the Manchester Scoring System for BRCA1 and BRCA2 testing. *J. Med. Genet.* **42**, e39.

20. Smith, A., Moran, A., Boyd, M.C., Bulman, M., Shenton, A., Smith, L., et al. (2007) The trouble with phenocopies: are those testing negative for a family BRCA1/2 mutation really at population risk? *J. Med. Genet.* **44**, 10–15.

21. Evans, D.G.R., Eccles, D.M., Rahman, N., Young, K., Bulman, M., Amir, E., et al. (2004) A new scoring system for the chances of identifying a BRCA1/2 mutation, outperforms existing models including BRCAPRO. *J. Med. Genet.* **41**, 474–480.

22. Evans, D.G., Lalloo, F., and Eccles, D. (2006) Optimal selection of individuals for BRCA mutation testing. *J. Clin. Oncol.* **10**, 3311–3112.

23. Thirthagiri, E., Lee, S., Kang, P., Lee, D., Toh, G., Selamat, S., et al. (2008) Evaluation of BRCA1 and BRCA2 mutations and risk-prediction models in a typical Asian country (Malaysia) with a relatively low incidence of breast cancer. *Breast Cancer Res.* **16**, R59.

24. James, P.A., Doherty, R., Harris, M., Mukesh, B.N., Milner, A., Young, M.A., et al. (2006) Optimal selection of individuals for BRCA mutation testing: a comparison of available methods. *J. Clin. Oncol.* **24**, 707–715.

25. Shannon, K.M., Lubratovich, M.L., Finkelstein, D.M., Smith, B.L., Powell, S.N., Seiden, M.V. (2002) Model-based predictions of BRCA1/2 mutation status in breast carcinoma patients treated at an academic medical center. *Cancer* **94**, 305–313.

26. Bodmer, D., Ligtenberg, M.J., van der Hout, A.H., Gloudemans, S., Ansink, K., Oosterwijk, J.C., et al. (2006) Optimal selection for BRCA1 and BRCA2 mutation testing using a combination of 'easy to apply' probability models. *Br. J. Cancer* **95**, 757–762.

27. Kang, H.H., Williams, R., Leary, J.; kConFab Investigators; Ringland, C., Kirk, J., Ward, R. (2006) Evaluation of models to predict BRCA germline mutations. *Br. J. Cancer* **95**, 914–920.

28. Barcenas, C.H., Hosain, G.M., Arun, B., Zong, J., Zhou, X., Chen, J., et al. (2006) BRCA carrier probabilities in extended families. *J. Clin. Oncol.* **24**, 354–360.

29. Simard, J., Dumont, M., Moisan, A.M., Gaborieau, V., Malouin, H., Durocher, F., et al. (2007) Evaluation of BRCA1 and BRCA2 mutation prevalence, risk prediction models and a multistep testing approach in French-Canadian families with high risk of breast and ovarian cancer. *J. Med. Genet.* **44**, 107–121.

30. Antoniou, A.C., Hardy, R., Walker, L., Evans, D.G.R., Shenton, A., et al. (2008) Predicting the likelihood of carrying a BRCA1 or BRCA2 mutation: validation of BOADICEA, BRCAPRO, IBIS, Myriad and the Manchester scoring system using data from UK genetics clinics. *J. Med. Genet.* **45**, 425–431.

31. Roudgari, H., Miedzybrodzka, Z.H., and Haites, N.E. (2008) Probability estimation models for prediction of BRCA1 and BRCA2 mutation carriers: COS compares favourably with other models. *Fam. Cancer* **7**, 199–212.

32. Antoniou, A.C., Cunningham, A.P., Peto, J., Evans, D.G.R., Lalloo, F., Narod, S.A., et al. (2008) The BOADICEA model of genetic susceptibility to breast and ovarian cancers: updates and extensions. *Br. J. Cancer* **98**, 1457–1466.

Chapter 15

Use of Splicing Reporter Minigene Assay to Evaluate the Effect on Splicing of Unclassified Genetic Variants

Pascaline Gaildrat, Audrey Killian, Alexandra Martins, Isabelle Tournier, Thierry Frébourg, and Mario Tosi

Abstract

The interpretation of the numerous sequence variants of unknown biological and clinical significance (UV for "unclassified variant") found in genetic screenings represents a major challenge in the molecular diagnosis of genetic disease, including cancer susceptibility. A fraction of UVs may be deleterious because they affect mRNA splicing. Here, we describe a functional splicing assay based on a minigene construct that assesses the impact of sequence variants on splicing. A genomic segment encompassing the variant sequence of interest along with flanking intronic sequences is PCR-amplified from patient genomic DNA and is cloned into a minigene vector. After transient transfection into cultured cells, the splicing patterns of the transcripts generated from the wild-type and from the variant constructs are compared by reverse transcription-PCR analysis and sequencing. This method represents a complementary approach to reverse transcription-PCR analyses of patient RNA, for the identification of pathogenic splicing mutations.

Key words: Cancer molecular diagnosis, Minigene construct, Splicing mutations, Unclassified genetic variants

1. Introduction

Functional splicing reporter minigene assays represent a powerful tool to assess the impact of sequence variants on splicing (*1, 2*). These assays are very useful to diagnostic laboratories for determining the biological and the pathological significance of certain sequence variations detected in genetic screenings of disease-predisposing genes. The protocol provided here is used routinely in our laboratory to evaluate whether unclassified variants (UVs) identified in genes associated with predisposition to Lynch syndrome (*MLH1/MSH2*) or to hereditary breast-ovarian cancer (*BRCA1/BRCA2*) lead to splicing defects (*3, 4*).

The assay relies on the use of a minigene vector, which contains a fragment of the *C1 inhibitor* gene (*SERPING1/C1NH*), with two exonic regions separated by an intron, cloned into the mammalian expression vector pcDNA3.1(–), downstream of the cytomegalovirus (CMV) promoter (3, 4) (see Fig. 1). The genomic segment encompassing the variant sequence of interest along with ~150 bp of the corresponding flanking intronic sequences is amplified by PCR from the genomic DNA of the patient and is cloned into the minigene expression plasmid by insertion into the *SERPING1/C1NH* intron (see Fig. 1). The resulting minigene constructs (variant and wild-type) are expressed by transient transfection into cultured cells. The splicing pattern of the chimeric transcripts generated from both constructs is then compared by RT-PCR analysis and sequencing (see Fig. 1).

The splicing reporter minigene assay presents many advantages. Patient blood RNA samples or lymphoblastoid cell lines are not always available to the diagnostic laboratories and the splicing reporter minigene assay, which is based on genomic DNA, circumvents this problem. In addition, the minigene approach facilitates the interpretation of the effect of sequence variant on splicing especially because it is monoallelic. Another significant advantage is the parallel analysis of the variant and wild-type construct in an identical cellular background. Moreover, each UV is tested within a defined sequence segment of the natural gene. This feature often allows one to rule out the alternative hypothesis that the defect observed in vivo may be due to a sequence alteration affecting, e.g., intronic regions that have not been sequenced. The splicing reporter minigene assay can nevertheless present some limitations. In the minigene assay, the expression of an artificial transcript is analyzed, whereas the RT-PCR analysis from patient blood RNA presents the advantage of assessing the natural endogenous expression of the gene of interest. In addition, the heterologous cellular system used in the minigene assay may not fully reflect the splicing regulatory process involved in the affected tissue. However, one should also note that even the observation of a splicing defect by RT-PCR analysis of patient blood RNA does not necessarily reflect its magnitude in the relevant tissue.

Fig. 1. (continued) the stretch of 114 bp derived from intron 1 of the *SERPING1/C1NH* gene has been removed, and the translation initiation site within exon A has been inactivated in order to prevent the induction of the NMD pathway. Genomic segments are inserted using BamHI and MluI cloning sites located within the intron 2. In this construct, the transcription is driven by the human CMV immediate-early promoter/enhancer (P CMV) from the pcDNA3.1(–) vector. (3) and (4) After transfection of the pCAS constructs into HeLa cells, total RNAs are extracted and the transcripts are analyzed by RT-PCR, using forward (F) and reverse (R) primers complementary to exon A and exon B of the minigene, respectively. The RT-PCR products are analyzed by electrophoresis on an agarose gel stained with ethidium bromide followed by direct sequencing of the different gel-excised bands. The effect of each variant is evaluated by comparison to the effect of the corresponding wild-type sequence. In this example, the variant sequence tested induces the complete skipping of the exon, while the wild-type exon is fully included in the mature transcript. Several other examples are presented in [*3, 4*].

Use of Splicing Reporter Minigene Assay to Evaluate the Effect on Splicing   251

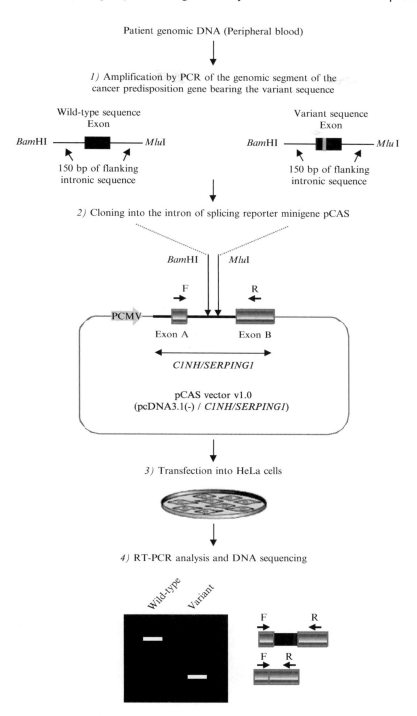

Fig. 1. Schematic representation of the functional splicing reporter minigene assay. (1) The wild-type and the variant exonic sequences of interest are PCR-amplified from patient genomic DNA together with ~150 bp of their 5′ and 3′ intronic flanking sequences, using specific primers carrying 5′ tails with BamHI and MluI restriction sites. (2) The amplicons are cloned into the pCAS1 reporter vector, which is based on the pcDNA3.1 plasmid and contains a minigene composed of two exons (here, named A and B). The minigene contains 114 bp of intron 1, exon 2, the entire intron 2, and exon 3, fused to partial exon 4 of the *SERPING1/C1NH* gene. In a recent version of the minigene construct, named pCAS2,

2. Materials

2.1. Splicing Reporter Minigene pCAS

The splicing reporter minigene pCAS (pCAS1) was constructed using the pcDNA3.1(–) vector (Invitrogen), by cloning into the EcoRI and BamHI sites an EcoRI-BglII fragment of the *C1 inhibitor* gene (*SERPING1/C1NH*, GenBank NM_000062), as described in (3–5) (see Fig. 1). It contains the last 114 bp of intron 1, exon 2, intron 2, and exon 3 fused to 122 bp of exon 4 of the *SERPING1/C1NH* gene. A MluI site was generated in the intron 2 of this construct, 118 bp downstream of a natural intronic BamHI site (see Fig. 1). In addition, the sequence of exon 3 was modified by site directed mutagenesis at three positions (underlined) resulting in the sequence AGCCAAGATCCAGA (5). These modifications inactivate an internal BamHI site and allow the discrimination between the endogenous *SERPING1/C1NH* mRNA and the one expressed from the transfected construct. The MluI site at position 229 bp of the pcDNA3.1(–) vector was also inactivated by site directed mutagenesis. In this construct, transcription is driven by the human CMV immediate-early promoter/enhancer from the pcDNA3.1(–) vector (see Fig. 1). A modified version of the pCAS1, named pCAS2, has recently been constructed in our laboratory and is currently under evaluation (unpublished). This new version differs from pCAS1 in that the stretch of 114 bp derived from intron 1 of the *SERPING1/C1NH* gene has been deleted, and the protein initiation codon in exon 2 of the *SERPING1/C1NH* gene has been inactivated.

2.2. Cloning Variant Sequences into the pCAS Vector

1. Amplification by PCR. Thermoprime plus DNA polymerase (ABgene) or a high fidelity DNA polymerase, such as the AccuPrime Taq DNA Polymerase High Fidelity, 100 mM dNTP Set PCR Grade (Invitrogen).
2. Electrophoresis. SeaKem LE Agarose (Tebu-bio), Tris Borate EDTA (TBE) buffer: 89 mM Tris-HCl, 89 mM Boric Acid, 2 mM EDTA (Euromedex), Ethidium bromide (Qbiogene), DNA size marker (New England Biolabs).
3. DNA purification from agarose gels. NucleoSpin Extract II kit (Macherey-Nagel).
4. Double digestion. Restriction endonucleases BamHI and MluI with NEBuffer 3 (New England Biolabs).
5. Ligation. T4 DNA ligase (New England Biolabs).
6. Transformation and bacterial culture. XL1B *E. Coli* competent cells (Stratagene), Bacterial growth Luria Bertani (LB) medium (MP Biomedicals), LB Agar (Invitrogen), Carbenicillin (Sigma).
7. Plasmid DNA purification. NucleoSpin plasmid kit (Macherey-Nagel).

8. Sequencing. ABI PRISM BigDye Terminator v3.1 cycle Sequencing kit (Applied Biosystems).

2.3. Transfection of the pCAS Vector into HeLa Cells

1. Cell Culture. HeLa cells (ATCC), Dulbecco's Modified Eagle's Medium (D-MEM) with L-Glutamine, 4,500 mg/L D-Glucose, without Sodium Pyruvate (Gibco), Fetal bovine serum (FBS) (Biowest).
2. Transfection. FuGENE 6 Transfection Reagent (Roche Applied Science).
3. Treatment by puromycin (Sigma-Aldrich).

2.4. RT-PCR Analysis

1. RNA extraction. TriPure Isolation Reagent (Roche Applied Science).
2. DNase treatment. Deoxyribonuclease Amplification Grade RNase-free (Sigma-Aldrich).
3. First-strand cDNA synthesis. SuperScript II Reverse Transcriptase (Invitrogen), Oligo(dT)$_{18}$ mRNA primer (New England Biolabs), 100 mM dNTP Set PCR Grade (Invitrogen), RNase OUT (Invitrogen).
4. Amplification by PCR. Thermoprime plus DNA polymerase (ABgene), 100 mM dNTP Set PCR Grade (Invitrogen).
5. Electrophoresis. SeaKem LE Agarose (Tebu-bio), TBE buffer: 89 mM Tris-HCl, 89 mM Boric Acid, 2 mM EDTA (Euromedex), Ethidium bromide (Qbiogene), DNA size marker (New England Biolabs).
6. DNA purification from agarose gel: NucleoSpin Extract II kit (Macherey-Nagel).
7. Sequencing: ABI PRISM BigDye Terminator v3.1 cycle Sequencing kit (Applied Biosystems).

3. Methods

3.1. Cloning of the Variant Sequence into the pCAS Vector

1. Amplification of the genomic fragments by PCR: The wild-type and the variant exonic sequences of interest are PCR-amplified from patient genomic DNA together with approximately 150 bp of their 5′ and 3′ intronic flanking sequences (see Notes 1 and 2). Specific forward and reverse primers carrying 5′ tails that contain sites for BamHI and MluI restriction enzymes are used (see Note 3). To a 0.2 mL Eppendorf tube, add 5 µL of 10× reaction buffer, 0.4 µM of each forward and reverse primers, 1.5 mM MgCl$_2$, 0.2 mM of each dNTP, 1.25 U Thermoprime plus DNA Polymerase (ABgene) (see Note 4), and 100 ng genomic DNA, and add

sterile distilled water to a final volume of 50 µL. Place Eppendorf tubes in the thermal cycler. The PCR program is divided into four steps: (1) initial denaturation step at 94°C for 5 min, (2) 30 cycles of 94°C for 20 s, 57°C for 30 s and 72°C for 30 s, and (3) final elongation step at 72°C for 10 min (see Note 5).

2. Separation of the PCR products, alongside the DNA size marker, by electrophoresis through an agarose gel containing ethidium bromide (0.5 µg/mL) in 1× TBE buffer (see Note 6). Purify the DNA bands from the agarose gel using NucleoSpin Extract II kit, according to the manufacturer's instructions (see Note 7).

3. Digestion of the purified PCR product by adding 10 U of the BamHI restriction enzyme and 10 U of the MluI restriction enzyme in NEBuffer 3 in the presence of BSA (1 µg/mL), add sterile distilled water to a final volume of 50 µL. Incubate at 37°C for 2 h for digestion. The double digestion reaction product is directly purified using NucleoSpin Extract II kit, according to the manufacturer's instructions.

4. Ligation of the digested and purified fragments (wild-type and variant sequences) into the BamHI and MluI restriction sites of the splicing reporter pCAS minigene (see Fig. 1) (see Note 8). Bacterial transformations are performed following standard protocols. Each transformed bacterial culture is plated onto an LB agar plate supplemented with carbenicillin (50 µg/mL). After incubation overnight at 37°C, isolated colonies are inoculated into 3 mL LB supplemented with carbenicillin (50 µg/mL) and grown at 37°C overnight under shaking. Plasmid DNA is prepared from colonies using a NucleoSpin plasmid kit, according to the manufacturer's instructions (see Note 9). Wild-type and mutant constructs are identified by sequencing. The sequence of the entire insert is verified to exclude the presence of unwanted PCR-generated mutations.

3.2. Cell Culture and Transfection

1. HeLa cells (see Note 10) are cultured as a monolayer at 37°C (95% air, 5% CO_2) in DMEM supplemented with 10% fetal calf serum. The cells are plated 1 day before transfection onto six-well plates at a density of approximately 5×10^5 cells/well.

2. Transfection is performed using FuGENE 6 transfection reagent, according to the manufacturer's instructions, using 1 µg/well of plasmid DNA and 3 µL of FuGENE 6 transfection reagent/well in OptiMEM medium. Wild-type and mutant constructs are transiently transfected into HeLa cells alongside each other. Two transfections are performed for each construct, one in the absence and the other in the presence of puromycin. For puromycin treatment, 10 µg/mL puromycin

is added to the culture 5.5 h before harvesting. Cells are collected 24 h post-transfection. Puromycin treatment inhibits translation, thus preventing the degradation of transcripts containing a premature stop codon that are targets of the nonsense-mediated mRNA decay (NMD).

3.3. RT-PCR Analysis

1. Total RNAs are isolated from transfected cells using the TriPure Isolation Reagent (Roche), according to the manufacturer's instructions. Total RNAs are quantified by spectrophotometry (optical density at 260 nm, OD_{260}). In order to eliminate contaminating DNA, RNAs are treated with Amplification Grade RNase-free DNase I (Sigma-Aldrich), as described by the manufacturer.

2. First-strand cDNAs are synthesized from 1 to 2 μg of each DNase-treated total RNA sample using oligo$(dT)_{18}$ mRNA primer and the SuperScriptTM II Reverse Transcriptase in a 20 μL reaction volume, as described by the manufacturer (see Note 11).

3. PCR amplifications are performed from 6 μL of the first-strand cDNA reaction mixture using primers F and R located, respectively, in exon A and exon B of the minigene pCAS1 (see Fig. 1). Thermoprime plus DNA Polymerase (ABgene) is used for the PCR reaction in a 50 μL volume, under the same conditions as described in step 1 of Subheading 3.1. PCRs are performed as follows: initial denaturation at 94°C for 5 min, followed by 30 cycles of 94°C for 10 s, 57°C for 20 s, and 72°C for 50 s, with a final elongation step at 72°C for 10 min (see Note 12).

4. RT-PCR products are separated, alongside the DNA size marker, by electrophoresis through an agarose gel containing ethidium bromide (0.5 μg/mL) in 1× TBE buffer and visualized by the exposure to ultraviolet light (see Note 6). Each DNA band is gel-purified using Nucleospin Extract II kit and sequenced using Big Dye Terminator cycle sequencing kit and ABI Prism 3100 automated sequencer, as described by the manufacturers (see Note 13).

4. Notes

1. In most cases studied, the sequence variant to be tested is present in the heterozygous state. Therefore, the wild-type and the variant exonic sequences are coamplified by PCR from patient genomic DNA and subsequently selected after molecular cloning and sequencing.

2. A genomic segment containing up to 150 nucleotides of flanking intronic sequences is a reasonable starting point. When one of the flanking intronic sequences is smaller than 150 nucleotides, a genomic DNA fragment containing two exons can be amplified and cloned into the pCAS vector. For example, we use this strategy to study UVs in the exons 17 and 18 of the *MLH1* gene.

3. When the region to be amplified contains one of these restriction sites, the restriction sites BglII or AscI can be included into the 5′ tails of the primers, in lieu of BamHI and MluI, respectively. These sites are compatible with BamHI and MluI sites, respectively, present in the splicing reporter minigene pCAS.

4. For genomic fragments smaller than 500 bp in size, standard thermophilic DNA polymerases can be used. For genomic fragments greater than 500 bp in size, we recommend using a high fidelity DNA polymerase, such as the Pfu Ultra High-Fidelity DNA polymerase, in order to ensure error-free amplification.

5. In our hands, these PCR reaction conditions work well for most of the amplicons tested. However, for some specific DNA target sequence, the PCR conditions could require optimization (see Ref. 6).

6. The concentration of agarose used, the voltage applied and the time of electrophoresis will vary according to the size of the PCR product to be resolved.

7. It is important to minimize ultraviolet light (UV) exposure in order to protect the DNA bands from UV-induced mutations.

8. The preparation of the splicing reporter minigene vector involves the following steps: double digestion by BamHI and MluI restriction enzymes, phosphatase treatment, and agarose gel purification. The ligation of the PCR product into the minigene vector is then performed according to a standard protocol. Typically, we use the T4 DNA ligase (New England Biolabs), according to the manufacturer's indications.

9. Typically, six plasmid DNAs are prepared and sequenced for each construct.

10. HeLa immortal cell line derived from human cervical cancer cells presents high transfection efficiency. Most in vitro studies on splicing are carried out using extracts from HeLa cells. Other cell lines can be used, taking into consideration that splicing regulation can be cell-type specific.

11. Alternatively, both reverse transcription and PCR amplification can be combined in a one-step reaction using commercial kit such as the "OneStep RT-PCR Kit" from Qiagen.

12. Typically, we use 30 cycles for PCR amplification in order to detect potential minor bands and to generate enough product for sequencing. In some cases, a semi-quantitative RT-PCR analysis can be useful to determine the ratio of the different mRNA splice variants. This requires using PCR conditions within the linear range of amplification, determined experimentally by using different number of cycles.

13. All wild-type *MLH1, MSH2, BRCA1, and BRCA2* exons that we have tested in the pCAS assay were predominantly included in the mature transcript (see (3, 4)). A sequence variant can induce different effects on splicing such as exon skipping, cryptic splice site activation, cryptic splice site disruption, or generation of a new splice site. The impact of the variants on splicing is determined by comparison of the splicing patterns obtained from the wild-type and variant minigene constructs (see Fig. 1). The RT-PCR products are first analyzed by electrophoresis to detect size differences, but the real identity of each band is determined by sequencing.

Acknowledgments

This work has been generously supported by the Foundation de France (including a fellowship to Pascaline Gaildrat) and is presently supported by the French North West Canceropole.

References

1. Baralle, D., and Baralle, M. (2005) Splicing in action: assessing disease causing sequence changes. *J. Med. Genet.* **42**, 737–748
2. Cooper, T.A. (2005) Use of minigene systems to dissect alternative splicing elements. *Methods* **37**, 331–340
3. Tournier, I., Vezain, M., Martins, A., Charbonnier, F., Baert-Desurmont, S., Olschwang, S et al. (2008) A large fraction of unclassified variants of the mismatch repair genes MLH1 and MSH2 is associated with splicing defects. *Hum. Mutat.* **29**, 1412–1424
4. Bonnet, C., Krieger, S., Vezain, M., Rousselin, A., Tournier, I., Martins, A., et al. (2008) Screening BRCA1 and BRCA2 unclassified variants for splicing mutations using reverse transcription PCR on patient RNA and an ex vivo assay based on a splicing reporter minigene. *J. Med. Genet.* **45**, 438–446
5. Duponchel, C., Djenouhat, K., Frémeaux-Bacchi, V., Monnier, N., Drouet, C., and Tosi, M. (2006) Functional analysis of splicing mutations and of an exon 2 polymorphic variant of SERPING1/C1NH. *Hum. Mutat.* **27**, 295–296
6. Kolmodin, L.A. and Birch, D.E. (2002) Polymerase chain reaction. Basic principles and routine practice. *Methods Mol. Biol.* **192**, 3–18

Chapter 16

Functional Analysis of Human BRCA2 Variants Using a Mouse Embryonic Stem Cell-Based Assay

Sergey G. Kuznetsov, Suhwan Chang, and Shyam K. Sharan

Abstract

We describe here a comprehensive and reliable assay to test the functional significance of variants of unknown clinical significance (VUS) identified in the human breast cancer susceptibility gene, *BRCA2*. The assay is based on the ability of human *BRCA2* to complement the loss of endogenous *Brca2* in mouse embryonic stem cells. The procedure involves generation of a desired mutation in *BRCA2* present in a bacterial artificial chromosome (BAC) and the introduction of the BAC into ES cells engineered for the assay. These ES cells have one null and one conditional allele of *Brca2*. First, the effect of the BRCA2 variants on the viability of ES cells is tested by Cre-mediated deletion of the conditional allele. Subsequently, variants that result in viable ES cells are examined for their effect on known functions of BRCA2 using a variety of functional assays such as sensitivity to genotoxic agents, in vivo and in vitro proliferation, effect on homologous recombination and genomic stability. The method described herein allows for the analysis of three to five sequence variants within 2–3 months. This approach can also be used for functional analysis of variants identified in other human disease genes that result in a phenotype detectable in ES cells.

Key words: Breast cancer, BRCA2, Variants of unknown clinical significance (VUS), Missense mutation, Mouse embryonic stem (ES) cells, Functional assay, DNA repair, Bacterial artificial chromosome (BAC), *HPRT1* minigene

1. Introduction

The identification of a number of human disease genes and advances in sequencing technologies have revolutionized the field of molecular diagnostics in the last decade (1). Among the genes that are routinely being tested are the breast cancer susceptibility genes *BRCA1* and *BRCA2*. For *BRCA1/2* mutation carriers, the lifetime risk of developing breast or ovarian cancer is 80% and 37%, respectively. Therefore, it is not surprising that individuals with a family history of these cancers are now opting to know if they have a mutation in one of these genes. One of the inherent weaknesses of sequencing-based approaches is the determination of the actual risk associated with any variant identified in the gene. This is highlighted by the fact that more than 800 variants of BRCA1 and 1,100 variants of BRCA2 are listed as variants of unknown clinical significance in the breast cancer information core (BIC) database (http://research.nhgri.nih.gov/projects/bic/). Segregation analysis in disease-afflicted families provides the most reliable information to distinguish between deleterious and neutral alterations identified in hereditary disease genes (2). However, there is an enormous need to have a functional assay to classify variants for which such information is not available because most mutations are rare and familial data are often insufficient (3).

The functional significance of nonsense and frame shifting mutations can be predicted with a high degree of confidence. In contrast, the functional significance of splicing, intronic, regulatory, and point mutations is more difficult to predict.

The functionality of some sequence variants can be tested in a complementation assay when a corresponding mutant gene is transfected into an established cell line in which its endogenous counterpart is inactive (4). However, such complementation assays have two caveats. First, they usually rely upon the delivery of a certain gene using cDNAs under the control of a heterologous promoter. This often results in a significantly higher expression level than the endogenous protein, which for many genes leads to apoptosis. In addition, cDNA expression vectors do not allow for testing mutations that affect splicing or map to regulatory regions. Second, established tumor cell lines are inherently prone to genomic instability and cell cycle deregulation, which sometimes complicates the interpretation of the results (5). ES cells are more suitable for such studies because they retain a normal karyotype, even after extensive genetic manipulations, which makes them suitable for the functional analysis of DNA repair genes like *BRCA2* (6). Instead of using cDNA expression vectors, BACs allow for gene expression at physiological levels under the control of their own promoter. More importantly, this allows the examination of regulatory mutations as well as splicing and intronic alterations in addition to those that alter the protein-coding sequence. Desired mutations in *BRCA2* can be rapidly generated in the BAC using the recombineering technology (7–10). We have demonstrated the suitability of mouse ES cells and BACs for the functional analysis of human mutations by analyzing sequence variants of the human *BRCA2* (11). Using this approach, as outlined in Fig. 1, 5 variants can be tested in 2–3 months.

The functional assay is based on the observation that BRCA2 is essential for ES cell viability and DNA double strand break repair (12). The ability of BRCA2 variants to rescue the lethality of *Brca2*-deficient ES-cells and complement DNA repair defect is

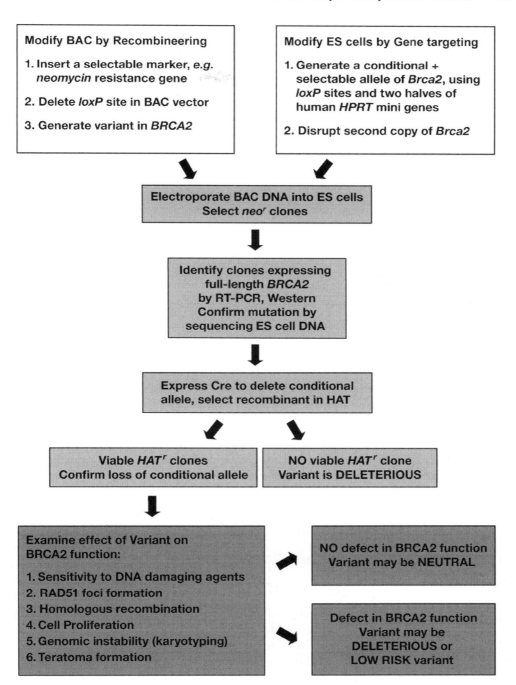

Fig. 1. Overall scheme to evaluate functional significance of human BRCA2 variants. Overview of the experimental design to examine the functional significance of BRCA2 variants in mouse ES-cells. Different steps are described in detail in the text.

used to evaluate their functional significance. The assay utilizes a mouse ES cell line, PL2F7, in which one allele is functionally null and the other allele is rendered conditional (see Fig. 2).

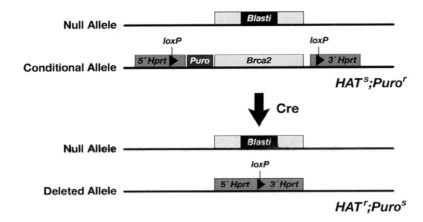

Fig. 2. Generation of ES cells with a conditional allele of *Brca2*. To generate a conditional allele of *Brca2* and to select the recombinants, two *loxP* sites were targeted upstream and downstream of the gene along with the 3′ or 5′ halves of the human *HPRT1* minigene and a Puromycin resistance gene by homologous recombination. To disrupt the other allele of *Brca2*, a Blasticidin resistance gene was targeted to exon 11. The conditional allele of *Brca2* can be deleted by transiently expressing Cre. ES cells become HAT^r and $Puro^s$. However, such cells do not survive because of the loss of functional BRCA2.

The allele that is functionally null has an insertion of the *Blasticidin* resistance gene in exon 11. The conditional allele has two *loxP* sites upstream and downstream of *Brca2*. In addition, a *puromycin* resistance gene is targeted next to the *loxP* site upstream of *Brca2* such that it would be deleted along with *Brca2* after the Cre-mediated recombination of the *loxP* sites. To allow for the selection of the recombinant clones, two halves of the human *HPRT1* minigene are targeted along with the *loxP* sites. The *HPRT1* minigene can be split into two fragments, a 5′ fragment containing sequences from exons 1–2 and intron 2, and the 3′ fragment containing intron 2 and exons 3–9 (13). A *loxP* site is present in intron 2 in both the fragments. The two halves of *HPRT1* can recombine in the presence of the Cre protein to generate a functional *HPRT1* minigene and the recombinants can be selected in the presence of HAT. The PL2F7 ES cell line is derived from an *Hprt*-deficient ES cell line (AB2.2), which allows the use of *HPRT1*-mediated selection.

When Cre is transiently expressed in PL2F7 cells, HAT^r clones do not survive due to the loss of BRCA2 (11). However, when a BAC clone expressing the wild type human BRCA2 is introduced into PL2F7 cells, viable HAT^r clones are obtained. BRCA2 variants can be generated in the BAC DNA and electroporated into PL2F7 cells before the conditional allele of *Brca2* can be deleted. When no HAT^r colonies are obtained after Cre expression, the BRCA2 sequence variant is likely to be deleterious. Variants that result in viable ES cells are tested for their effect on the known functions of BRCA2 such as DNA repair, in vitro proliferation, RAD51 foci formation, homologous recombination, genomic stability, in vivo proliferation and differentiation by teratoma formation in mice (see Fig. 1). We describe here in detail various steps involved in the generation of a BRCA2 variant in BAC, introducing the BAC into ES cells and performing various functional assays.

2. Materials

2.1. Bacterial Strain

The *Escherichia coli* SW102 strain harboring the defective lambda prophage and used for recombineering can be obtained from NCI recombineering resource (http://recombineering.ncifcrf.gov/). This strain is temperature sensitive and must be grown at 32°C.

2.2. Cell Lines

1. PL2F7 ES-cells generated from *Hprt*-deficient AB2.2 (129S7/SvEvBrd-Hprt$^{b\text{-}m2}$) mouse ES cells (13). PL2F7 cells have one functionally null and one conditional allele of *Brca2* (available upon request).
2. SNL 76/7 STO feeder cells (14).

2.3. Equipment

Standard laboratory equipments are used, some of which are described below:

1. An incubator set at 32°C, a shaking incubator set at 32°C and shaking water bath (200 rpm) set at 42°C
2. CO_2 incubators
3. Electroporator (Genepulser II with Pulse Controller II, BioRad) and cuvettes with 0.1 and 0.4 cm gap (BioRad)
4. High speed centrifuge and a refrigerated microcentrifuge
5. PCR machine
6. Spectrophotometer
7. Microplate reader
8. Coulter particle counter Z1 (Beckman Coulter)
9. Inverse microscope with a phase contrast (Leica)
10. Hybridization oven (VWR)
11. UV crosslinker 1800 (Stratagene)
12. ^{137}Cs γ-irradiator

2.4. Antibodies

1. Rabbit anti-Rad51 (Calbiochem)
2. Mouse anti-γ-H2AX antibody (Upstate)
3. FDAR (Fluorescein (FITC) AffiniPure Donkey Anti Rabbit IgG, Jackson Labs)

4. RDAM (Rhodamine (TRITC) AffiniPure Donkey Anti-Mouse IgG, Jackson Labs)
5. Rabbit Anti-BRCA2 (Ab-2, Calbiochem)
6. Goat anti-rabbit IgG-HRP (Santa Cruz)

2.5. Other Reagents

1. BAC Clone RPCI-11 777 19I (for simplicity referred to as BAC777, 250 kb genomic fragment containing human BRCA2 in *pBACe3.6* vector, in which *loxP511* site was deleted and the second loxP site replaced with a PGK-Neo cassette, available upon request)
2. Plasmid DNA purification reagents (Qiagen)
3. Gel extraction kit or reagents to purify DNA from Agarose gel (Qiagen)
4. Expand High Fidelity (HiFi) PCR System (Roche)
5. D-PBS (Gibco)
6. DMEM without phenol red (Gibco)
7. Trypsin-EDTA (Invitrogen)
8. HAT supplement (Gibco)
9. HT supplement (Gibco)
10. G418 (Geneticin®, Gibco)
11. Puromycin (Sigma)
12. Prime-It® II Random Primer Labeling Kit (Stratagene)
13. LB Medium
14. LB Agar
15. M15 medium: To make 600 mL of M15 medium, add 90 mL of Fetal Bovine Serum (HyClone ES cell quality, final conc. 15%), 6 mL of 10 mM β-mercaptoethanol (Sigma, final conc. 0.1 mM) and 6 mL of 100× GPS (glutamate, penicillin/streptomycin, Gibco) to 500 mL of Knockout-DMEM (Invitrogen)
16. ES-cell Lysis Buffer: 10 mM Tris-HCl, pH 7.5, 10 mM EDTA, pH 8.0, 10 mM NaCl, 0.5% Sarcosyl, 1 mg/mL Proteinase K
17. 1× TAE buffer
18. 1× TBE buffer
19. TBS buffer
20. RIPA buffer
21. NuPAGE MOPS SDS running buffer
22. 1× NuPAGE transfer buffer
23. Antibody blocking solution

2.6. Mice

1. Immunocompromised athymic nude mice (C3H/HeNCr-nu)

3. Methods

3.1. Generation of a Desired Mutation in BRCA2 in the BAC DNA by Recombineering Technology Using a Two-Step "Hit and Fix" Method

The use of oligonucleotides to generate subtle alterations in a BAC, without the use of any selectable marker by recombineering in *E. coli* strains harboring a defective lambda prophage, such as DY380 or SW102, has been described in detail previously (9, 15, 16). Recombinants can be identified by a mismatch amplification mutation assay (17). While this approach is helpful, it can occasionally result in false positive clones. A two-step "hit and fix" method allows for a rapid generation of any mutation in BACs, and recombinants can be easily identified using standard PCR-based methods (9). The two-step "hit and fix" procedure involves the introduction of 20 unique nucleotides (unique heterologous sequence) to the site where a mutation has to be generated in the first "hit" step (see Fig. 3).

The original sequence is then restored with the exception of the point mutation in the second "fix" step. In both steps, 180-bases-long single-stranded DNA fragments generated by PCR are used as targeting vectors. The 20 nucleotide sequence can be used for initial screening by PCR; however, the hybridization approach allows screening of more than 5,000 individual colonies from a single 15 cm agar plate (10). It also allows the simultaneous screening of multiple mutations ("hit" step) by using the same hybridization probe. In addition, the "hit" cassette is designed to contain several restriction sites that facilitate rapid confirmation of the correct targeting.

3.1.1. Introduction of the BAC DNA into SW102 Strain to Provide the Lambda Recombination Function

1. To prepare electro-competent SW102 cells, pick an isolated colony of SW102 strain of *E. coli* from a LB plate and grow overnight in 3 mL of LB at 32°C.
2. Next morning add 1 mL of the culture to 50 mL of LB in a 250 mL flask and grow at 32°C to an OD_{600} of 0.50–0.60. Transfer 10 mL of the culture to a 50 mL Oak Ridge tube and centrifuge at $6,000 \times g$ in a prechilled rotor for 10 min at 1°C.
3. Wash the cell pellet once with 10 mL of ice-cold water, resuspend in 1 mL of water and transfer to a chilled 1.5 mL tube. Centrifuge at $18,000 \times g$ for 20–30 s at 1°C.
4. Wash the cells two more times with 1 mL of ice cold water. Resuspend the cell pellet in water to a final volume of 50 µL and keep on ice.
5. Mix 1 µL of BAC DNA (100 ng) with 50 µl of electro-competent *E. coli* cells and chill on ice for 5 min and then transfer into a 0.1 cm gap cuvette. Set the Gene Pulser at 1.8 kV, 25 µF capacitance and 200 ohm resistance.
6. Electroporate the BAC DNA into the cells and immediately add 1 mL of LB medium.

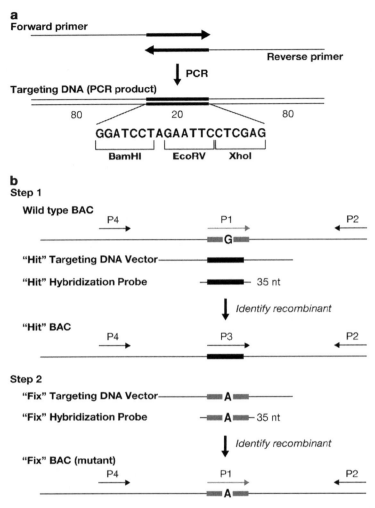

Fig. 3. Two-step "hit & fix" method to generate subtle mutations using single stranded short PCR product or oligonucleotides as targeting vector. (**a**) The single-stranded oligonucleotides containing 160 bases of homology and 20 unique bases are generated by using two 100-mer oligonucleotides in a PCR reaction. The two 100-mer oligonucleotides have 20 complementary bases (in this case the 20 bp contains restriction sites *Bam*HI, *Eco*RV, *Xho*I) at the 3′ end. The 180 bp PCR product can be denatured to obtain single-stranded oligonucleotides that can be used as the targeting construct. (**b**) Schematic representation of the two steps involved in the "hit and fix" method to generate subtle alterations (e.g. G to A) without the use of a selectable marker. In step 1, a 180-mer single-strand oligonucleotide is used to replace 20 nucleotides (*gray box*) around the target site with 20 heterologous nucleotides (*black box*). Recombinants can be identified by colony hybridization using an end-labeled 35-mer oligonuclotide that can specifically anneal only to the recombinant DNA. A primer set specific for the heterologous "hit" sequence (P3 and P2) can be used to confirm the presence of recombinant clones by PCR. A second primer set (P1 and P2) can be used as a control to amplify only the nonrecombinant DNA. Generation of a correct recombinant clone can be confirmed by digesting the PCR product (~300–500 bp) produced using primers P2 and P4 with *Bam*HI, *Eco*RV or *Xho*I. In step 2, the 20 nucleotides are restored to the original sequence, except for the desired mutation. Such clones can be identified by colony hybridization using a 35-mer oligonucleotide as a probe and further confirmed by PCR amplification using primers P1 and P2, by testing for the loss of the restriction sites inserted in step 1, by digesting the PCR product of primers P2 and P4, and by sequencing. (Reproduced from ref. 10).

7. Grow cells at 32°C for 1 h. Centrifuge the cells and resuspend in 200 µL of LB medium.

8. Plate the cells on an LB agar plate containing chloramphenicol (12 µg/ml). Incubate overnight at 32°C.

9. Pick isolated colonies for recombineering. Confirm the integrity of the BAC DNA by digesting the BAC with a few restriction enzymes (e.g. *Bam*HI, *Eco*RI, *Hin*dIII, *Eco*RV) and comparing the restriction pattern with the original BAC clone by running the two samples in parallel on a 0.8% agarose gel. Make glycerol stocks and freeze at –80°C.

3.1.2. Generation of a Targeting Cassette to Introduce a Desired Mutation in a BAC

A targeting cassette to generate a point mutation in a BAC is synthesized by PCR using two 100-mer oligonucleotide primers overlapping by 20 nucleotides at their 3'-end. The resulting targeting vector contains two homology arms that are 80 bases in length, flanking a 20-mer heterologous sequence in the middle (see Fig. 3a). This heterologous sequence (5'-GGATCCTAGAATTCCTCGAG-3') is the same for all "hit" targeting vectors allowing for a highly efficient and simultaneous screening of targeted clones of any number of mutated genes or regions. "Fix" targeting cassettes are composed of the same homology arms as the corresponding "hit" vectors, while the heterologous middle region of the "hit" vector is replaced with the final sequence including a desired mutation. At this point, a 20–35-mer oligonucleotide encompassing this region can serve as a probe to differentiate "fix"-recombinants from the "hit" (see Fig. 3b).

1. Set up the following reaction using the Expand High Fidelity (HiFi) PCR System (Roche, cat.# 11732641001). In general, use 6 µL of each 100-mer oligonucleotide (10 µM) and 10 µL of 2 mM dNTPs, 2 µL of HiFi Taq Polymerase (3.5 U/µL) in a 100 µL PCR reaction. Conditions for the PCR cycle include an initial denaturation at 94°C for 1 min followed by 40 cycles of 94°C for 30 s, 55–60°C for 30 s, and 72°C for 30 s and a final extension at 72°C for 2 min.

2. Examine 1 µL of the reaction on a 1.0–1.5% agarose gel in 1× TAE buffer. A 180 bp product should be observed (see Note 1).

3. Purify the targeting vector using a Qiagen PCR Purification Kit and elute in 30 µL of Qiagen Elution Buffer or ethanol-precipitate and dissolve in 20–30 µL dH$_2$O.

3.1.3. Induction of the Lambda Recombination Genes and Preparation of Electrocompetent Cells

1. Inoculate SW102 cells containing the BAC from a frozen glycerol stock or a single colony into 3–5 mL LB medium. Shake at 32°C overnight.

2. Add 0.5 mL of the overnight culture to 35 mL of LB medium in a 250-mL (baffled) Erlenmeyer flask.

3. Grow cells at 32°C for about 2 h. The cells are ready when the OD_{600} is between 0.5 and 0.6. It is important not to overgrow the cells.

4. Transfer 10 mL of the culture to a 50 mL Erlenmeyer flask and place that flask in the 42°C water bath. Shake for 15 min at 200 rpm to induce the lambda recombination genes. Leave the remainder of the culture on ice (see Note 2).

5. Immediately after inducing for 15 min at 42°C, rapidly cool the flask on ice with gentle swirling for 10–15 min. As a control, use 10 mL of uninduced cells and process them exactly as the induced cells. While the cells are on ice, precool the centrifuge to 4°C and chill two labeled 50 mL Oak Ridge tubes.

6. Transfer 10 mL of both the induced and uninduced cultures to the Oak Ridge tubes. Centrifuge for 10 min at $4,600 \times g$ at 4°C. Carefully discard the supernatant.

7. Add 1 mL ice-cold distilled water to the cell pellet in the bottom of each tube and gently resuspend the cells with a large pipet tip (do not vortex). Add 30 mL ice-cold distilled water to each tube and mix gently. Centrifuge tubes again as in the previous step.

8. Decant the supernatant very carefully from the soft pellet in each tube and resuspend each cell pellet in 1 mL ice-cold distilled water. (Remove tubes from the centrifuge promptly. Because the pellet is very soft, care should be taken not to dislodge it, especially when processing multiple tubes).

9. Transfer the resuspended cells to prechilled microcentrifuge tubes. Centrifuge 30–60 s at a maximum speed at 4°C. Carefully aspirate the supernatant.

10. Wash the cells two more times with 1 mL of ice cold water.

11. Resuspend the cell pellet in the cold distilled water to a total volume of 50 µL.

3.1.4. Electroporating the Targeting Vector into SW102 Cells Containing the BAC

1. Chill the desired number of 0.1-cm electroporation cuvettes on ice.

2. In a 0.5 mL tube, mix appropriate volume of DNA (200–300 ng of salt-free PCR fragment) with 50 µL of electro-competent induced or uninduced cells. Leave the tubes on ice for 5 min.

3. Electroporate the DNA into the cells using 1.8 kV, 25 µF capacitance, and 200 ohm resistance. Immediately add 1 mL LB medium to the cuvette and transfer the electroporation mix to sterile culture tubes and incubate the tubes with shaking at 32°C for 1.5 h.

4. Serially dilute the cell suspension in LB medium and plate 200 µL of 10^{-2} and 10^{-3} dilutions onto a 15 cm LB agar plate containing an appropriate antibiotic (Chloramphenicol

at 12 μg/mL or Kanamycin at 25 μg/mL). Use sterile glass beads instead of a bacteriological spreader to achieve a uniform distribution of colonies throughout the plate. Incubate agar plates for 18–22 h at 32°C.

3.1.5. Identifying the Recombinant Clones

1. Pick the plate with approximately 3,000–6,000 colonies. Colony density should be such that individual colonies can be identified. Transfer the colonies to a charged nylon membrane (Hybond) by standard methods and hybridize with γ-^{32}P-labeled oligonucleotide probe for 2–3 h at 50°C. Hybridizing for more than 4 h results in high background. This oligonucleotide probe corresponds to the heterologous sequence that is being inserted in the "hit" step.

2. After positive clones are identified, they should be subcloned by a second round of hybridization to obtain a pure recombinant clone that does not contain the original nonrecombinant BAC.

3. Confirm by testing for restriction sites present in the heterologous sequence or by sequencing.

4. Once the correctly targeted pure "hit" colonies are identified, repeat the targeting step (fix targeting) to replace the 20-nucleotide heterologous sequence with the desired mutation exactly as described above for the "hit" step.

5. Confirm the mutation by sequencing.

3.2. Electroporating the BAC DNA into ES Cells

1. Prepare BAC DNA, using a QIAGEN Maxi Prep kit from bacteria cultured overnight at 32°C in 250 mL LB medium according to a manufacturer's protocol. Dissolve the DNA pellet in 100 μL dH$_2$O. The usual yield is between 50 and 150 μg of DNA.

2. Expand PL2F7 ES cells by growing them on SNL feeder cells in M15 medium using standard ES cell culturing techniques as described previously (18).

3. Split PL2F7 cells at 1:2 ratio one day prior to BAC electroporation. 1.0×10^7 cells are needed for each electroporation. The usual yield from one 80–90% confluent 10 cm dish is $2.5–3 \times 10^7$ cells.

4. Change the M15 medium 3–4 h prior to the electroporation.

5. Wash the plates two times with PBS, add 2 ml trypsin, incubate 15 min at 37°C, add 2 mL M15, disaggregate the cells by vigorous pipetting 25–30 times using a plastic disposable transfer pipette, pellet cells by centrifugation at $250 \times g$ for 5 min, wash once with 10 mL PBS, pellet cells as before, resuspend in 1 ml PBS and count 20 μL aliquot using a Coulter counter. Adjust cell concentration to 1.1×10^7 cells/ml with PBS.

6. Transfer 0.9 mL cell suspension into an electroporation cuvette.
7. Add 25 µg BAC DNA. Mix by inverting several times. Leave the cuvette at room temperature for 5 min.
8. Set the electroporator (BioRad GenePulser II) at 230 V, 500 µF and electroporate the BAC into ES cells. The time constant should be between 5.6 and 7.3 msec.
9. Leave the cuvette at room temperature for 5 min. Transfer the electroporated cells to a 10 cm feeder plate containing 15 mL of M15 medium. After 36 h, add G418 (180 µg/mL) to M15 medium.
10. Change the medium daily with fresh M15 medium containing G418 for 5 days. After 5 days, add M15 without G418.
11. Once colonies become visible (usually takes 2–3 days), pick 24–36 colonies in a 96-well plate (one colony/well) for each BAC construct as described previously (18) (see Note 3).
12. Once cells are about 80% confluent, split them into three 96-well plates (one plate with feeders and two gelatinized plates without feeders).
13. When cells are about 80% confluent, freeze the plates with feeders using freezing medium (60% DMEM, 20% FBS, 20% DMSO; freshly prepared) as described previously (18).
14. Wash the plates without feeders twice with PBS, remove PBS, and transfer at −80°C.
15. Plates can be stored at −80°C for up to 6 months.

3.3. Select BRCA2 BAC Transgenic ES Cell Clones by Southern Hybridization

Identify ES cell clones that have full-length *BRCA2* gene by Southern blot analysis using probes from the 5′ and 3′ ends of the gene. Subsequently, test the "Southern positive" clones for BRCA2 expression by Western blot analysis. When a variant is predicted to result in no detectable protein product, RT-PCR should be performed to detect mRNA expression.

1. Remove one of the 96-well plates from step 14 of Subheading 3.2, add 50 µL of ES-cell Lysis Buffer per well, incubate overnight at 60°C.
2. Extract DNA, digest with *Eco*RI restriction enzyme as described previously (18).
3. Load the DNA samples on a 0.8% agarose gel (1× TBE buffer). 96 DNA samples can be analyzed on a 20×25 cm^2 gel with three rows of 36-wells. Run the gel long enough to separate 1.8 kb and 4.3 kb *Eco*RI fragments corresponding to 5′- and 3′-ends of *BRCA2*, respectively.
4. Transfer the DNA to a nylon membrane using Southern blotting procedure and hybridize the membrane with ^{32}P-labeled both 5′- and 3′-BRCA2 probes (see Note 4) using standard procedures (19).

5. Identify ES cell clones positive for both probes. Usually 50% of such clones express the BRCA2 protein.

3.4. Western Blot Analysis to Identify BRCA2 Expressing Clones

1. Thaw the 96-well plate containing frozen ES cells from step 14 of Subheading 3.2 at 37°C. Transfer Southern positive ES cells identified above into a 24-well plate with a feeder layer containing 2 mL M15 medium in each well. The entire well content including the oil should be transferred into 24-well plates. Incubate the plate until the wells become 80% confluent. Change the M15 medium daily.
2. To obtain cells for the Western blot, trypsinize ES cells growing in 24-well plates with 250 µL trypsin-EDTA.
3. Add 250 µL M15 medium, dissociate cells by pipetting and transfer 100 µL aliquot in to a new 6-well plate pretreated with gelatin and containing 4 mL M15 medium. Freeze the rest of the cells in individual freezing vials after adding 400 µL of 2× freezing medium.
4. Once the 6-well plate is almost 100% confluent, lyse the cells for Western analysis.
5. Wash plates twice with PBS, add 200 µL RIPA buffer, scrape cells using a plastic scraper and transfer into 1.5 mL Eppendorf tubes.
6. Rotate the cell lysates at 4°C for 40 min. Clear the lysates by centrifuging at $12,000 \times g$ for 10 min.
7. Transfer the supernatant into a new tube and estimate the protein concentration in the lysates using the BCA method according to manufacturer's procedure.
8. Prepare samples for Western blot. Take 35 µg protein, bring up the lysate volume to 15 µL with RIPA buffer, add 5.5 µL of 4× loading dye solution (Invitrogen), and 2 µL Sample Reducing Agent (Invitrogen).
9. Heat protein samples at 70°C for 10 min and chill on ice.
10. Assemble a precast NuPAGE 4–12% Bis-Tris gel cassette (Invitrogen) in a corresponding gel box with NuPAGE MOPS SDS Running buffer. Add 500 µL antioxidant in 200 mL running buffer in the upper chamber.
11. Load the samples and SeeBlue Plus 2 size marker (Invitrogen) in gel slots and run a gel at 200 V for 1 h.
12. Set up protein transfer onto a PVDF membrane in 1× NuPAGE Transfer Buffer containing 10% methanol, according to manufacturer's instructions. Transfer at 22 V overnight at 4°C. Results are more consistent when one blot is transferred per transfer module.
13. Next day, disassemble the transfer module, mark the wells, and label the blot with a pencil. Soak the membrane in two changes of TBS.

14. Transfer the membrane into blocking buffer (1× TBS, 0.05% Tween20, 5% Milk) and incubate for 1 h at room temperature with agitation.
15. Wash in 1× TBS, 0.05% Tween20 three times for 5 min.
16. Incubate the membrane with the primary antibody (Rabbit-anti-human BRCA2) in the blocking buffer overnight on a rocking platform at 4°C.
17. Wash the blot three times for 30 min in 1× TBS, 0.05% Tween20 at room temperature.
18. Incubate with the secondary antibody for 30 min at room temperature (HRP-labeled goat-anti-rabbit IgG antibody).
19. Wash four times, 30 min each in 1× TBS, 0.05% Tween20 at room temperature.
20. Detect the chemiluminescent signal using ECL Plus system, according to the manufacturer's procedure. Identify "Western-positive" ES cell clones (see Note 5).

3.5. Excision of the Conditional Brca2 Allele

1. Thaw Western-positive ES cell clones in 6 cm feeder plates. Test at least two clones for each sequence variant. Select clones that express BRCA2 at a level comparable to the endogenous levels (e.g., in human ES cells).
2. Split 80% confluent plates 1:2 one day prior to electroporation.
3. Electroporate 25 µg *Pgk-Cre* plasmid for each clone as described in steps 7–9 of Subheading 3.2.
4. Plate 10 µL (10^5 cells) of the electroporated cells into a 10 cm feeder plate.
5. Freeze the remaining unelectroporated cells into two freezing vials at approximately 5×10^6 cells per vial.
6. Select for recombinant clones in HAT containing M15 medium, 36 h after electroporation. Maintain HAT selection for 5 days. Change HAT containing M15 medium everyday.
7. Replace HAT supplement with HT for an two additional days.
8. Culture the cells in M15 medium for additional 3–4 days until colonies are ready to be picked. When a BAC containing wild-type *BRCA2* is used, 1,000–3,000 HAT^r colonies are obtained on one 10 cm dish. PL2F7 cells yield less than 10 colonies, which represent background colonies. Therefore, hypomorphic BRCA2 variants may yield less than 1,000 colonies depending on the mutation.

See Note 6 for an alternative approach.

3.6. Confirming the Cre-mediated Loss of the Conditional Allele

1. Pick 12–24 colonies for each electroporated clone and transfer them into a 96-well feeder plate and expand them to one 96-well feeder plate and two 96-well plates without feeders as described above. Sensitivity of ES cell clones to puromycin

can be used to determine the loss of the conditional allele. However, clones must be genotyped to confirm the loss of the conditional allele. Use one of the plates without feeders for genotyping by Southern analysis as described above in Subheading 3.3.

2. Use *Eco*RV enzyme to digest the DNA and probe "144/145" for hybridization (see Note 7).

3. Identify clones that have lost the wild type (conditional) *Brca2* allele (see Note 8).

4. Expand 3–5 correctly targeted HAT^r ES cell clones for each variant from a frozen 96-well feeder plate and freeze stocks in liquid nitrogen.

5. Proceed with functional analysis using two clones for each variant.

3.7. Functional Analysis of ES Cell Clones Expressing BRCA2 Variants

Test the DNA repair function of BRCA2 sequence variants by challenging them with various DNA-damaging compounds.

3.7.1. Testing Sensitivity to DNA Damaging Compounds

1. Seed 8,000 ES cells per well in a gelatinized 96-well plate. Clones with poor plating efficiency or proliferation defect may need to be seeded at a higher density to compensate for lower growth and seeding efficiency (see Note 9). Designate seven rows for increasing drug concentrations with three columns for each clone being tested (triplicates). Leave the last row empty as a blank control.

2. Eighteen hours after seeding the cells, replace the M15 for medium containing increasing doses of each of the DNA damaging compounds (see Note 10).

3. Maintain treatment for 3 days without changing the medium.

4. Estimate relative cell survival using XTT metabolic assay (20). Wash the plates twice with PBS. Leave the plates with the last change of PBS at 37°C while mixing warm XTT solution with PMS. Replace PBS with 100 µL of XTT reagent per well.

5. Incubate for 2.5–3 h at 37°C, and then measure the absorbance at wavelength 450 nm for 0.1 s per well.

3.7.2. Testing Sensitivity to Ionizing Radiation

1. To test the cell sensitivity to ionizing radiation, seed each tested clone in five 96-well plates at 8,000 cells per well, one column per clone, one plate per one radiation dose.

2. Next day expose each plate without changing the medium to a ^{137}Cs source to achieve a designated γ-radiation dose (0, 0.5, 1, 2 and 4 Gy).

3. Measure cell survival 72 h later, using the XTT assay as described above (step 4 of Subheading 3.7.1).

3.7.3. Testing Sensitivity to UV Light

1. Seed 32,000 ES cells (64,000 cells for mutant cells with severe proliferation defect) in gelatinized 24-well plates in triplicates.
2. Eighteen hours later remove the medium and the plate lid, and irradiate with 0, 5, 10, or 15 J/m^2 using a UV crosslinker (Stratagene) or any other suitable UV source. Replace the M15 medium.
3. Seventy-two hours later, wash the plates twice with PBS, add 400 µL XTT reagent, incubate for 2.5–3 h. Transfer 100 µL of developed color solution from each well into a 96-well plate for measurement as described above (step 4 of Subheading 3.7.1).

3.7.4. Measuring In Vitro Proliferation

1. To determine the effect of a BRCA2 variant on in vitro proliferation, seed 3 sets of each clone at 50,000 cells per well in triplicates in 24-well feeder plates. Leave a few wells empty with only feeder cells as a background control.
2. After 24 h, wash the plates twice with PBS, trypsinize with 200 µl trypsin-EDTA for 15 min at 37°C, add 200 µL M15 medium and pipette vigorously up and down 20 times to achieve a single cell suspension.
3. Count a 200 µL aliquot using a Coulter counter.
4. Repeat the procedure with the second and third set of cells on the second and third day after seeding, respectively.
5. To estimate the cell proliferation, subtract the average feeder cell count from each value and express the resulting numbers as multiples of the average cell number (or a concentration) recorded at the first day after seeding.

3.7.5. Measuring In Vivo Proliferation

1. To measure the in vivo proliferation, harvest ES cells from three confluent 10 cm plates. Resuspend ES cells in PBS at 10^8 cells/ml.
2. Inject 0.1 mL of this cell suspension (5×10^6 cells) subcutaneously in flanks of 1-month-old immuno-compromised nude mice. 3–5 males and 3–5 females should be injected for each ES cell clone.
3. Monitor teratoma growth by measuring the length and width of the tumor for 3 weeks (or until the tumor reaches 1.5 cm in any dimention), starting on day 7 after injection. Calculate the tumor size as a product of $2 \times \text{length} \times \text{width}$ in cm^3.

3.7.6. Evaluating Genomic Instability

To examine the effect of a BRCA2 variant on genomic stability, measure chromosomal aberrations by karyotypic analysis.

1. Plate $3–5 \times 10^6$ ES cells in 6 cm gelatinized dishes without feeders.

2. Next day treat cells with 10 μg/mL colcemid for 1.5 h to arrest cells at metaphase and prepare metaphase spreads using standard procedures (21).
3. Stain slides in a Giemsa solution as described elsewhere (22). Blindly score 200 well-spread metaphases containing at least 40 chromosomes for structural aberrations classified according to the ISCN scheme into chromosome and chromatid gaps, breaks and other anomalies (23).

3.7.7. Homologous Recombination Assay

1. To test ES cells directly for homologous recombination, electroporate them with 25 μg of linear *Rosa26-Puro* targeting vector (11) as described above (steps 7–9 of Subheading 3.2).
2. Select on puromycin for 5 days starting 36 h after electroporation.
3. Pick 96 colonies for each cell line and expand them for Southern blot analysis as described above (steps 10–14 of Subheading 3.2), except that there is no need for a duplicate 96-well plate with feeders because these cells are not intended to be cultured any further.
4. Perform Southern blot analysis as described above (Subheading 3.3), except that the DNA should be digested with SpeI and hybridized with the *Rosa26*-specifi probe. Clones that underwent a homologous recombination will reveal a 4.5 kb band and their proportion relative to the total number of clones indicates the efficiency of the homologous recombination.

3.7.8. RAD51 Foci Formation Assay

BRCA2 is required for the recruitment of RAD51 to the sites of DNA double strand breaks (24). RAD51 foci at the sites of DNA damage can be visualized by immunofluorescence staining.

1. Seed 40,000 cells per well in gelatinized SonicSeal plastic slides (see Note 11).
2. Forty-eight hours later, γ-irradiate the cells with 10 Gy.
3. Incubate the cells at 37°C for 6 h.
4. Fix the cells with 4% paraformaldehyde for 5 min.
5. Wash twice with PBS and permeabilize in PBS-buffered 0.1% Triton X-100 solution for 10 min.
6. Wash twice with PBS and block overnight in antibody blocking solution at 4°C.
7. Wash once with PBS for 5 min at room temperature, add rabbit anti-Rad51 antibody (PC130 diluted 1:200) and mouse anti-γ-H2AX antibody (Upstate) diluted 1:1,000 in antibody blocking solution and incubate overnight at 4°C.
8. Wash four times for 30 min with 1× PBS, 0.05% Trion X-100.

9. Incubate with secondary antibodies FDAR and RDAM diluted in antibody blocking solution 1:100 and 1:150, respectively, for 2 h at room temperature in the dark.
10. Wash as in step 6 of this Subheading, stain with DAPI, and mount in Vectashield mounting medium.
11. Evaluate preparations under a fluorescent microscope equipped with a proper filter set and count the number of RAD51 foci per nucleus (see Note 12).

4. Notes

1. The 180 bp band is quite frequently not a single clean band, instead it appears to be fuzzy. Such products have worked well in our hands and therefore should be used for targeting.
2. It helps induce 20 mL of bacterial culture that yields 100 μL of electrocompetent cells. Although only 50 μL are needed for each electroporation, it is good to have cells for an additional electroporation should something go wrong with the first set.
3. If very few G418^r colonies are obtained after electroporating BAC DNA into ES cells, try linearizing the BAC DNA using a unique *Asc*I restriction site. Digest DNA with *Asc*I enzyme for 1 h at 37°C. Purify DNA by phenol:chloroform extraction. Precipitate DNA by adding 0.1 vol. of 3 M sodium acetate and 2 vol. of absolute ethanol. Spool DNA precipitated with ethanol and dissolve in 100 μL TE buffer.
4. Southern hybridization probes from the 5′ and 3′ ends of human BRCA2 can be generated by PCR using BAC 777 as template. To generate 5′ specific probe (581 bp), use primers: HB2UTR5F1, 5′-GAACTGCACCTCTGGAGCG-3′, HB2in1R1, 5′-AAGCACTCGAAACGTGGCTA-3′; and for 3′ probe (287 bp) use primers: HB2ex25F1, 5′-GTGAGTAACCTTGTTCATAGGTG-3′, and HB2ex25R1, 5′-AATGACCTGTTGCTTACAGTG-3′.
5. If no full-length protein is detected by Western analysis of multiple independent ES cells containing a BRCA2 variant in a BAC, it may suggest that the mutant BRCA2 protein is unstable. In such cases, the expression of the *BRCA2* transcript can be examined by RT-PCR or Northern blot analysis.
6. To reduce the time involved in testing whether a variant can rescue the lethality of *Brca2 null* ES cells, we have developed

an alternative method, which relies on testing the expression of the transgene by RT-PCR and the use of the Adeno-Cre virus to deliver Cre. The steps involved in the alternative method are:

(a) After electroporating the BAC into ES cells as described in Subheading 3.2, pick G418^r clones and expand them into three 96-well plates (one plate for RT-PCR analysis, the second one will be frozen as a master plate, and the third will be used to expand RT-PCR positive clones).

(b) Use one 96-well plate for expression analysis by RT-PCR to select clones with the full-length BAC. Use commercially available kits (such as, RNaeasy-96 from Qiagen) to extract RNA from cells in 96-well plates. Lyse the cells in 100 μL for easy handling in 96-well plates and elute the RNA once with 40 μL of water to ensure a high concentration of RNA. Use Titan one step RT PCR kit (Roche) to perform RT-PCR using 1 μL of total RNA from the step above. For PCR, use primers specific to human *BRCA2*, hBRCA2_Ex11F, 5′-ACAT GTCCCGAAAATGAGGA-3′, and hBRCA2_Ex18R, 5′-GCCGATCTTCTGCTTCTATCA-3′. The 1,250 bp PCR product spans through exons 11–18 of *BRCA2*.

(c) Passage RT-PCR-positive ES cell clones from one of the 96-well plates (from a above) to a 24-well plate.

(d) Transduce 10^5 cells with adenovirus expressing Cre to delete the conditional allele and freeze the rest of the cells. In general, 10^6 ES cells are obtained from a 80–90% confluent well of a 24-well plate. Resuspend one-tenth of the cells in 100 μL of M15 medium. For Adenoviral-Cre transduction, use MOI of 100. If the viral titer is 10^{10} pfu/mL, use 1 μL of the virus for 10^5 cells. After infection, bring up the volume of transduced cells to 1 mL with M15 medium and plate 10 μL and 100 μL of the cell suspension in two separate 6-cm plates such that the numbers of cells plated will be 10^3 and 10^4, respectively.

(e) Select Adeno-Cre-transduced ES cells in the HAT medium to select for recombinant clones.

(f) Pick clones, expand and genotype to confirm the loss of the conditional allele. If viable clones are obtained, perform drug sensitivity assay as described in Subheading 3.7.

This approach is faster and saves about 4 weeks in evaluation time for each set of mutants. However, this approach has a disadvantage; if *HAT*^{r} clones are not obtained after Cre expression, it is difficult to conclude if the variant is deleterious or the clones failed to survive because of the lack of expression of the full-length protein. In such cases, it is recommended to test clones individually to confirm protein expression. This disadvantage is off-set by the fact that 6–12 independent G418^r & RT-PCR positive clones for each variant can be easily tested at a time. It is highly unlikely that none will express the full-length protein, unless reduction or the lack of protein expression is linked to the mutation. We believe that the number of such cases will be relatively small and should not hinder the overall progress.

7. The Southern hybridization probe 144/145 (1,250 bp) to genotype ES cells for the loss of conditional allele can be generated by PCR using BAC 777 as a template and PCR primers: SKS-144, 5′-TGTCATTGTGATGACATGCA-3′, and SKS-145, 5′-CAGTCACTCCTCCTCTTTTC-3′.

8. Occasionally, genotyping of HAT^r ES cell clones show the presence of the conditional allele. This is likely to be due to a spontaneous trisomy of chromosome 5 containing the conditional *Brca2* allele. Partial Cre-mediated recombination of only one of the conditional alleles will generate HAT^r clones, while the "unrecombined" allele will show the presence of the conditional allele.

9. For some hypomorphic mutants, we have observed cell numbers and OD values in the XTT assay to be significantly lower compared with controls. This is due to the severe growth retardation associated with a defect in BRCA2 function. In such cases, plating more cells than control samples compensates for lower seeding efficiency and growth rate.

10. The suggested concentrations of different DNA damaging agents used in the study are:

    MMC (Mitomicin C): 0, 5, 10, 20, 30, 40, 60 ng/mL

    MMS (Methyl-methanesulfonate): 0, 5, 10, 15, 20, 30, 40 µg/mL

    Cisplatin (cis-Diammineplatinum(II)dichloride): 0, 0.1, 0.2, 0.4, 0.5, 0.6, 0.8 µM

    MNNG (N-Methyl-N′-Nitro-N-Nitrosoguanidine): 0, 1, 2, 8, 15, 20, 30 µM.

11. Mouse ES cells poorly adhere to glass slides or cover slips. Therefore, only plastic slides suitable for tissue culture can be used to grow ES cells for immunofluorescence.

12. Images of 50–100 nuclei should be taken and evaluated for the numbers of gamma H2AX and Rad51-positive foci. Rad51 foci not overlapping with gamma H2AX are likely to be unspecific and should be disregarded. Depending on the cell cycle stage, not all nuclei will show the foci.

Acknowledgments

We thank Jiro Wada for help with illustrations. Research was sponsored by the Center for Cancer Research, National Cancer Institute, National Institutes of Health.

References

1. Beaudet, A.L., and Belmont, J.W. (2008) Array-based DNA diagnostics: let the revolution begin. *Annu. Rev. Med.* **59**, 113–129.
2. Thompson, D., Easton, D.F., and Goldgar, D.E. (2003) A full-likelihood method for the evaluation of causality of sequence variants from family data. *Am. J. Hum. Genet.* **73**, 652–655.
3. Easton, D.F., Deffenbaugh, A.M., Pruss, D., Frye, C., Wenstrup, R.J., Allen-Brady, K., et al. (2007) A systematic genetic assessment of 1,433 sequence variants of unknown clinical significance in the BRCA1 and BRCA2 breast cancer-predisposition genes. *Am. J. Hum. Genet.* **81**, 873–883.
4. Carvalho, M.A., Couch, F.J., and Monteiro, A.N. (2007) Functional assays for BRCA1 and BRCA2. *Int. J. Biochem. Cell Biol.* **39**, 298–310.
5. Roschke, A.V., Tonon, G., Gehlhaus, K.S., McTyre, N., Bussey, K.J., Lababidi, S., et al. (2003) Karyotypic complexity of the NCI-60 drug-screening panel. *Cancer Res.* **63**, 8634–8647.
6. Amit, M., Carpenter, M.K., Inokuma, M.S., Chiu, C.P., Harris, C.P., Waknitz, M.A., et al. (2000) Clonally derived human embryonic stem cell lines maintain pluripotency and proliferative potential for prolonged periods of culture. *Dev. Biol.* **227**, 271–278.
7. Copeland, N.G., Jenkins, N.A., and Court, D.L. (2001) Recombineering: a powerful new tool for mouse functional genomics. *Nat. Rev. Genet.* **2**, 769–779.
8. Swaminathan, S., Ellis, H.M., Waters, L.S., Yu, D., Lee, E.C., Court, D.L. et al. (2001) Rapid engineering of bacterial artificial chromosomes using oligonucleotides. *Genesis* **29**, 14–21.
9. Yang, Y., and Sharan, S.K. (2003) A simple two-step, 'hit and fix' method to generate subtle mutations in BACs using short denatured PCR fragments. *Nucleic Acids Res.* **31**, e80.
10. Sharan, S.K., Thomason, L.C., Kuznetsov, S.G., and Court, D.L. (2009) Recombineering: a homologous recombination-based method of genetic engineering. *Nat. Protoc.* **4**, 206–223.
11. Kuznetsov, S.G., Liu, P., and Sharan, S.K. (2008) Mouse embryonic stem cell-based functional assay to evaluate mutations in BRCA2. *Nat. Med.* **14**, 875–881.
12. Sharan, S.K., Morimatsu, M., Albrecht,U., Lim, D., Regel, E., Dinh, C., et al. (1997) Embryonic lethality and radiation hypersensitivity mediated by Rad51 in mice lacking Brca2. *Nature* **386**, 804–810.
13. Ramirez-Solis, R., Liu, P., and Bradley, A. (1995) Chromosome engineering in mice. *Nature* **378**, 720–724.
14. Friedrich, G., and Soriano, P. (1993) Insertional mutagenesis by retroviruses and promoter traps in embryonic stem cells. *Methods Enzymol.* **225**, 681–701.
15. Warming, S., Costantino, N., Court, D.L., Jenkins, N.A., and Copeland, N.G. (2005) Simple and highly efficient BAC recombineering using galK selection. *Nucleic Acids Res.* **33**, e36.
16. Yu, D., Ellis, H.M., Lee, E.C., Jenkins, N.A., Copeland, N.G., and Court, D.L. (2000) An efficient recombination system for chromosome engineering in *Escherichia coli*. *Proc. Natl. Acad. Sci. U.S.A.* **97**, 5978–5983.
17. Cha, R.S, Zarbl, H., Keohavong, P., and Thilly, W.G. (1992) Mismatch amplification mutation assay (MAMA): application to the c-H-ras gene. *PCR Methods Appl.* **2**, 14–20.
18. Ramirez-Solis, R., Davis, A.C., and Bradley, A. (1993) Gene targeting in embryonic stem cells. *Methods Enzymol.* **225**, 855–878.
19. Sambrook, J., Fritsch, E.F., and Maniatis, T. (1989) *Molecular Cloning: A Laboratory Manual*, Cold Spring Harbor Laboratory Press, NY.
20. Scudiero, D.A., Shoemaker, R.H., Paull, K.D., Monks, A., Tierney, S., Nofziger, T.H., et al. (1988) Evaluation of a soluble tetrazolium/formazan assay for cell growth and drug sensitivity in culture using human and other tumor cell lines. *Cancer Res.* **48**, 4827–4833.

21. Barch, M.J., Knutsen, T., and Spurbeck, J.L. (*ed.*) (1997) *The AGT Cytogenetics Laboratory Manual*, Lippincott-Raven Publishers, Philadelphia, PA.
22. Sonoda, E., Sasaki M.S., Buerstedde, J.M., Bezzubova, O., Shinohara, A., Ogawa, H., et al. (1998) Rad51-deficient vertebrate cells accumulate chromosomal breaks prior to cell death. *EMBO J.* **17**, 598–608.
23. Mitelman, F. (*ed.*) (1995) *ISCN: An International System for Human Cytogenetic Nomenclature*, Karger, Basel.
24. Chen, J., Silver, D.P., Walpita, D., Cantor, S.B., Gazdar, A.F., Tomlinson, G., et al. (1998) Stable interaction between the products of the BRCA1 and BRCA2 tumor suppressor genes in mitotic and meiotic cells. *Mol. Cell* **2**, 317–328.

Chapter 17

Developing Functional Assays for BRCA1 Unclassified Variants

Michelle Webb

Abstract

Women with a family history of breast cancer have mutations in one of the breast cancer susceptibility genes, *BRCA1 or BRCA2*. Since the discovery of these two genes, around 100,000 women worldwide have undergone genetic testing. The decisions they make based on the results are usually life changing and may involve radical preventive surgeries such as prophylactic mastectomy and oophorectamy. However, not all mutations will lead to breast cancer, and to prevent unnecessary surgery, we are developing assays to determine which mutations adversely affect the functions of the protein encoded by the *BRCA1* gene. The functions of BRCA1 are mediated by numerous interactions that are required for cell-cycle and centrosome control, transcriptional regulation and the DNA damage response. Missense mutations that perturb the interactions of BRCA1 will adversely affect these functions and are, therefore, likely to lead to breast cancer. Determining the effect missense mutations have on the interaction of BRCA1 with DNA will form the basis of the assay described in this chapter.

Key words: BRCA1, Functional assay, DNA binding

1. Introduction

Individuals carrying mutations in the *BRCA1* gene have an increased risk of developing breast and ovarian cancer. Screening these patients for *BRCA1* mutations began almost immediately after the discovery of the gene in 1994 (1). Once a mutation is identified in a family, pre-symptomatic genetic screening is now offered to all at risk relatives. While in many cases this is informative, in others it is frustratingly ambiguous because the result depends upon the nature of the mutation found. *BRCA1* is an exceptionally large gene containing 5,592 (22 exons) nucleotides (1) and since its discovery over 1,600 distinct mutations, polymorphisms and variants have been identified throughout the entire coding region (2). Approximately 70% of mutations are frame-shift, splice site or nonsense mutations, all of which lead to truncated protein products and are predicted to be pathogenic. A further 10% are large exonic deletions or insertions, which would have a similar effect on the protein. The remaining mutations are mostly missense variants resulting from single amino acid substitutions and occasionally in frame deletions that result in the loss of a single amino acid. The pathogenicity of these mutations is difficult to determine due to limited knowledge regarding the functional outcome of the substitutions.

Some of missense variants have been successfully classified using a combination of clinical, pathological and functional features (3–5). However, these methods can only classify a small number of variants all of which are located in two established functional domains (6), the N-terminal RING finger domain and the C-terminal BRCT containing domain. These domains, however, account for only 15% of the total protein and the pathogenicity of almost all missense mutations located in the central region of BRCA1 remain to be classified.

There are around 120 missense mutations in the central region of BRCA1 that have been submitted to the Breast Cancer Information Core (BIC) database (2) three times or more. These sites are high priority for functional analyses. However, as the *BRCA1* gene encodes a large protein that performs a multifaceted role in maintaining genome integrity and transcriptional regulation (7), it is unlikely that a single assay will be developed to account for the functional effects of all these missense variants.

The different functions of BRCA1 are mediated by around 50 interactions that take place throughout the protein (8, 9). A significant number of them locate to the central region of BRCA1, for example, DNA (10–12), p53 (13, 14) c-Myc (15), RAD50 (16), RAD51 (17), FANCA (18) and RB (19). To assess the pathogenicity of missense mutations located in this region, a number of functional assays capable of determining their effect on each interaction are being developed. This chapter will focus on an assay developed to determine the effects missense mutations have on the DNA-binding activity of BRCA1. Many of the techniques described can, however, be applied for the analysis of other interactions that mediate BRCA1 function.

2. Materials

2.1. Preparation of Recombinant pET22b Containing DNA Encoding Residues of BRCA1

1. *Pfu* DNA polymerase (Promega; 2.5 U/μL), 10× *Pfu* polymerase buffer (Promega).

2. dNTP set, 100 mM solutions of dATP, dCTP, dGTP, dTTP (GE healthcare).

3. Primers diluted to a concentration of 5 pmol/μL in 10 mM Tris–HCl, pH 7.5 (MWG-Biotech).
4. QIAquick PCR Purification Kit (QIAGEN).
5. Restriction Enzymes Nde1 and Xho (New England Biolabs® Inc), NEBuffer 2 (New England Biolabs® Inc).
6. QIAquick gel extraction kit (QIAGEN).
7. T4 DNA Ligase (Roche; 1 U/μL), 10× ligase buffer (Roche).
8. *E. coli* XL-1 blue competent cells (Stratagene).
9. LB medium (1 L): 10 g tryptone peptone, 5 g yeast extract, 5 g NaCl.
10. QIAprep spin Miniprep Kit (QIAGEN).
11. *E. coli* pulser (Bio-Rad).

2.2. Site Directed Mutagenesis

1. QuikChange Site Directed Mutagenesis Kit (Stratagene).
2. Mutagenic Primers (MWG-Biotech).

2.3. Protein Expression

1. 2× YT medium (1 L): 16 g tryptone peptone, 10 g yeast extract, 5 g NaCl.
2. pET 22b expression vector (Novagen).
3. *E. coli* BL21-CodonPlus (DE3)-RIPL competent cells (Stratagene).
4. Isopropyl β-D-thiogalatosidase, IPTG (Melford).

2.4. Protein Purification

1. Y-PER, Yeast Protein Extraction Reagent (Pierce) (see Note 1).
2. Ni-NTA Agarose (QIAGEN).
3. Complete™ Protease Inhibitor Cocktail Tablet, EDTA free (Roche) (see Note 2).
4. Wash buffer 1: 10 mM immidazole, 10 mM Tris–HCl, pH 8, 300 mM NaCl.
5. Slide-A-Lyzer (10K MWCO) dialysis cassette (Pierce)

2.5. DNA Binding Analysis

1. Four-way junction oligonucleotide (F1, F2, F3, and F4) (MWG-Biotech)

   F1 5´-GAATTCAGCACGAGTCCTAACGCCAGATCT-3´
   F2 5´-AGATCTGGCGTTAGGTGATACCGATGCATC-3´
   F3 5´-GATGCATCGGTATCAGGCTTACGACTAGTG-3´
   F4 5´-CACTAGTCGTAAGCCACTCGTGCTGAATTC-3´

2. DNA binding buffer: 10 mM Tris–HCl, pH 8.0, 1 mM dithiothreitol (DTT), 25 mM NaCl, 5% (v/v) glycerol.

2.6. Agarose Gel Electrophoresis

1. 50× TAE: 0.1 M EDTA and 2 M Tris titrated to pH 8.5 with approximately 11 mL of glacial acetic acid per litre.
2. Agarose gel loading buffer (6×): 30% glycerol (v/v), 0.25% Bromophenol blue (w/v), 0.25% xylene cyanol (w/v).
3. HyperLadder 1 molecular weight marker (BioLine).
4. Ethidium bromide (BioRad) (see Note 3).

2.7. SDS Polyacrylamide Gel Electrophoresis

1. SDS-PAGE loading dye: 10% glycerol (v/v), 3% SDS (w/v), 0.0125% bromophenol blue (w/v), 60 mM Tris–HCl, pH 6.8 and 50 mM DTT (added on day of experiment, see Note 4).
2. Ammonium persulfate: prepare a 10% w/v solution in dH_2O and use immediately.
3. N,N,N,N'-Tetramethyl-ethylenediamine (TEMED; Sigma Aldrich).
4. SDS-PAGE Running Buffer (10×): 0.1% SDS (w/v), 190 mM glycine, 27 mM Tris.
5. SDS-PAGE Solution A: 30% Acrylamide (w/v), 0.5% bis-acrylamide (w/v).
6. SDS-PAGE Solution B: 1.5 M Tris–HCl, pH 8.8, 0.4% SDS (w/v).
7. SDS-PAGE Solution C: 0.5 M Tris–HCl, pH 6.8, 0.4% SDS (w/v).
8. Low-range molecular weight marker (Sigma).
9. BioSafe Coomasie Stain (Bio-Rad).

2.8. Native Gel Electrophoresis

1. 29:1(w/w) acrylamide: N,N' methylene-bis acrylamide (Bio-Rad).

3. Methods

For all binding assays, relatively large amounts of protein are required but because of the difficulties associated with purifying full length BRCA1, functional assays are made easier if small domains are used. A recognised feature of the central region of BRCA1 is, however, that it is intrinsically disordered with only transient-folded regions and no obvious domain structure (10, 11). Fortunately, peptide fragments containing the interaction sites for all the molecules that associate with the central region can be produced in soluble form after expression in *E. coli*. Although, in this chapter, we will describe the cloning expression and purification of a fragment of BRCA1 containing the binding site for DNA, the methods described can also be used for the production of other protein fragments of BRCA1 that can be used in further interaction studies.

3.1. Preparation of Recombinant pET22b Containing DNA Encoding Residues of BRCA1 That Interact with Four-Way Junction DNA

1. To a 0.2 mL thin-walled centrifuge tube add 1 µL of *pfu* polymerase, 5 µL 10× *pfu* Buffer, 200 ng template DNA, 5 µL of both the forward and reverse primers (see Note 5), 5 µL dNTPS and make up to 50 µL with dH$_2$O.
2. Perform the PCR reaction using the following cycle

Initial denaturation	95°C, 60 s
Amplification (16 cycles)	95°C, 20 s denaturation
	55°C, 60 s annealing
	68°C, 60 s extension
Extension	72°C, 420 s

3. Following the manufacturer's instructions, remove primers, nucleotides, polymerase and salts from the amplified DNA using the QIAquick PCR purification kit.
4. Analyse the purified PCR product in a 1% agarose gel. The size and concentration of resolved DNA fragments can be determined by comparison of the position and band intensity to those of the HyperLadder I marker.
5. In separate reactions, digest ~500 ng of the purified PCR product and pET22b with 20 units of the restriction enzymes: *Nde*I and *Xho*I. Carry out the reactions in final volumes of 100 µL containing 1× NEB Buffer 2 at 37°C for 2 h.
6. Heat inactivate the digests at 70°C for 20 min and analyse in a 0.1% agarose gel.
7. Following the manufacturer's instruction, purify the digestion products by gel extraction using a QIAquick gel extraction kit.
8. Ligate the PCR product into pET22b using an insert to vector molar ratio of 2:1. In a mix final volume of 15 µL, containing: 1× ligation buffer, 2 nM pET22b, 4 nM insert DNA and 1 unit T4 DNA Ligase. Ligate at 16°C for 10 h and heat inactivate at 70°C for 20 min.
9. Transform into *E. coli* XL-1 blue competent cells either by electroporation or heat sock. To induce electroporation, we used a 2.5 kV pulse generated with an *E. coli* pulser.
10. Pick five transformed colonies and inoculate five separate 50 mL Falcon tubes containing 15 mL of LB medium supplemented with ampicillin (50 µg/mL). Culture at 37°C for 16 h.
11. Purify the recombinant pET22b plasmids using the QIAGEN miniprep protocol.
12. Confirm insertion by automated DNA sequencing.

3.2. Site-Directed Mutagenesis

1. Missense mutations can be generated using the QuikChange protocol essentially as described in the Stratagene manual. Briefly purify recombinant pET22b following the QIAGEN

miniprep protocol. To a 0.2 mL thin-walled centrifuge tube add 1 μL of *pfu* polymerase, 5 μL of 10× *pfu* Buffer, template DNA, 5 μL of both the forward and reverse mutagenic primer, 5 μL dNTPS and make up to 50 μL with dH$_2$O.

2. Use the following program carry out the PCR

Initial denaturation	95°C, 30 s
Amplification (16 cycles)	95°C, 30 s denaturation
	55°C, 60 s annealing
	72°C, 1 min extension

3. Cleave the methylated strand by incubation with dpn1 at 37°C over night.
4. Transform, by heat sock or electroporation, *E. coli* XL-1 blue with 1 μL of the cleaved mutagenesis reaction.
5. Pick five transformed colonies and inoculate five separate 50 mL Falcon tubes containing 15 mL of LB medium supplemented with ampicillin (50 μg/mL). Culture at 37°C for 16 h.
6. Purify the recombinant pET22b plasmids using the Qiagen miniprep protocol.
7. Confirm correct mutation be DNA sequencing.

3.3. Expression and Purification of Wild Type and Mutant BRCA1 Protein Fragments

1. Inoculate 150 mL of 2×YT with 1.5 mL of an overnight culture of *E. coli* BL21 (DE3) codon plus cells harboring the recombinant pET22b.
2. Grow the cells to mid log phase at 37°C whereupon induce expression by the addition of 1 mM 5 isopropyl β-D-thiogalatosidase (see Note 6).
3. Grow the cells for an additional 4 h and harvest by centrifugation. The cells can be used immediately or stored at −20°C until required.
4. Lyse the cells by re-suspension in 4 mL of Y-PER containing one dissolved complete protease inhibitor tablet and incubating for 1 h with gentle rocking at room temperature.
5. Prepare the soluble extract by centrifugation at 5,000×g for 1 h at 4°C. Discard the pellet and incubate the supernatant with 1.5 mL Ni^{2+}-NTA agarose equilibrated in wash buffer 1.
6. Wash the immobilized proteins three times with 10 mL of wash buffer 1. After the final wash re-suspend the Ni^{2+}-NTA agarose beads in 3 mL of wash buffer 1 and pack into a 5 mL syringe plugged with glass wool.
7. Wash the immobilized proteins by application of 6 mL of 50 mM immidazole, 10 mM Tris–HCl pH 8, 300 mM NaCl to the column. Discard the eluent.

8. Immobilised proteins are eluted in 5×1 mL fractions of 300 mM immidazole, 10 mM Tris–HCl, pH 8, 300 mM NaCl.

9. Analyse the eluted fractions in 12% SDS polyacrylamide gels (see Subheading 3.6) by comparison to molecular weight standards. An example of the results are displayed in Fig. 1.

10. Pool the fractions containing the desired proteins and dialyse overnight against 10 mM Na phosphate, pH 7, 50 mM NaCl, 1 mM DTT, 1 mM EDTA.

11. To determine protein concentrations, record the Protein absorbance at 280 nm. Reference each measurement against the dialysis buffer and calculate the protein concentrations using the Beer–Lambert law (Eq. 17.1). We used a Varian CARY UV/Vis spectrophotometer.

$$A = \varepsilon c l \tag{1}$$

A = absorbance, ε = extinction coefficient (L/mol/cm), c = concentration (mol/L), l = path length (1 cm)

3.4. DNA Binding Assay

3.4.1. Preparation of Four-Way Junction DNA

1. Dilute each of the oligonucleotides F1, F2, F3, and F4 with 10 mM Tris–HCl, pH 7.5 to 100 μM. To prepare 10 μM four-way junction DNA, mix 10 μL each of the oligonucleotide solutions and make up to 100 μL with 10 mM Tris–HCl, pH 7.5.

2. Heat to 90°C for 15 min and cool slowly to 4°C (see Note 7).

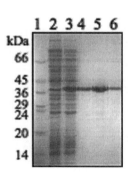

Fig. 1. An example of purified BRCA1 330-554 and some of the mutants generated. All proteins were expressed in E. coli BL21 (DE3) codon plus cell after induction with 1 mM IPTG. The cells were lysed and soluble extract prepared by centrifugation. Proteins were purified using Nickel NTA agarose and then analysed in 12% SDS polyacrylamide gels. Lane 1 contains a molecular weight marker, lane 2 contains un-induced E. coli BL21 (DE3 cells), lane 3 contains cells induced with IPTG for 4 h, showing the expression of wild type BRCA1 330-554 and lanes 4–6 contain purified wild type BRCA1 330-554 and mutants R496A and R496C, respectively.

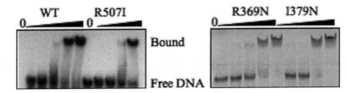

Fig. 2. An example of the DNA binding analysis of BRCA1 mutant proteins. The affinity of each mutant for four-way junction DNA was analysed and compared to that of the wild type protein by gel retardation assays. Four-way junction DNA (1 µm) was incubated with increasing concentration (0.5, 1, 5, and 10 µM) of each of the mutants and analysed in 8% polyacrylamide gels. Lanes labelled 0 contain no protein.

3.4.2. Gel Retardation Assay

1. Mix 1 µM of the four-way junction DNA with increasing concentrations of the BRCA1 proteins (500 nM, 1 µM, 2 µM, and 5 µM), 2 µL 5× binding buffer and make up to 10 µL with dH$_2$O.
2. Incubate at room temperature for 30 min.
3. Analyse samples in a pre-electrophoresed 6.5% non-denaturing polyacrylamide gels (see Subheading 3.7). An example of the results is displayed in Fig. 2.

3.5. Agarose Gel Electrophoresis

1. Agarose gel electrophoresis is carried out in submarine gel system.
2. Dissolve 1 g of agarose in 100 mL of 1× TAE by heating in a microwave.
3. Cool to about 60°C and add 1 µL of 10 mg/mL ethidium bromide and pour in to a gel tray, which has been sealed with autoclave tape. Leave to set for about 30 min.
4. Resuspended in 6× agarose gel loading buffer and electrophorese at 100 V in 1× TAE running buffer.
5. Analyse by comparison to DNA molecular weight markers (HyperLadder I). Gels were stained with 0.5 µg/mL ethidium bromide and destained in dH$_2$O.
6. Ethidium-stained DNA is visualised under the UV light of wavelength 365 nm and images captured through a red filter on a UVP High Performance Transilluminator.

3.6. SDS Polyacrylamide Gel Electrophoresis

1. Assemble the glass plates and cast gels according to the manufacturer's description. We used the Bio-Rad mini PROTEAN tetra electrophoresis system.
2. Prepare a 12% resolving gel solution by mixing 4 mL of SDS solution A, 2.5 mL of SDS solution B, 3.5 mL of dH$_2$O and polymerise by adding 100 µL of ammonium persulphate and 20 µL TEMED (see Note 8). Pour the solution into the plates leaving space for the stacking gel and overlay with dH$_2$O. The gel should polymerise within 20 min.
3. Prepare the stacking gel solution by mixing 0.67 mL of SDS solution A, 1 mL of SDS solution C, 2.3 mL of dH$_2$O, 50 µL

ammonium persulfate solution and 10 µL TEMED. Pour on top of the resolving gel, insert the comb and leave to polymerase for 20 min.

4. Once the stacking gel has polymerised carefully remove the comb and use a 5 mL syringe fitted with a 22-gauge needle to rinse the wells with 1× running buffer.

5. Prepare samples to be analysed in 1× SDS loading dye and denature by heating at 95°C for 5 min.

6. Add the running buffer to the upper and lower chambers of the gel tank and load 20 µL of each sample into each well. A low molecular weight marker should also be loaded in to one of the wells.

7. Electrophorese towards the cathode at a constant current of 45 mA until the bromophenol blue reaches the bottom of the gel.

8. Stain the proteins by immersion in 200 mL of BioSafe Coomassie stain for 30 min and destain in 10% (v/v) methanol and 10% (v/v) acetic acid. Images can be visualised and recorded using a UVP High Performance Transilluminator.

3.7. Non-denaturing Polyacrylamide Electrophoresis

1. Rinse all the gel electrophoresis equipment thoroughly with distilled water and assemble gel plates according to the manufacturer's instructions. We used the Bio-Rad mini PROTEAN tetra electrophoresis system.

2. Prepare gel solution for an 8% gel by mixing 0.6 mL 50× TAE, 8 mL 29:1(w/w) acrylamide: N,N' methylene-bis acrylamide, 21.4 mL H_2O and polymerise with 0.07% (w/v) APS and 0.035% (v/v) TEMED. Pour the solution into the plates and insert 10 well gel comb. The gel should polymerise within 20 min.

3. Add 1× TAE to the upper and lower chambers of the gel tank, remove combs and rinse well with 1× TAE using a fine-gauge syringe needle. Pre-electrophorese at 100 V until the current stops dropping. Replace with fresh running buffer then flush the wells again and load the sample into each of the wells

4. Electrophorese the DNA–protein samples at 100 V towards the cathode for 40 min at 4°C.

5. Stain in ethidium bromide and visualise under UV light.

4. Notes

1. Y-PER is a mild detergent lysis reagent and although it is designed to efficiently release functionally active solubilised proteins from Yeast it is also very effective for lysing *E. coli* cells.

2. Protease inhibitors without EDTA should be used to prevent stripping of the Ni-NTA agarose resulting in reduced protein binding.

3. Ethidium Bromide is a known mutagen and should be handled with considerable caution.
4. DTT has a half life of 10 h at pH 7.5 and, therefore, should be made fresh on the day of use.
5. Primers were designed to anneal to the 5′ and 3′ of the DNA sequence of interest in the template DNA, providing an adequate length of complementary bases for efficient annealing. To aid cloning, unique restriction sites that were absent from the region of interest were incorporated at the 5′ of each primer. Six additional base pairs at the 5′ end of each primer increase the affinity of the restriction enzymes for their recognition sequences.
6. *E. coli* cells are usually in mid log phase when the optical density at 600 nm is between 0.4 and 0.8.
7. To prepare four-way junction DNA, the mixture must be cooled slowly to promote base pairing. If the sample is cooled too quickly, more of the DNA will remain in the single stranded form.
8. Care must be taken while working with TEMED, Acrylamide and Ammonium Persulphate. TEMED is very destructive to tissue of the mucous membranes and upper respiratory tract, eyes and skin. Acrylamide monomer is a neurotoxin. When working with these compounds wear gloves at all times.

Acknowledgements

The author would like to thank the Breast Cancer Campaign for funding the studies described in this chapter.

References

1. Miki, Y., Swensen, J., Shattuck-Eidens, D., Futreal, P.A., Harshman, K., Tavtigian, S., et al. (1994) A strong candidate for the breast and ovarian cancer susceptibility gene BRCA1. *Science* **266**, 66–71.
2. Breast Cancer Information Core (BIC) dataset for BRCA1 (http://research.nhgri.nih.gov/bic/)
3. Easton, D.F., Deffenbaugh, A.M., Pruss, D., Frye, C., Wenstrup, R.J., Allen-Brady, K., et al. (2007) Systematic genetic assessment of 1,433 sequence variants of unknown clinical significance in the BRCA1 and BRCA2 breast cancer-predisposition genes. *Am. J. Hum. Genet.* **81**, 873–883.
4. Tavtigian, S.V., Greenblatt, M.S., Lesueur, F., Byrnes, G.B; IARC Unclassified Genetic Variants Working Group. (2008) In silico analysis of missense substitutions using sequence-alignment based methods. *Hum. Mutat.* **29**, 1327–1336.
5. Fleming, M.A., Potter, J.D., Ramirez, C.J., Ostrander, G.K., and Ostrander, E.A. (2003) Understanding missense mutations in the BRCA1 gene: an evolutionary approach. *Proc. Natl. Acad. Sci. U. S. A.* **100**, 1151–1156,
6. Koonin, V.F., Altschul, S.F., and Bork, P. BRCA1 protein products: Functional motifs (1996) *Nat. Genet.* **13**, 266–267.
7. Yoshida, K., and Miki, Y. (2004) Role of BRCA1 and BRCA2 as regulators of DNA

repair, transcription, and cell cycle in response to DNA damage. *Cancer Sci.* **95**, 866–871.

8. Wang, Y., Cortez, D., Yazdi, P., Neff, N., Elledge, S.J., and Qin, J., (2000) BASC, a super complex of BRCA1-associated proteins involved in the recognition and repair of aberrant DNA structures. *Genes Dev.* **14**, 927–939.

9. Cortese, M.S., Uversky, V.N., and Keith Dunker, A. (2008) Intrinsic disorder in scaffold proteins: getting more from less. *Prog. Biophys. Mol. Biol.* **98**, 85–106.

10. Mark, W.Y., Liao, J.C., Lu, Y., Ayed, A., Laister, R., Szymczyna, B., et al. (2005) Characterization of segments from the central region of BRCA1: an intrinsically disordered scaffold for multiple protein-protein and protein-DNA interactions? *J. Mol. Biol.* **345**, 275–287.

11. Sturdy, A., Naseem, R., and Webb, M. (2004) Purification and characterisation of a soluble N-terminal fragment of the breast cancer susceptibility protein BRCA1. *J. Mol. Biol.* **340**, 469–475.

12. Paull, T.T., Cortez, D., Bowers, B., Elledge, S.J., and Gellert, M. (2001) Direct DNA binding by BRCA1. *Proc. Natl. Acad. Sci. U. S. A.* **9**, 6086–6091.

13. Naseem, R., and Webb, M. (2008) Analysis of the DNA binding activity of BRCA1 and its modulation by the tumour suppressor p53. *PLoS ONE* **3**, e2336.

14. Hohenstein, P., and Giles, R.H. (2003) BRCA1: a scaffold for p53 response? *Trends Genet.* **19**, 489–494.

15. Wang, Q., Zhang, H., Kajino, K., and Greene, M.I. (1998) BRCA1 binds c-Myc and inhibits its transcriptional and transforming activity in cells. *Oncogene* **17**, 1939–1948.

16. Zhong, Q., Chen, C.F., Li, S., Chen, Y., Wang, C.C., Xiao, J. et al. (1999) Association of BRCA1 with the hRad50-hMre11-p95 complex and the DNA damage response. *Science* **285**, 747–750.

17. Scully, R., Chen, J., Plug, A., Xiao, Y., Weaver, D., Feunteun, J., et al. (1997) Association of BRCA1 with Rad51 in mitotic and meiotic cells. *Cell* **88**, 265–275.

18. Folias, A., Matkovic, M., Bruun, D., Reid, S., Hejna, J., Grompe, M., et al. (2002) BRCA1 interacts directly with the Fanconi anemia protein FANCA. *Hum. Mol. Genet.* **11**, 2591–2597.

19. Aprelikova, O.N., Fang, B.S., Meissner, E.G., Cotter, S., Campbell, M., Kuthiala, A., et al. (1999) BRCA1-associated growth arrest is RB dependent. *Proc. Natl. Acad. Sci. U. S. A.* **96**, 11866–11871.

INDEX

A

Adenomatous polyposis coli (APC) 9, 142
Affected sib-pairs 4–6
Allelic heterogeneity 9–10
Alternative splicing 120
Ancestry informative markers 11
Aneuploidy 73–84
Array comparative genomic hybridization
 (aCGH) 221–234
Ashkenazi 5, 244
Autosomal inheritance 9
Autosomes 9, 65

B

Bacterial artificial chromosomes (BACs) 36, 69,
 124, 260, 262–265, 267–270, 272, 276–278
Batch Gene Finder 123
BioMercator 111–113
BOADICEA 245, 246
Bonferroni correction 14
BRCA1 .... 5, 23–32, 77, 134,
 147–181, 188, 221, 225–227, 237–246, 249, 259,
 260, 281–290
BRCA2 .... 5, 23–32,
 147–181, 221, 226, 227, 231, 232, 238–243, 245,
 249, 257, 259–279
BRCAPRO 238, 239, 243, 245, 246
Breast cancer information core (BIC) 260, 282

C

Cancer gene anatomy project (CGAP) 116,
 117, 119, 120, 123–124
Cancer outlier profile analysis (COPA) 121–122
Candidate gene 11, 23–32, 35, 93, 98, 99, 105–126
Capillary electrophoresis (CE) 147–180,
 182, 187–189, 208
Case control designs 5–7, 12, 13
CDKN2A 226, 227
cDNA microarrays 36, 38, 39, 42
cDNA xProfiler 123
CGAP database 116, 119, 120, 123–124
Clone Finder 123
Colorectal cancer 3, 5, 91, 100, 116, 193–204
Comparative genomic hybridization (CGH) 35–45,
 47–70, 221–234

Complex traits
 oligogenic 8
 polygenic 8, 107
Conformation sensitive gel electrophoresis (CSGE) 134
Couch model 243
Cre protein 262
Cyanine dyes
 Cy3 .... 26, 29, 37, 38, 40, 42, 229, 233
 Cy5 .... 37, 38, 40, 42, 229, 233

D

Denaturing gradient gel electrophoresis
 (DGGE) 137, 143, 193–204
Denaturing high performance liquid
 chromatography (DHPLC) 133–144,
 148, 149, 208, 211–216, 218
DHPLC melt program 137
Digital candidate gene approach (DigiCGA) 105–126
Digital differential display (DDD) 116, 119, 120
Digital gene expression displayer (DGED) 123, 124
Discordant sib pairs 4, 6
DNA extraction 36, 43, 138, 210, 217
DNA isolation from lymphocytes 194–195
Dominant 8, 9, 91, 99, 238

E

EIGENSTRAT 11
Electroporation 268–270, 272, 275, 276, 286
Endeavour 111, 112, 114
Enhanced mismatch mutation analysis
 (EMMA) 147–180
Ensembl 43, 44, 51, 98, 113, 114, 122
Epistasis 8
Epstein Barr virus-transformed lymphoblastoid
 cell lines 25
eVOC 111–113
Expression based SNP Imagemaps 124
Expression sequence tags (ESTs) 38
Extraction of genomic DNA 212

F

False discovery rate 14, 27
False positive report probability 14
Family based study designs 4–7
FAP 5
FISH-mapped BACs 124

Index

Fluorescence in situ hybridization (FISH) 63, 124
Founder populations 4, 5, 244

G

GC-clamp 135, 143, 193, 197, 198, 203, 209, 210, 212
Gel retardation 288
Gene environment interactions 6, 13, 14
Gene expression preprocessing analysis suite (GEPAS) 38, 41
Gene finder 123
Gene gene interactions 14
GeneHub-GEPIS 122
Gene modifiers 23–32, 73
Gene ontology database 84, 98, 109–111, 120, 121
GenomeMasker 50, 53, 54
Genome wide association 3, 11, 15, 25, 26, 32, 238
Genome wide linkage 10, 107
Genomic control 10, 74
Genomic DNA extraction 36, 217
Genomic DNA labeling 37, 40
Genomic instability 74, 77, 80, 81, 84, 260, 274–275
Genorama™ genotyping software 53, 62
Glioblastomas 35–45
GO browser 123

H

HaploRec 95
Haplotype 6, 13, 87–89, 92, 93, 95–99, 101, 102, 108
Haplotype tests 13
HapMap 12, 13, 15, 87, 190
Hardy–Weinberg principle 89
Haseman–Elston regression equation 5
Hereditary nonpolyposis colorectal cancer syndrome (HNPCC) 193, 204, 221, 227
Heteroduplex 134, 137–141, 144, 148, 149, 171, 181–191, 194, 208, 211, 213, 217, 314
Heteroduplex analysis (HDA) 148, 181–191, 194
Heterozygous chromosome regions 95
Hirschsprung disease 8
Homoduplex 134, 138, 139, 141, 148, 149, 182, 189
Homologous recombination 224, 262, 263, 275
HPRT1 minigene 262

I

Imputation 15, 17
Insertional mutagenesis 75, 77, 79, 82, 83
Inverse PCR 76, 82
Ionizing radiation 24, 273

K

KEGG database 115, 116, 121

L

LC-GREEN™ 209
Linkage disequilibrium 8, 88
Linkage genome-wide scan 10
Long interspersed nuclear elements (LINEs) 224
Lymphoblastoid cell lines 224
Lymphocytes 194–195, 199
Lynch syndrome 249

M

MAPHDesigner 51, 53
MAPH hybridization 49, 57, 69
MAPHStat 53, 63
MegaBLAST 54
Mendelian traits 8
MGC sequences 124
Microarray
 aCGH array 228, 229
 array-MAPH 48, 49, 51–52, 57–66, 69
 cDNA microarrays 36, 38, 39, 42
 SNP microarrays 88–91, 108
Minigene vector 250, 256
Mismatch repair (MMR) 5, 9, 193, 221, 226
Mitelman database tool 124
MLH1 .... 181, 221, 226, 227, 249, 256, 257
Module maps 119–121
Mouse embryonic stem (ES) cells 259–279
MSH2 .... 181, 221, 225–228, 249, 257
Multigenerational family pedigrees 4–5
Multiplex amplifiable probe hybridization (MAPH) 47–70
Multiplicative 9

N

Ni^{2+}-NTA agarose 286
Non-denaturing polyacrylamide electrophoresis 289
Nucleotide blast 123

O

Online mendelian inheritance in man (OMIM) 5, 8, 9, 16, 114, 134, 135, 142

P

PamGene 48
pCAS minigene 251, 252, 254, 256
Penetrance 8
Permutation testing 14
PLINK 11–15
Polyacrylamide gel electrophoresis 195–197, 200–204, 284, 288–289
Population stratification 10–11

Power calculations 4, 7
Principal components 10–12
Proband 4, 91, 141
PROSPECTR 112–114
Protein truncation test (PTT) 134, 194, 239
PTEN 134, 143, 208, 226, 227

Q

Quantile-quantile (Q-Q) plots 13, 29
Quantitative trait loci 113

R

Rad5 .... 1, 23, 24, 263, 275, 276, 278, 282
Real time PCR (RT-PCR) 63, 69,
    148, 180, 208–211, 213, 214, 216
Recessive 8, 9, 77, 88, 89, 91–93, 96, 99, 101
Recurrent aberrations CGAP 124
Repair-FunMap 122–123
Risk modifiers 24, 31
RNA amplification 28, 32
RNA isolation 27, 28

S

Saccharomyces cerevisiae 73–84
SAGEmap 116
Shattuck–Eidens model 238
Short interspersed nuclear elements (SINEs) 224
Single nucleotide polymorphisms (SNP) 13–15,
    17, 23, 24, 27, 30–32, 88–96, 98, 99, 101, 106, 108,
    112, 117, 120, 123, 124, 184, 190, 223, 224, 228
Single-strand conformational polymorphism
    (SSCP) 134, 137, 182–184,
    186–188, 190, 191, 194, 239
Site directed mutagenesis 252, 283, 285–286
SNP500Cancer 117, 124
SNP gene viewer 124
SNP maps
    genetic 124
    physical 124
Snyder mTn-lacZ/LEU2-mutagenized library 77

Southern hybridization 270–271, 276, 278
Splicing reporter minigene assay 249–257
s-RT-MELT 207–218
SSAHA program 54
SSCP-HD 182–184, 186–188
Surveyor™ nuclease 208, 211, 213
SYBR-GREEN™ 209

T

TOM 111, 112
TOPO TA cloning 50, 55, 56, 66, 67
Transfection 250, 251, 253–256
Transmission disequilibrium test 6
Trios 5, 6
Two dimensional gene scanning (TDGS) 134
Tyrer–Cuzick 238

U

Unclassified variants (UVs) 249, 256
UNPHASED 13
UV light 256, 274, 288, 289

V

Vectorette PCR 76, 82
von Hippel Lindau disease 135, 141

W

WAVE® System 135, 136, 139
Western blot 270–272

X

X-linked 9

Y

Y-PER 283, 286, 289

Z

Zoom-in aCGH 222–228, 230–232